A Complete Guide To Primary Care Mental Health

'The Primary Care Mental Health CD-Rom toolkit makes a unique and very valuable contribution to the field as it focuses on the needs and preferences of mental health service users – an area in which all providers need additional skills. The quality of the materials is really outstanding and the instructions for best utilizing the toolkit make it easy for learners and facilitators alike. Overall, this multimedia toolkit is an excellent teaching-learning program that can help better prepare providers to render sensitive, compassionate, respectful and effective care. As such, it should be integrated into as many service settings as possible.'

Gail W. Stuart, PhD, APRN, FAAN,
Dean and Professor, College of Nursing, Medical
University of South Carolina

'I like the visual aspects of the CDs, and how it is thematically structured into specific areas very helpful. I like the ease of navigation and the exercises. Excellent references and reading list that you can download and print, plus glossary and web hyperlinks are really useful. It is user friendly and the written transcripts utility is very valuable.'

Mary Steen, Royal College of Midwives

'It is excellent as a reference tool and gives me the knowledge and confidence to work with mothers with mental health issues.'

Indrah Carter, Health Visitor

'The toolkit is a must for Primary Care Mental Health Workers in training but also of use to anyone developing or refreshing knowledge and training in mental health.'

Suzanne Bamber, Primary Care Mental Health
Practitioner

'I think it is a great package. It is well presented, and the content is comprehensive and detailed . . . I particularly liked the wide range of issues covered. Overall, I was really impressed.'

Daisy Forster, Graduate Mental
Health Worker

'This would be very useful for GP Registrars (and some GPs who are rusty on their knowledge base in this area) as we have to learn the same and here it is all on one CD. I think the whole CD set would be very useful for the graduate workers in mental health.'

Dr Dilip Patel, GP, Middlesex

A Complete Guide To Primary Care Mental Health

A toolkit for professionals working with common mental health problems

Edited by: Pamela Myles and David Rushforth

Written by: Julie Attenborough, Barbara Goodfellow, Nigel Harrison, Eifion Ingham, Caroline Johnson, Ian Light, Nick Moor, Pamela Myles, Sonia Ramdour, Susan Ramsdale, David Richards and Roger Rowlands

ROBINSON
London

Constable & Robinson Ltd
3 The Lanchesters
162 Fulham Palace Road
London W6 9ER
www.constablerobinson.com

First published in the UK by Robinson,
an imprint of Constable & Robinson Ltd 2007

ISBN: 978–1–84529–596–7

Printed and bound in the EU

1 3 5 7 9 10 8 6 4 2

1/3/08

This book is dedicated to Ian Light 1961–2007

Contents

Illustrations

Tables

Figures

Foreword

Primary care services are under enormous pressure. Worldwide, depression is projected to be the second-most common cause of disability, after heart disease, by 2020. In the United Kingdom, nine out of ten patients with mental health problems seek help from their family doctor and it comes as no surprise that mental health problems are collectively the second-most common reason for consulting a general practitioner.

The Layard report (2006)[1] signalled the determination to address the national economic burden and stark personal financial costs of unemployment and extended sick leave for people with anxiety and depression, and this has influenced the target client group and service models deployed.

Government policy fully recognizes the challenge facing front-line workers in primary care, and is committed to modernizing primary care service provision through investment in skills training for both new workforce and primary care disciplines with an interest in mental health. Some progress has been made, with close to a thousand primary care mental health workers recruited by Primary Care Trusts since January 1994.

As we go to publication, the two national demonstration sites at Doncaster and Newham are preparing to publish initial outcome data. The interim report will provide a clearer appreciation of the competencies required by primary care staff to deliver on improvements in the health and social functioning of people with common mental health problems.

Training in evidence-based skills is the key to improving both clinical outcomes and social functioning for people seeking help to overcome mild to moderate anxiety or depression. Core to this book are skills-based units of study which develop patient-centred skills in interviewing, risk management, problem formulation and brief, low-intensity interventions based on tried and tested psychological therapies.

The Centre for Clinical Academic Workforce Innovation at the University of Lincoln has invested heavily in higher education training programmes to prepare the new graduate workers. Now, with the publication of this book, this ambition has widened. This volume with its accompanying CD-ROMs provides primary care disciplines with a learning resource which can also be accessed on a personal computer. The CD-ROMs include a wealth of training materials supported by high-quality video and audio clips, web-links, information leaflets, diaries and other clinical tools.

A Complete Guide to Primary Care Mental Health is above all a flexible learning programme which offers a comprehensive teaching resource designed for post-qualified primary care staff who seek to update or advance their skills in the management of anxiety-related conditions and depression. With education and training budgets under immense strain, and where funding to attend conventionally delivered training programmes is scarce, this learning resource is both timely and welcome.

Professor Tony Butterworth CBE
Centre Director, University of Lincoln,
and Senior Policy Advisor to NHS Employers

1 Layard R (2006). *The Depression Report. A new deal for depression and anxiety disorders.* The Centre for Economic Performance, London School of Economics.

Introduction and rationale

The programme provided by this book, and by the accompanying set of CD-ROMs, is the product of an invitation to tender from the former Trent NHS Workforce Development Confederation, now the Centre for Clinical and Academic Workforce Innovation at the University of Lincoln.

This training package offered an opportunity for stakeholders to work together to provide a bespoke educational programme for learners. The programme aims to contribute to the improvement of primary care mental health services within the modernisation agenda, in order to enhance the quality of care received by individuals with mental health problems.

Rationale

This programme aims to develop the knowledge and skills of primary care workers who have an interest in improving the mental health of people presenting with common mental health problems in general practice and other community settings. The investment in education and training in primary care mental health is a product of a raft of Government policies and initiatives, most notably the structural reform of the NHS, trailed in the *NHS Plan* (Department of Health, 2000). Primary Care Trusts (PCTs) are now at the cornerstone of the NHS, as both commissioners and providers of mental health services, and are charged with delivering the targets set out within the *National Service Framework (NSF) for Mental Health* (Department of Health, 1999a). One of the targets within the NHS Plan was the recruitment, training and employment within PCTs of 1000 new mental health workers who could support primary care (Department of Health, 2002).

The subsequent collaborative development of the programme is underpinned by empirical evidence which demonstrates that bespoke training of non-specialist workers, such as mental health workers in primary care, can deliver effective mental healthcare for people with common mental health problems (Gilbody et al, 2003; Katon et al, 1999; Lovell et al, 2003; NHS Centre for Reviews and Dissemination, 2002; Richards et al, 2002; Richards et al, 2003; Simon et al, 2000).

The education and training available within the book and the three CD-ROMs is appropriate for these new mental health workers and other healthcare professionals who work in primary care and have a role in working with patients with common mental health problems.

Philosophically, the programme is based on some core propositions. These include:

Self-management and self-help

Primary care is a unique environment and requires a service designed and tailored to the needs of patients accessing services in primary care. Traditional secondary care models lack flexibility and responsiveness and are inappropriate for primary care settings. They result in: long waiting lists; frustration on the part of patients, staff and GPs; inefficient use of resources; and unwelcome pathologising of common mental health experiences. In short, this narrows access to effective care, disempowers patients, results in services that either become very selective or operate merely as triage services which signpost patients to other providers. It is necessary, therefore, to understand the culture and processes of primary care before designing and providing mental health services in primary care. The education of mental health workers must be clearly focused within an understanding of the unique culture and process of the primary care environment.

Patients are generally the best managers of their personal and family mental health problems. However, people often lack the information and support to manage their problems effectively. The provision of high-quality health information, within a graduated system of healthcare access by workers using patient-centred and flexible approaches to mental healthcare, is the most desirable way of empowering patients in the self-management of their mental health problems (Rogers et al, 1999).

New workers can deliver

Workers with no experience of mental healthcare can be trained to support self-management health technologies. This can be achieved by innovative, focused and skill-based education programmes. Evidence suggests that skills and attitudes to patients with mental health problems can be significantly improved through such skill-based and focused training courses, even where this training is delivered over a short space of time (Payne et al, 2002; Richards et al, 2002).

The unique primary care environment

Finally, but most significantly: primary care is a unique environment that requires service designs and associated education opportunities to fully appreciate the needs of patients accessing services within this generalist environment (Department of Health, 2001a).

We have learnt much over the past few years and now recognise that applying a secondary care model of good practice to a primary care setting is unhelpful. We are able to identify specific models that better suit the delivery of mental health and social support, advice and treatment in primary care communities.

Louis Appleby, in *The National Service Framework for Mental Health – Five Years On* (Department of Health, 2004a), called for a clear vision for mental health services in primary care to guide national service developments. He reminds us that the vision should include an emphasis on the health and well-being of the community as a whole, and, amongst other things:

- an increase in the numbers of new primary care mental health workers to support people with common mental health problems
- a broader choice of therapy providers with an overall increase in talking therapy skills of frontline staff
- an improved response to physical and mental co-morbidity with enhanced primary care support for those with longer-term mental health problems
- an increase in the self-management ethos and the availability of self-help technology

This reinforces how essential it is to understand the process and culture of primary care, ensuring that our service vision clearly recognises this unique environment.

Acknowledgements

The editors would like to acknowledge the work undertaken by many people and organisations who have greatly influenced the production of the book and the three interactive CD-ROMs. The collaboration between the University of Central Lancashire, the University of Manchester and Liverpool John Moores University, in the development of a taught Post Graduate Certificate in Primary Care Mental Health Practice in 2003, has shaped the overall approach and values that are included within the model adopted for mental health practice in primary care and the corresponding practice-based examples and interactive exercises within the three CD-ROMs. The writing of Book 1 would not have been possible without the collaboration between the University of Central Lancashire and the Primary Care Trusts within the North West, NIHME North West and a range of service user and carer organisations, particularly Lancashire Advocacy Service and Preston Service Users Forum, who have shared information and insightful experiences contributing to the development of the curriculum. Our thanks also to Nick Moor at Mental Health Strategies for writing the learning materials on policy, legal and ethical framework.

We wish to further acknowledge the contribution of City University, in partnership with local voluntary agencies and service users, who co-authored Part 2 on practice-based working with users, carers and support agencies.

The editors are indebted to Professor David Richards, who gave generously of his time to assist Pamela Myles in the development and editing of Part 3 on clinical skills for primary care mental health practice.

This book would not be possible without the support and guidance of the project management team, steering group, editing team, and actors, with a special thank you to the writing teams.

Finally, we wish to acknowledge the expertise of the team which undertook the final edit of the original CD-ROM content material. A special thanks to Ivy Blackburn, Paul Brewer, Nigel Harrison, Lancashire Advocacy Service, Mick McKeown, Jackie Prosser, Patricia Ronan, David Richards, Graham Russel and Jean Taylor.

The full list of contributers, in alphabetical order, is as follows:

Writers: Julie Attenborough, Barbara Goodfellow, Nigel Harrison, Eifion Ingham, Caroline Johnson, Ian Light, Nick Moor, Pamela Myles, Sonia Ramdour, Susan Ramsdale, David Richards and Roger Rowlands.

Editors: Ivy Blackburn, Paul Brewer, Nigel Harrison, Lancashire Advocacy Service, Mick McKeown, Pamela Myles, Preston Mental Health Service User Forum, Jackie Prosser, David Richards, Patricia Ronan, David Rushforth, Graham Russell and Jean Taylor.

Project Management Team: Julie Attenborough, Tim Bilham, Nigel Harrison, Nick Moor, Pamela Myles, David Rushforth and Richard Walne.

Steering Group: Julie Attenborough, Tim Bilham, Colin Gell, Nigel Harrison, Duncan Henderson, Aiden Houlders, Ian Light, Nick Moor, Pamela Myles, Jackie Prosser, David Richards, Patricia Ronan, David Rushforth, Graham Russell, Gina Smith and Richard Walne.

Actors: Rueban Anderson, Laurel Andrews, Julie Attenborough, Laura Blackender, Paul Chapman, Anne Crowley, Sue Dawson, Sarah Eales, Deborah Ellis, Chloe Foster, Gordon Fraser, Nick Gauntlet, Debbie Green, Phil Hamarack, Louise Harrison, Patrick Hyland, Stephen James, Victoria Jeffrey, Ian Light, Eddie McCann, Peter Mann, Guy Marsden, Pamela Myles, Ranj Nagra, Prashant Phillips, Polly Tidyman, Lynny Turner, Anita Waite, Dominic Walker, Steve Walker, Lesley Warner and Emma Way.

Our thanks also to: Ian Baguley, Patrick Callaghan, Gary Freeman, Peter Lindley, Christina Lyons, Jit Patel, John Playle, Preston Mental Health User Forum, David Richards, Jan Robinson and Jan Thomson.

The CD-ROMs were designed, programmed and produced by Rare Sense Ltd.

References

Department of Health (1999a). *A National Service Framework for Mental Health.* London: HMSO.

Department of Health (2000). *The NHS Plan: a Plan for Investment, a Plan for Reform.* London: HMSO.

Department of Health (2001a). *Mental Health National Service Framework (and the NHS Plan) workforce planning, education and training underpinning programme: adult mental health services – final report by the Workforce Action Team.* London: Department of Health.

Department of Health (2002). *Fast Forwarding Primary Care Mental Health: 1000 New Graduate Workers to Support Primary Care Mental Health.* London: Department of Health.

Department of Health (2004a). *The National Service Framework for Mental Health – Five Years On.* London: Department of Health.

Gilbody, S., Whitty, P., Grimshaw, J. & Thomas, R. (2003). Educational and Organizational Interventions to Improve the Management of Depression in Primary Care: A Systematic review. *JAMA*, 289, 23, 3145-3151.

Katon, W., Von Korff, M., Lin, E., Simon, G., Walker, E., & Unutzer, J. (1999). Stepped collaborative care for primary care patients with persistent depression: A randomised trial. *Archives of General Psychiatry*, 56, 1109-1115.

Lovell, K., Richards, D.A. & Bowers, D. (2003). Improving access to primary care mental health:

uncontrolled evaluation of a pilot self-help clinic. *British Journal of General Practice*, 53, 133-135.

NHS Centre for Reviews and Dissemination (2002). Improving the recognition and management of depression in primary care. *Effective Health Care Bulletin*, 7, 5, 1-12.

Payne, F., Harvey, K., Jessopp, L., Plummer, S., Tylee, A. & Gournay, K. (2002). Knowledge, confidence and attitudes towards mental health of nurses working in NHS Direct and the effects of training. *Journal of Advanced Nursing*, 40, 549-559.

Richards, D., Richards, A., Barkham, M., Williams, C. & Cahill, J. (2002). PHASE: a health technology approach to psychological treatment in pri-mary mental health care. *Primary Health Care Research and Developments*, 3: 159-168.

Richards, D.A., Lovell, K. & McEvoy, P. (2003). Access and effectiveness in psychological therapies: self-help as a routine health technology. *Health and Social Care in the Community*, 11, 175-182.

Rogers, A., Flowers, J. & Pencheon, D. (1999). Improving access needs a whole systems approach. *British Medical Journal*, 319, 866-7.

Simon, G.E., Von Korff, M., Rutter, C. & Wagner, E. (2000). Randomised trial of monitoring, feedback and management of care by telephone to improve treatment of depression in primary care. *British Medical Journal*, 320, 550-554.

How to use this book

The programme contained in this book is adapted from the accompanying set of three CD-ROMs. It is intended to be used by those who do not have free and constant access to a PC, and for those who prefer a more tradition-al approach to learning than that provided by the interactive environment of the CD-ROMs.

Nevertheless, it does make use of external resources. For example, the case histories make extensive use of consultations and interactions between healthcare professionals and their clients. The histories always include full tran-scripts, but the reader will find video or audio recordings of these sessions on the CD-ROMs. These are indicated in the text by symbols – an arrow for a video recording and a speaker for audio. Where the session is an introductory meeting, the symbol is included within the client's photograph.

Indicates   *Indicates*
video   *audio*

Video and audio recordings are found in the Resources section of the Main Menu on each CD-ROM, listed under Audio/Video.

The programme also makes frequent refer-ence to printed documents which are available for the reader to download from the CD-ROMs. These are in Adobe PDF format. They are indicated in the text by a PDF symbol, and can be found in the Resources section of the Main Menu on each CD-ROM, listed under Print Room.

Indicates PDF file

To read and print these downloaded docu-ments on a PC requires Adobe's Acrobat Reader, which can be obtained online from www.adobe.com/uk/products/acrobat/readstep2.html.

In each case, as an alternative source for these documents, an internet address is given from which they can be downloaded. However, unlike a book, the internet is a medium which is constantly subject to change and development, and so these addresses, in common with internet data in general, may not remain current. None the less, all internet addresses mentioned in this book have been checked, and were current in December 2006.

Terms which may be unfamiliar to the reader are included in a Glossary at the back of the book.

If you would like to test your progress, the CD-ROMs contain self-test exercises. These are found at the end of each section. Though not included in the book (in most cases they make use of interactive graphics), their presence is indicated with a symbol at the appropriate parts of the book.

Indicates self-test exercise on CD–ROM

CD-ROMs: Minimum system requirements

You must have:
- Windows XP/2000
- 8x CD-ROM drive
- A video card capable of at least 800x600 and 16-bit colour
- A 16-bit sound card
- 300MHz+ processor
- 128Mb+ RAM

To use the CD-ROMs

Insert the disc in your CD-ROM drive. The CD-ROM should start automatically after a few seconds. If this does not happen, navigate to your CD-ROM drive and double-click the 'Start.exe' icon.

If you still experience problems consult the README.txt file on the CD-ROM for answers to common questions and trouble-shooting tips.

Important note for readers on clinical supervision

Primary care professionals learning new skills in cognitive behavioural interventions will benefit from structured supervision of their practice when working with people seeking help.

We strongly advise early and careful reading of the unit on 'Clinical Supervision' in Part 1.2.4 on page 21. The appointment of a clinical supervisor, together with a schedule of regular meetings, is essential and should be arranged well in advance of contact with service users and carers. The supervisor should have appropriate experience in cognitive behavioural interventions and a recognized qualification to practise in this field.

New workers in primary care will require formal guidance from a qualified professional trainer or lecturer to support their learning and use of the accompanying resource material in this book.

Part 1

Culture and processes in primary mental healthcare

Co-editor: Nigel Harrison

Authors: Eifion Ingman, Nigel Harrison, Caroline Johnson, Nick Moor, Sonia Ramdour, Susan Ramsdale and Roger Rowlands

Chapter 1.1

Culture and processes in primary mental healthcare

'As we approach the fiftieth anniversary of the NHS, it is time to reflect on the huge achievements of the NHS. But in a changing world, no organisation, however great, can stand still. The NHS needs to meet the demands of today's public. The NHS will start to provide new and better services for the public.'

Tony Blair, December 1997

Aims

- To enable the development of a coherent understanding of the health and social policy agenda influencing primary mental healthcare since 1989
- To provide an opportunity to critically examine primary care services, roles and responsibilities
- To facilitate the appraisal of the integration of primary care with other mental health service providers

Learning outcomes

At the end of this Chapter, the reader will be able critically to:
- Evaluate the development of health and social care policy in relation to primary care
- Evaluate the value of key developments from the perspective of both the health professional and the patient
- Examine the consequences of re-engineering a range of mental health services from specialist services, and of incorporating them into the primary care arena
- Evaluate the effectiveness of primary care teams with regard to individual roles and responsibilities and overall approach to mental healthcare

- Appraise local mental healthcare, treatment and support services

Chapter 1.1 content is as follows:

1   The history and development of primary care services
2   Profiles of primary care services
3   Roles and responsibilities of the primary care team
4   The patient's perspective of primary care

Section 1: The history and development of primary care services

In 1989, the NHS experienced the most significant cultural shift since its inception. The 'internal market' was introduced in the White Paper, *Working for Patients* (Department of Health, 1989). This passed into law as the NHS and Community Care Act (Department of Health, 1990). The Conservative Government had been confronted with numerous problems within the NHS, such as growing waiting lists, and demand for services was far exceeding the resources available. In a bid to address these issues, the government introduced the internal market system. Prior to this, the NHS was run via a massive and complex bureaucracy. With the introduction of the internal market, the service was split into purchasers and providers.

In order to become a provider within the internal market, the existing health organizations had to evolve and became NHS Trusts. These were independent organizations with their own management systems, competing with each other for business.

The first wave of NHS Trusts came into being in 1991, and by 1995 all healthcare was provided in this way. The NHS and Community Care Act (1990) (Department of Health, 1990) introduced GP fund holding and family doctors were given the opportunity to manage their own budgets and buy healthcare from the NHS Trusts. Those who did not join the scheme still had their budgets controlled by the health authorities, which bought healthcare in bulk from the NHS Trusts.

In 1997, a Labour government was elected, which brought with it a new approach to the NHS. The government felt that some aspects of the internal market system had been successful, in that the NHS had at last become cost conscious, but it had also served to create a duplication of services in the drive for competition between providers. The White Paper, *The New NHS: Modern, Dependable* (Department of Health, 1997a) introduced a 'third way' of running the NHS and promised to abolish the internal market system and move away from direct competition to a more collaborative approach to working. It described this approach as 'a new model for a new century' and was based on six key principles. These were:

1   To renew the NHS as a genuinely **national** service. Patients will get fair access to consistently high quality, prompt and accessible services, right across the country
2   To make the delivery of healthcare against these new national standards a matter of **local** responsibility. Local doctors and nurses who are in the best position to know what patients need will be in the driving seat in shaping services
3   To get the NHS to work in **partnership**. By breaking down organizational barriers and forging stronger links with Local Authorities, the needs of the patient will be put at the centre of the care process
4   To drive **efficiency** through a more rigorous approach to performance and by cutting bureaucracy, so that every pound in the NHS is spent to maximize the care for patients
5   To shift the focus onto quality of care so that **excellence** is guaranteed to all patients, and quality becomes the driving force for decision-making at every level of the service
6   To rebuild **public confidence** in the NHS as a public service, accountable to patients, open to the public and shaped by their views

As a vehicle to deliver the six principles effectively, the Government introduced the concept of Primary Care Groups (PCGs) in the White Paper, *The New NHS: Modern, Dependable* (Department of Health, 1997a). It highlighted three areas. Primary Care Groups should:

1   Develop around natural communities and try to work alongside the boundaries of social services
2   Cover a population of about 100,000
3   Restore public confidence in the NHS

When introducing Primary Care Groups (PCGs), the government was already paving the way for the larger Primary Care Trusts (PCTs). They were first introduced in the NHS (Primary Care) Act 1997 (Department of Health, 1997b), and in more detail in the Annex of the aforementioned White Paper. The idea was that successful PCGs could apply for Trust status to integrate primary and community healthcare. The focus of the Trusts would be on improving rehabilitation and recovery services and making services more accessible to the community that they served. They would not be responsible for specialist mental health services or learning disabilities services. A condition for the transition from PCG to PCT was that the PCG was able to clearly demonstrate an active and successful approach to the NHS commitment to Clinical Governance. This is discussed in the consultation document *A First Class Service* (Department of Health, 1998a).

'Clinical Governance is a framework through which NHS organizations are accountable for continuously improving the quality of their services and safeguarding high standards of care, by creating an environment in which excellence in clinical care will flourish' (Department of Health, 1999b).

The national and local priorities for Clinical Governance were identified by the National Institute for Health and Clinical Excellence (NICE) (www.nice. org.uk).

Summary

- The NHS has experienced considerable change in recent years. It has seen the introduction and abolition of the internal market system and the evolvement of NHS Trusts
- The introduction of GP fund holding gave doctors the opportunity to manage their own budgets and buy healthcare from NHS Trusts
- In 1997 a 'new model for a new century' was introduced. This brought the concept of Primary Care Groups, with an emphasis on delivering more services via primary care; the eventual development was the formation of Primary Care Trusts, with a remit to make services more accessible

References

Department of Health (1989). *Working for Patients*. London: HMSO.

Department of Health (1990). *The NHS and Community Care Act*. London: HMSO.

Department of Health (1997a). *The New NHS: Modern, Dependable*. London: HMSO.

Department of Health (1997b). *NHS (Primary Care) Act 1997*. London: HMSO.

Department of Health (1998a). *A First Class Service: Quality in the new NHS*. London: HMSO.

Department of Health (1999b). *Clinical Governance: quality in the new NHS*, HSC 99/065. London: HMSO.

Useful websites

www.dh.gov.uk (Department of Health)
www.nice.org.uk (National Institution for Health and Clinical Excellence)

Test yourself

 To check your progress, locate this section on CD-ROM 1 and work through the interactive questions at the end.

Section 2: Profiles of primary care services

Primary Care Trusts (PCTs) manage all aspects of primary care and receive 75% of the NHS budget. They are local organizations, and so are in a position to understand the needs of their community (for information on NHS England see online at www.nhs.uk/england/authoritiestrusts/pct/default.aspx).

Primary care is the care and treatment provided by people you normally see when you first have a health problem (e.g. the dentist, optician, pharmacist, doctor or nurse). NHS Direct and NHS Walk-In Centres are also part of primary care. PCTs are responsible for the continued improvement of the health and well-being of their residents, and ensuring that there are adequate services for the people within their locality and that the services are accessible. They are now also responsible for providing cover out of hours and for ensuring that health and social services work collaboratively in the best interests of patients.

Most people with mental health problems are cared for in a primary care setting, with support provided by specialist services when needed. Increasingly, services are seeking to provide integrated health and social care. In order to build on the work initiated in the documents *The New NHS* (Department of Health, 1997a) and *Modernising Social Services* (Department of Health, 1998b), the government detailed in *A First Class Service* (Department of Health, 1998a) how the NHS standards would be:

- Set by the National Institute for Health and Clinical Excellence (NICE) and National Service Frameworks (NSFs)
- Delivered by clinical governance
- Monitored by the Commission for Health Improvement (CHI)

Following the publication of the Health and Social Care Act 2003, CHI was abolished and replaced by the Health are Commission on 1 April 2004.

The *National Service Framework (NSF) for Mental Health* (Department of Health, 1999a) focuses on the mental health needs of working-age adults (up to 65 years), and aims to:

- Set national standards and define service models for promoting health and treating mental illness
- Put in place underpinning programmes to support local delivery
- Establish milestones and a specific group of high-level performance indicators against which progress within agreed time-scales will be measured

Its focus is on health promotion, assessment, diagnosis, treatment, rehabilitation and care, encompassing primary and specialist care and the roles of partner agencies.

In order to guide this development, seven standards have been set in five areas:

Standard one: Mental health promotion

Standards two and three: Primary care and access to services

Standards four and five: Effective services for people with severe mental illness

Standard six: Caring about carers

Standard seven: Preventing suicide

Primary care standards from the *National Service Framework for Mental Health*

Standards two and three of the *National Service Framework for Mental Health* (Department of Health, 1999a) emphasize the importance of primary care in addressing mental health problems:

- Any patient who contacts their primary healthcare team with a common mental health problem should:
  - Have their mental health needs identified and assessed
  - Be offered effective treatments, including referral to specialist services for further assessment, treatment and care, if required
- To achieve this standard, each Primary Care Trust will need to work with the support of specialized mental health services to:
  - Develop the resources within each practice to assess mental health needs
  - Develop the resources to work with diverse groups in the population

- Develop the skills and competencies to manage common mental health problems
- Agree the arrangements for referral for assessment, advice or treatment and care
- Have the skills and necessary organizational systems in place to provide the physical healthcare and other primary care support needed, as agreed in their care plan, for people with severe mental illness

The demands of the NSF to provide effective and accessible interventions are compromised at the present time by the current nature of psychological delivery. Richards et al (2003) believe there is strong evidence to promote self-help to the centre of primary mental healthcare, so as to address the volume of referrals. This appears to be a pragmatic move forward, with the mental health worker placed in a strong position to facilitate 'self-help approaches'.

Delivering the NSF for Mental Health requires new patterns of working. Social care organizations have to work in partnership with mental health services across the five areas to achieve the standards successfully. For primary care mental health, the improvement of partnership working (i.e. health, social and voluntary-sector) will help provide faster access to effective treatments for common mental health problems and improved education and development for staff.

In order for this process to happen, most health authority functions had to be devolved to the newly emerging PCTs, as determined in the document *Shifting the Balance of Power* (Department of Health, 2001b). The PCTs then had the responsibility to develop and modernize services in line with the NSF and the NHS Plan (Department of Health, 2000). This change process is led by the Mental Health Local Implementation Teams (LITs), and the key document for consolidating investment and service development is *The Mental Health Policy Implementation Guide* as converted into Local Implementation Plans (Department of Health, 2001c).

Exercise

Search online at www.doh.gov.uk/mentalhealth/implementationguide
- What groups and service providers are represented on the LIT in your area?
- Read the local implementation plan for your area. What does it say about mental health in primary care settings?

Management of long-term conditions

The move to improve and increase healthcare provision in primary care, and to manage chronic disease more effectively within the community, has led to the introduction of new ways of allocating funds to GP practices. These are the most ambitious changes to primary care services since the inception of the NHS in 1948. The *General Medical Services contract (GMS)* (NHS Confederation & BMA, 2003; Department of Health, 2004b) was introduced, which aims to incentivize general practices to improve patient care and services, and to reward primary care professionals for the outcomes they achieve. Funding in these new contracts does not rely on how many doctors are engaged in a practice, but on what the patients' needs are. The contract is between the practice and the PCT, giving the whole primary care team more flexibility in designing services to meet local needs.

A voluntary Quality and Outcomes Framework will allow practices that opt in to earn financial rewards by caring for patients to set standards, rather than by the number of patients that they treat. Practices will also be able to transfer some of their services to other providers (e.g. out-of-hours care).

The GMS contracts also embrace the needs of individuals with severe long-term mental illness – primarily, but not exclusively, schizophrenia and bipolar affective disorder. About 40% of patients in this category are not in contact with specialist services (Murie, 2004).

The new GMS contract has provided a vehicle with which to address these concerns and seeks to introduce Serious Mental Illness Registers (SMI Registers) of people with severe and enduring mental illness who require and have agreed to regular follow-up to improve their physical health.

Who should be on the SMI Register?

This is open to each practice to decide; but it is recommended that, as a minimum, people with psychotic illness are included, as there is a wealth of evidence to support the fact that the physical health needs of this vulnerable patient group are a high priority (Cohen & Hove, 2001). This issue is also addressed in Chapter 1.3, Section 8. However, it is important that patients are given an 'informed choice' and are able to decide whether or not they wish to receive the care that is offered. Registers are kept in primary care for other types of disorders as a method of monitoring the health of the local population (e.g. for diabetes and coronary heart disease).

Exercise
- What reasons might there be for a patient to decline being placed on a register?
- Cardiovascular and respiratory disease and diabetes mellitus are common in people with severe mental health problems such as schizophrenia and bipolar disorder. Why do you think this is?
- How might patients with any of the above physical health needs benefit from being included on a register?

The new contract is part of major investment into primary care. UK expenditure in this area rose from £6.1bn in 2002–2003 to £8.0bn in 2005–2006 – an increase of 33%.

Exercise

- What would you consider to be the main implications for patients and staff under the new GMS contracts?

Exercise

Visit your local Primary Care Trust website and download a profile of the services provided.

Primary care profile

The aim of developing a primary care profile is for you to become more familiar with what mental health provision is available to patients and carers needing assessment, treatment, education, housing and support. Mental health services are routinely provided by the Health Service, Social Services, the voluntary sector and independent sector organizations. It is important that you identify services typically provided by Primary Care Trusts, Mental Health Trusts, Social Services and Independent Sector organizations, as well as the unique range of local services and resources provided which may only be available within your locality. These are often offered by charitable organizations, the church, Further Education and Higher Education Institutions and housing departments.

A pro-forma primary care profile is available on CD-ROM 1 in PDF format to enable you to complete your own personal Primary Care Profile. Keep this as a resource that you can refer to on a day-to-day basis. It would be useful for you to keep this updated as services change and develop.

Having explored and discovered what type of mental health-related services are available in your local area, it may be helpful to convert information gathered, when building up the profile, into a mental health resource directory, including contact details and a summary of the type of service and type of patients the service is for. There are likely to be resource directories developed by neighbouring organizations that could contribute to the development of a primary care directory. For more information contact the information officers in your local Mental Health Trust, Social Services and independent sector organizations, Mental Health Advocacy Services and Council for Voluntary Services.

Summary

- Most people with mental health problems are cared for in a primary care setting, with access to specialist services if needed
- Mental health provision is becoming more integrated, combining health and social care services, to deliver standards of care as detailed in the National Service Framework for Mental Health (Department of Health, 1999a)
- New patterns of working have been needed, and social care and voluntary organizations have had to work in partnership with health services to achieve these standards successfully
- Primary Care Trusts have been given the responsibility to develop and modernize services, and a new General Medical Contract has increased flexibility in service provision in general practice

References

Cohen, A. & Hove, M. (2001). *Physical Health of the Severe and Enduring Mentally Ill: A Training Pack for GP Educators*. London: Sainsbury Centre for Mental Health.

Department of Health (1997a). *The New NHS: Modern, Dependable*. London: HMSO.

Department of Health (1998a). *A First Class Service: Quality in the new NHS*. London: HMSO.

Department of Health (1998b). *Modernising Social Services*. London: HMSO.

Department of Health (1999a). *A National Service Framework for Mental Health*. London: Department of Health.

Department of Health (2000). *The NHS Plan: a Plan*

for Investment, a Plan for Reform. London: HMSO.

Department of Health (2001b). *Shifting the Balance of Power within the NHS: Securing Delivery.* London: Department of Health.

Department of Health (2001c). *The Mental Health Policy Implementation Guide.* London: Department of Health.

Department of Health (2004b). *The General Medical Services Contract.* London: HMSO.

Murie, J. (2004). Contract will address needs of patients with severe mental illness. *Guidelines in Practice,* 7, 3, 35-42.

NHS Confederation & British Medical Association (2003). *New General Medical Services Contract 2003 – Investing in general practice.* London: NHS Confederation & BMA.

Richards, D.A., Lovell, K. & McEvoy, P. (2003). Access and effectiveness in psychological therapies: self-help as a routine health technology. *Health and Social Care in the Community,* 11, 175–182.

The Health and Social Care Act 2003

Useful websites

www.doh.gov.uk/mentalhealth/ implementationguide (Department of Health)

www.natpact.nhs.uk (National Primary Care Trust)

www.nhs.uk/england/authoritiestrusts/pct/default.aspx (National Health Service in England Primary Care Trusts UK)

www.primarycarecontracting.nhs.uk/3.php (Primary Medical Services)

www.scmh.org.uk (Sainsbury Centre for Mental Health)

Test yourself

 To check your progress, locate this section on CD-ROM 1 and work through the interactive questions at the end.

Section 3: Roles and responsibilities of the primary care team

The primary care team is made up of a number of professionals, and one of these will probably be the first point of contact for someone needing medical or nursing help. The team is generally comprised of GPs, midwives, health visitors, practice nurses, mental health workers, health promotion officers, district nurses, school nurses, counsellors, pharmacists, allied health professionals and receptionists. These professionals work together to provide assessment and treatment that will resolve or improve common mental health problems. If further treatment or investigations are needed, they will refer the patient to a hospital, an appropriate specialist service or some other local support agency. A patient may be seen by several members of the primary care team to meet individual needs. It is, therefore, important that each team member has an understanding of the roles and responsibilities of other team members.

The primary care team encompasses a range of disciplines, working in close proximity to each other and within each of their respective professional groups. Each healthcare professional will have undertaken academic and professional education, and qualifications developing their knowledge, skills and evidenced-based practice to prepare them for their role. While there are discrete differences between roles of the members of the primary care team, there may also be some sharing of resources and facilities and overlaps between roles, for the benefit of patients.

 CD-ROM 1 includes two video clips (Team Meeting - National Mental Health Day: Parts 1 and 2) which show a primary care team meeting in progress.

Evidence shows that, in a typical working day, a GP expects a significant psychological component in 70% of consultations and, in 20–25% of patients a mental health problem would be their sole reason for consultations. Criticism has been made when patients have been categorized as 'the worried well', since they can be just as disabled as those with chronic physical conditions, generating major social and financial burdens to families, friends and employers and consuming large amounts of health resources (Melzer et al, 1995).

It has been recognized that primary care workers working in the field of mental health

Exercise

Imagine that you are the Practice Manager. Provide a brief outline of the roles and responsibilities of the primary care team in your practice. How would you ensure that individual team members understand each other's roles and responsibilities?

still have many of their needs, relating to knowledge, interventions and effective partnerships with specialists, unmet.

This has been reviewed by the primary care subgroup of the Mental Health Workforce Action Team and has resulted in the production of *Ten Essential Shared Capabilities* within a guideline for the knowledge, skills and values needed to work effectively in mental healthcare (NIMHE, NHSU & SCMH, 2004. The Ten Essential Sharing Capabilities have been produced by the National Institute for Mental Health England (NIMHE) which publishes key documents to help local health and social care systems develop and take forward their workforce issues, with the needs of service users and carers being at the forefront of their recommendations. They are:

1 Working in Partnership.
2 Respecting Diversity.
3 Practising Ethically.
4 Challenging Inequality.
5 Promoting Recovery.
6 Identifying People's Needs and Strengths.
7 Providing Service User Centred Care.
8 Making a Difference.
9 Promoting Safety and Positive Risk Taking.
10 Personal Development and Learning.

Details of the Ten ESCs can be found online at www.skillsforhealth.org.uk/mentalhealth/esc.php.

An aspiration of primary care services is the improved education and development of primary care staff able to recognize and screen for symptoms of common mental health problems using recognized diagnostic criteria and screening tools such as the Diagnostic Statistical Manual (DSM-IV-TR) (American Psychiatric Association, 2000). Evidence suggests that skills and attitudes to patients with mental health problems can be significantly improved through such skill-based and focused training courses, even where this training is delivered over a short space of time (Payne et al, 2002; Richards et al, 2002). A practice nurse may manage a number of clinics including those for patients with diabetes, hypertension, or asthma, and come into contact with many patients who have chronic physical illness. It is important that all professionals within the primary care team be mindful that such patients form a vulnerable group and may experience depression and/or anxiety. *The Enhanced Services Specification for Depression* (NIMHE North West Development Centre, 2004a) offers guidance on suitable screening tools.

Liaison with mental health workers in the primary care team and referral to them will also improve early detection of serious mental health problems and ensure that treatment is offered within primary care. Failure to do this may result in patients living with mental health problems that could be treated and eventually deteriorate.

Summary

- The primary care team is probably the first point of contact for someone needing medical or nursing help and is comprised of a variety of healthcare professionals, including mental health practitioners
- The team works together to provide treatment that will resolve both physical health problems and common mental health problems. It is important, therefore, that each team member understands the roles and responsibilities of other members within the team

References

American Psychiatric Association (2000). *Diagnostic and Statistical Manual of Mental Disorders: DSM-IV-TR: Fourth Edition Text Revision*. Washington DC: American Psychiatric Association.

Melzer, H., Gill, B., Petticrew, M. & Hinds, K. (1995).

The prevalence of psychiatric morbidity among adults living in private households. London: HMSO.

National Institute for Mental Health in England, National Health Service University & Sainsbury Centre for Mental Health (2004). *The Ten Essential Shared Capabilities. A framework for the whole of the mental health workforce.* London: Department of Health.

National Institute for Mental Health in England North West Development Centre (2004a). *Enhanced Services Specification for depression under the new GP contract.* Hyde, Cheshire: NIMHE North West Development Centre.

Payne, F., Harvey, K., Jessopp, L., Plummer, S., Tylee, A. & Gournay, K. (2002). Knowledge, confidence and attitudes towards mental health of nurses working in NHS Direct and the effects of training. *Journal of Advanced Nursing,* 40, 549–559.

Richards, D., Richards, A., Barkham, M., Williams, C. & Cahill, J. (2002). PHASE: a health technology approach to psychological treatment in primary mental health care. *Primary Health Care Research and Developments,* 3: 159–168.

Useful websites

www.nimhe.org.uk (National Institute for Mental Health in England)

www.nimhenorthwest.org.uk (NIMHE North West Development Centre)

www.psych.org. (American Psychiatric Association)

www.scmh.org.uk (Sainsbury Centre for Mental Health)

www.skillsforhealth.org.uk (Skills For Health)

Test yourself

 To check your progress, locate this section on CD-ROM 1 and work through the interactive questions at the end.

Section 4: The patient's perspective of primary care

Often when a patient enters primary care with a mental health problem, they are unaware of what the problem is. They could be experiencing

Meet Andrew

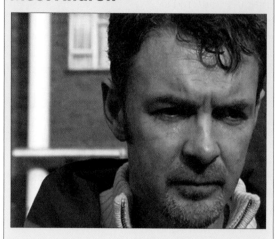

Andrew is a 34-year-old single man who lives alone. He is rather lonely, but has difficulty rectifying this problem as he is very nervous about meeting new people because of his worries that he will not know what to say and that people will think he is stupid because of this. Even when meeting people who appear friendly, he worries that they are noticing his discomfort and tension and generally concludes that they do not like him. In social situations he is prone to sweating, shaking and nausea; he has actually vomited occasionally. He spends most evenings at home, watching television. He works as a clerk at a local firm that supplies office equipment, where he generally avoids interacting with colleagues for fear of their negative evaluation. He has two close male friends who occasionally manage to persuade him to go down to the local pub. Andrew gets anxious about doing this and usually drinks a couple of beers in the house before venturing out with his friends.

 There are video and audio clips on CD-ROM 1 in which Andrew introduces himself, speaks to his mother about his pending visit to the health centre, waits in the centre's reception area, and then meets his GP. Transcripts of the clips follow.

a variety of symptoms, such as lethargy, loss of appetite or altered sleep pattern, which could be masking the real problem.

Failure or delay in diagnosing mild to moderate mental health problems can result in the patient being passed from one service to another, which can in turn exacerbate the situation. The NHS Modernisation Agency places a lot of emphasis on improving the patient's journey through services, including primary care. They have developed a mapping process to track and analyse what happens to people from referral to discharge, with the aim of analysing this and improving areas that cause distress through prolonged waiting times or poor service. This part of the improvement programme has been incorporated into the work of the National Primary Care Development Team.

Further information is available on the following websites: www.modern. nhs.uk (Modernisation Agency); www.npdt.org (National Primary Care Development Team).

Most health centres now have information booklets explaining the range of services offered and the process of making an appointment and obtaining repeat prescriptions. Many health centres have information available to patients through display boards, posters and leaflets introducing patients to the clinics offered and services available within the health centre, and groups and help available in the local area.

Some health centres also attempt to manage the waiting time by creating a relaxed atmosphere in the reception area, with easy listening music playing in the background, and having magazines and drinks machines available and/or play areas for children.

There are video and audio clips on CD-ROM 1 in which Andrew introduces himself, speaks to his mother about his pending visit to the health centre, waits in the centre's reception area, and then meets his GP. Transcripts of the clips are given below.

Video: Introducing Andrew (Social Phobia)

Andrew: I guess I'm kind of shy. The thing I find toughest though is meeting people for the first time. I never know what to say, I get all tongue-tied, my mind goes completely blank and I end up making a complete fool of myself. People just end up thinking I'm really stupid. You know, they can come across as the nicest person in the world and I'll still be like some kind of gibbering wreck. I try to avoid eye contact these days to reduce the chance that anyone will talk to me. I can just feel all the tension inside and start to shake really noticeably. I also start sweating like a pig. Sometimes I blush too, which I really hate. I can see how they must see me and just want to get away. There's no way they'll want to give me the time of day.

I've been sick a couple of times too, which is horrendous. Both were on family meals out when I just felt really self-conscious, being with all these aunties and uncles that I hadn't seen for ages, and I just couldn't eat while I was talking to them. It was a nightmare.

One of the times I remember, I'd ordered fish and chips because I thought that'd be easier to eat, but it came with peas. I plucked up the courage to eat some peas, but my hands shook that much that they went everywhere. I just ended up feeling sick and I had to go to the toilets where I actually vomited.

My mates drag me out every now and again, but I usually have to drink a couple of beers before I go out as I worry about my hand shaking in the pub. That does help, but I don't think it's good that I have to do that. I just try to avoid going if I can, or make some excuse and come away after an hour or so. I'm hoping that the person Dr Mehra has referred me to will be able to help.

Audio: Andrew's mother talks to him on the phone

Mum: I'm just phoning to check that you're going to see Dr Mehra today as arranged.

Andrew: Actually, I've been thinking about cancelling to be honest. I'll not know what to say. I feel like I'd be wasting his time.

Mum: Now Andrew, you've had this problem for quite some time now, and it is interfering in your life. It's stopping you doing lots of things, and look what an ordeal the family meal out last week was for you. We've talked about this. I'm worried about you.

Andrew: I know.

Mum: Tell you what, what if I come with you?

Andrew: NO! I'll go myself.

Mum: Oh well, alright, but the appointment's at 10 isn't it?

Andrew: Yes.

Mum: Right, well I'll give you time to get home then ring you.

Andrew: Okay I'll go and I'll talk to you later.

Mum: Now, you're sure you don't want me to come too?

Andrew: YES, I'm very sure. I promise I'll go and I'll speak to you later.

Mum: Well alright then, I'll talk to you later. Bye.

Andrew: Bye Mum.

Video: Andrew's experience of entering his health centre

Andrew: I'm here to see Dr Mehra at 10 o'clock.

Receptionist: Sorry, can you speak up, I can't hear you.

Andrew: Dr Mehra. I have an appointment at 10 o'clock.

Receptionist: Okay, what's the name please?

Andrew: Andrew Dutton.

Receptionist: Okay. Dr Mehra is running about 20 minutes late this morning. If you take a seat, I'll call you when he's ready.

Andrew: Thank you.

Andrew's thoughts: I made a mess of that. She thinks I'm stupid and wasting the doctor's time. She must have been able to see how much I'm sweating, and I can feel that I'm bright red. They're obviously too busy, I shouldn't be bothering them. Some of these people look really ill. What am I going to do for the next 20 minutes? Maybe I should go and come back. I could sit in the toilets. I'm feeling sick. Those two people waiting closest to reception must have heard that, they must think I'm really stupid too. They must be wondering what's wrong with me, that I'm sweating so much and so red. I shouldn't have listened to my Mum, or maybe it would have been better if she was here too.

Video: Andrew being called to see his GP

Receptionist: Andrew Dutton? Dr Mehra, Room 3.

Andrew: (Distracted with own thoughts and doesn't hear)

Receptionist: MR DUTTON? Dr Mehra is waiting in Room 3.

Andrew: I'm sorry. I'm sorry, I'm sorry.

Video: Andrew discussing his problem with his GP

Andrew's thoughts: What am I supposed to do? Am I supposed to just go in? What if he's still busy? Does the door being open mean I should go in? Perhaps I should knock. Maybe he'll be annoyed if I knock, and he's busy on the telephone. Maybe I should just wait.

Dr Mehra: Come in. Come in, sit down. How can I help?

Andrew: Sorry, I feel sick.

Dr Mehra: Okay, are you going to be sick now?

Andrew: No, I'll be alright. I've come because I haven't been coping too well around people, especially strangers.

Dr Mehra: Can you tell me a bit more about that?

Andrew: Ermmm, well I get anxious and I never know what to say, and it all comes out wrong, and I end up making a fool of myself. People can see that I'm blushing and sweating. I get very shaky and I know that I must look really stupid. When this happens, I feel sick and I just want to get away. I'm sorry, you must think I'm wasting your time.

Dr Mehra: No, no, not at all, you're not wasting my time. How often is this happening?

Andrew: Well, two or three times in the last week I've been like a gibbering wreck when

Exercise

- What are the potential barriers/obstacles that might impede a patient receiving the assessment and treatment they need?
- What measures has your own practice taken to mitigate these barriers/obstacles?
- What systems and information/resources are in place in your practice to help patients such as Andrew cope with visiting the practice and sitting in the waiting area?

I've been out, and that's not including this morning.

Dr Mehra: And how long has it been a problem?

Andrew: Well, I suppose I've always been a bit shy; I mean, even when I was at school, I found it difficult to make friends, but things were not so bad at college because I could just lose myself in the crowd. But I work for a small company, and my job has just changed, and I've got to speak to colleagues and customers, and it's becoming increasingly more difficult for me.

Dr Mehra: Has anything helped with the problem so far?

Andrew: I feel less anxious if I can get my head down and busy myself, and not attract any attention. But I don't go out with colleagues, I don't go to work dos, and I don't go to the pub on a Friday afternoon for drinks or anything.

Dr Mehra: So, what sort of help do you want?

Andrew: I'm not sure. My Mum seems to think that if I could talk to somebody, maybe a counsellor, that might help, but I'm not sure.

Dr Mehra: Well, we have a mental health worker based within the health centre who specializes in the kind of problems that you're describing. I could make an arrangement for her to see you at the centre if you like.

Andrew: Yes, if you think I wouldn't be wasting her time.

Dr Mehra: No, no, not at all.

Andrew: Thank you.

Dr Mehra: I'll arrange for an appointment to be sent to you. Is that okay?

Andrew: Thank you.

It is useful to consider the barriers and obstacles to a patient's journey through primary care, using a time line from the beginning to the end of contact, and then to generate solutions to each of the identified barriers and obstacles that enhance choice, speed of treatment and flexibility of service.

More information on a patient's perspective is available throughout Chapter 2.

Summary

- By reading this section, you will have considered the political and public influences that have united to change the face of healthcare delivery since 1989
- The introduction of Primary Care Trusts has greatly affected the way primary mental healthcare is delivered and has resulted in a wide range of services becoming available in primary care that had previously been available only in secondary care
- You should now be in a position to discuss the roles and responsibilities of PCTs and the individual roles and responsibilities within primary care teams, and demonstrate an understanding of how this integrates with secondary mental health services
- It is useful to consider the barriers and obstacles to a patient's journey through primary care using a time line and then generate solutions to each of the barriers and obstacles that enhance choice, speed of treatment and flexibility.

References

www.modern.nhs.uk (Modernisation Agency)

www.npdt.org (National Primary Care Development Team)

Test yourself

 To check your progress, locate this section on CD-ROM 1 and work through the interactive questions at the end.

Chapter 1.2
Policy, legal and ethical frameworks influencing primary mental healthcare

Introduction

Chapter 1.2 provides an overview of the concepts underpinning healthcare law. It is not intended to be a complete and comprehensive study of medico-legal law. It does not constitute legal advice. Significant cases of common law are included. Further details can be found by searching relevant law libraries or textbooks.

Aims

- To provide an overview and opportunity to examine the principles that underpin UK mental health law
- To provide an opportunity to evaluate frameworks that ensure standards of safe and competent care within the NHS including the maintenance of accurate records
- To enhance knowledge and understanding of the process of clinical supervision

Learning outcomes

At the end of Chapter 1.2 the reader will be able to critically:
- Appraise law affecting healthcare and mental health practice
- Examine the legal context of the mental health workers
- Appraise legal issues and related ethics pertaining to health and mental healthcare
- Evaluate the legislation that underpins the provision of quality care in the NHS
- Reflect on personal experience gained in structured reflection and clinical supervision

Chapter 1.2 content is as follows:

1 Frameworks for safe and competent practice: Clinical governance
2 Accountability
3 Record keeping
- Access to records
- Record retention
- Storage of records
- Principles of good record keeping
4 Clinical supervision
- Models of supervision
- Types of supervision
- The contracting process in supervision
- Overcoming barriers to successful supervision
5 English law
- Defining terms and acts of parliament
- Context of law
6 Common law
- Tort
- Negligence
- Duty of care
- Vicarious liability
- The Bolam Test and best interests
7 Consent
- Consent and mental health
- Children and consent
- Capacity and lawful consent
8 Capacity
- The Mental Capacity Bill
9 Confidentiality
- Confidentiality related to healthcare practice
- Data protection
10 The Human Rights Act 1998

Section 1: Frameworks for safe and competent practice: Clinical governance

When the NHS was first established in 1948, little emphasis was placed on quality. It was assumed

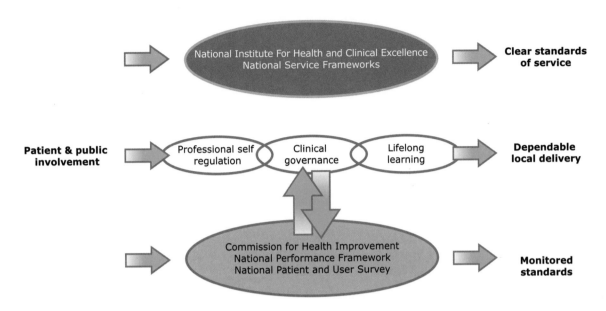

Figure 1: Setting, delivering, monitoring standards for a first class service – quality in the new NHS (Department of Health, 1998a)

that the overall infrastructure and emphasis on education and training would naturally improve quality (Freedman, 2002). It was not until the publication of *The New NHS: Modern, Dependable* (Department of Health, 1997a) that emphasis was formally placed on the improvement and maintenance of quality in the NHS. This document acknowledged that quality was highly variable and pledged to develop a National Health Service that offers people prompt, high-quality treatment and care when they need it.

This shift in focus towards the maintenance of quality was brought about in the wake of catastrophic failures in bone tumour diagnosis in Birmingham, paediatric cardiac surgery in Bristol, and cervical screening in Kent and Canterbury (Department of Health, 1998a). Equally catastrophic failures also occurred within the mental health field. One such incidence was the murder of Jonathan Zito in 1992 by Christopher Clunis, who had a diagnosis of schizophrenia. The subsequent report into the homicide revealed a catalogue of errors and missed opportunities in the patient's care, stretching back over many years. He had a long history of violence, institutional care and non-compliance with treatment programmes (Ritchie, 1994).

These cases received high-profile media

coverage resulting in public outcry. The White Paper – *A First Class Service: Quality in the new NHS* (Department of Health, 1998a) acknowledged that these high-profile cases have been one of three factors that had resulted in a reduction in public confidence in the NHS. The other two factors were:

1   Inequity of services available to patients (postcode lottery)
2   Speed of access to services

In an attempt to redress the imbalance in both access to, and quality of, care provision, the government introduced the National Service Frameworks (NSFs) (Department of Health, 1999a) and the National Institute for Health and Clinical Excellence (NICE) (www.nice.org.uk).

The NSFs aimed to stress that services should be organized to cater for patients with particular conditions, and to spell out the standards that services should meet. In addition, NICE produces information for clinicians about which treatments work best for which patients.

Clinical governance is seen as central to ensuring the continued improvement of the NHS (*see* Figure 1).

Clinical governance is a systematic approach to quality assurance and provides a framework for bringing together all local activity for assessing and improving clinical quality into a single programme. It is defined as:

'A framework through which NHS organisations are accountable for continuously improving the quality of their services and safeguarding high standards of care, by creating an environment in which excellence in clinical care will flourish.'

Department of Health, 1999b

The Commission for Health Improvement (CHI) was established in 1999. Its function was to support the delivery of high-quality care across the NHS. CHI was to conduct a programme of reviews, in which evidence would be sought to ensure that clinical governance arrangements were working and that national standards produced by NICE were adhered to.

Following the publication of the Health and Social Care Act 2003, CHI was abolished and replaced by the Healthcare Commission on 1 April 2004. The Healthcare Commission is responsible for promoting an improvement in the quality of healthcare in England and Wales; this includes regulation of the independent sector in England.

The Healthcare Commission has also assumed responsibility for reviewing complaints that have not been resolved at local level.

Exercise

- Find out about the clinical governance structure within your PCT
- What clinical governance groups exist within your PCT?

Summary

- Clinical governance is a systematic approach to quality assurance and provides a framework for bringing together, into a single programme, all local activity for assessing and improving clinical quality
- Clinical governance is seen as central to ensuring the continued improvement of patient care in the NHS
- *A First Class Service: Quality in the new NHS* (1998a) highlighted three factors that had resulted in a reduction in public confidence in the NHS:
    1. High-profile cases such as catastrophic failures in bone tumour diagnosis in Birmingham, paediatric cardiac surgery in Bristol, and cervical screening in Kent and Canterbury
    2. Inequity of services available to patients (postcode lottery)
    3. Speed of access to services
- In an attempt to redress the imbalance in both access to and quality of care provision, the government introduced the National Service Frameworks (NSFs) and the National Institute for Health and Clinical Excellence (NICE)
- The Commission for Health Improvement (CHI) was established in 1999 to ensure clinical governance arrangements were working and that national standards produced by NICE were adhered to. This was replaced by the Healthcare Commission in March 2004
- The Healthcare Commission promotes improvement in quality of healthcare in England and Wales, including the regulation of the independent sector in England. It also assumes responsibility for reviewing unresolved complaints

References

Department of Health (1997a). *The New NHS: Modern, Dependable*. London: HMSO.

Department of Health (1998a). *A First Class Service: Quality in the New NHS*. London: HMSO.

Department of Health (1999a). *The National Service Framework for Mental Health*. London: HMSO.

Department of Health (1999b). *Clinical governance: Quality in the new NHS*, HSC 99/065, London: HMSO.

Freedman, D.B. (2002). Clinical governance – bridging management and clinical approaches to quality in the UK. *Clinica Chimica Acta*, 319, 133–141.

Ritchie, J. (1994) *The report of the inquiry into the case and treatment of Christopher Clunis.* London: The Stationery Office.

The Health and Social Care Act 2003

Useful website

www.nice.org.uk (National Institute for Health and Clinical Excellence)

Test yourself

 To check your progress, locate this section on CD-ROM 1 and work through the interactive questions at the end.

Section 2: Accountability

Whilst responsibility is about being answerable for what you do, accountability is about being answerable for the consequences of what you do (Semple & Cable, 2003).

The Health Professions Council, in *The standards of conduct, performance and ethics* (HPC, 2003), states that 'as a health professional, you must protect the health and well-being of people who use or need your services in every circumstance.'

At present, mental health workers assuming new roles as assistant practitioners in line with the modernization agenda in primary care are not aligned to any professional body, which has raised issues regarding accountability. Each health profession holds its own code of professional conduct to ensure standards of conduct are maintained. For example, nurses adhere to the Nursing and Midwifery Code of Professional Conduct (NMC, 2004) which can be found online at www.nmc-uk.org/nmc/main/publications/CodeOfProfessionalConduct.pdf, and psychologists adhere to the *Code of Conduct, Ethical Principles and Guidelines* (The British Psychological Society, 1993) which can be found online at www.bps.org.uk/documents/Code.pdf. The Department of Health recognizes that large gaps exist in the regulation of healthcare staff and has recently published a consultation document which aims to address the issue of regulation of all healthcare staff (Department of Health, 2004c).

Three main reasons for regulating healthcare support staff are identified:

1   To protect the public by requiring these staff to meet standards of practice, conduct and training, and by dealing with those who do not meet the standards

2   To provide a regulated workforce of practitioners who can safely fill jobs vacated by professional practitioners as they take on extended medical roles, and who can build on this to go on to professional practice if they so wish

3   To plug the gaps in the overall regulatory framework, so that all staff in health and social care, whose work could impact on patients or carers, are subject to similar regulation

The Department of Health proposes that healthcare assistants, assistant practitioners, therapy assistants and those undertaking similar roles be regulated by means of a Statutory Committee within the Health Professions Council – the Health Occupations Committee.

Exercise

Read the Health Professions Council's *Standards of Conduct, Performance and Ethics* (available online at www.hpc-uk.org/aboutregistration/standards/standardsofconductperformanceandethics/index.asp) and consider the following:
• How do you intend to keep your knowledge and skills up to date?
• What are the factors that would assist or prevent you from keeping up to date?
• What do you understand by respecting the confidentiality of your patients?

Summary

• Accountability relates to being answerable for the consequences of your actions
• As a health worker you must protect the

health and well-being of those who use your service
- Each health profession has its own code of conduct; however, at present, mental health workers in primary care are not aligned to any professional body. The Department of Health proposes that the Health Professions Council will fulfil this role in the future

References

British Psychological Society (1993). *Code of Conduct, Ethical Principles and Guidelines.* Leicester: British Psychological Society.

Department of Health (2004c). *Regulation of Health Care Staff in England and Wales: A consultation document.* London: HMSO.

Health Professions Council (2003). *Standards of Conduct, Performance and Ethics. Your Duties as a Registrant.* London: Health Professions Council.

Nursing and Midwifery Council (2004). *The NMC Code of Professional Conduct: Standards for Conduct, Performance and Ethics.* London: Nursing and Midwifery Council.

Semple, M. & Cable, S. (2003). The New Code of Professional Conduct. *Nursing Standard,* 17, 23, 40–48.

Useful websites

www.bps.org.uk/documents/Code.pdf (British Psychological Society)

www.hpc-uk.org/publications/standards_of_conduct_ performance_and_ethics.htm (Health Professions Council)

www.nmc-uk.org/nmc/main/publications/CodeOf ProfessionalConduct.pdf (Nursing and Midwifery Council)

Test yourself

 To check your progress, locate this section on CD-ROM 1 and work through the interactive questions at the end.

Section 3: Record keeping

The Report on the Review of Patient-Identifiable Information (Department of Health, 1997c) was commissioned by the Chief Medical Officer of England in response to increasing concern about the ways in which patient information is used in the NHS.

A key recommendation of the review was the establishment of 'Guardians' of patient information throughout the NHS. It was recommended that each Health Authority, Special Health Authority, NHS Trust and Primary Care Trust should appoint a 'Caldicott' Guardian. The Guardian should be at board level, be a senior health professional and have responsibility for promoting clinical governance within the organization.

An essential requirement of all Codes of Professional Conduct is the maintenance of accurate patient and user records. Record keeping is defined by Young (1995) as 'Any permanent form of information recorded about a patient'.

The Nursing and Midwifery Council (2002) published guidelines for records and record keeping, updated in 2005 and available online at: www. nmc-uk.org/aFrameDisplay.aspx? DocumentID=516. These assert that good record keeping helps to protect the welfare of patients by promoting:
- High standards of clinical care
- Continuity of care
- Better communication and dissemination of information between members of the inter-professional healthcare team
- An accurate account of treatment and care planning and delivery
- The ability to detect problems, such as changes in the patient's condition, at an early stage

It is important to recognize that all information recorded about a patient's care can be:
- Called upon by a court as evidence
- Can be used as evidence in an investigation or complaints procedure

Tingle (1998) asserts that 'poor records mean a poor defence and no records means no defence'.

Common flaws that have been identified in record keeping are:

- Incomplete recording of information
- Use of jargon
- Assumptions being made on incomplete or inaccurate information
- Recording opinion rather than fact
- Use of abbreviation
- Offensive or subjective statements
- Failure to include dates and times
- Omission of a signature or use of initials
- Illegible writing

Access to records

The Access to Health Records Act 1990 gives patients the right of access to manual records made about them after 1 November 1991.

The Data Protection Act 1998 gives patients the right of access to their computer-held records. This act also regulates the storage and protection of information held on computer.

 CD-ROM 1 includes a video clip which explores the issue of managing a record system that serves all the disciplines working in a Primary Care Team. A transcript of the clip is shown below.

Video: Integrated clinical record system

Practice manager: Thanks. Now that everyone has introduced themselves, it's great to welcome Alan. We've been waiting such a long time for a counsellor. Perhaps I can just clarify the purpose of today's meeting. The Trust has recently produced a draft document and policy on implementing an integrated system of record keeping. Each team within the Trust has been asked to meet, and make comment on, the proposals within the policy and its implications for practice. So, what we need to do today is to consider how it is going to work in our team within this health centre, and raise any issues of concern we might have for discussing by the policy implementation group.

Practice nurse: So this is the document that you circulated two weeks ago, and asked us to make comment on?

Practice manager: Yes, yes, that's right. Has everyone had a chance to read it, and consider how it is going to affect the way they currently make records?

(Most people nod)

District nurse: I've only had a chance to glance briefly at it. I've been on holiday.

Practice manager: That's okay. Perhaps it would be useful to start by looking at how it's actually going to work in this health centre?

Health visitor: Can I just check: does this involve me putting all my patients' details and visits on an electronic record keeping system using a computer?

Practice manager: Yes, that will be part of the integrated system.

Counsellor: I'm feeling uncomfortable with this and confidentiality. My code of practice requires me to keep sensitive information confidential.

Practice manager: Actually, we are all required to keep sensitive information confidential. It is Trust policy and part of the Data Protection Act.

GP: Can I just say that I think it would be really useful if people's records were centrally kept. There seem to be some obvious benefits to implementing an integrated record system.

Mental health worker: So where would I write up in my records the face-to-face and telephone sessions with my patients in the patient notes?

Practice nurse: I currently write up all of my patient notes from the clinics that I run, electronically, as I see the patient. So I don't see how it would be any different for you than it is for me.

Practice manager: I can see that there are a number of issues here, but there appear to be a number of benefits to implementing an integrated system. So why don't we start writing things up on the flip chart?

Exercise

- Find out if your Trust uses an integrated record system
- What impact does this have on your role?

Record retention

The Health Service Circular (Department of Health, 1999c) provides guidance in its Appendix B, outlining retention periods for NHS records. The Health Service Circular can be accessed online at: www.dh.gov.uk/assetRoot/ 04/01/20/36/04012036.pdf. The length of retention depends on the type of record. Generally, case records should be kept for eight years after the conclusion of treatment, except in the following cases:

- Children's and young persons' records should be kept until the patient's 25th birthday, or 26th birthday if the young person was 17 years old at conclusion of treatment
- The records of 'mentally disordered persons' should be kept for 20 years after no further treatment was deemed necessary, or eight years after the patient's death, if they died while receiving treatment
- Where legal action has commenced

Storage of records

It is good practice to:
- Store patients' records in the environment designated by your PCT
- Book patients' records out as per local protocol
- Return patients' records as soon as possible
- Not leave patients' records unattended
- Always log off from the computer if not in use
- Avoid using short passwords or familiar names, birthdays, etc.
- Change passwords regularly
- Not share passwords
- Not give patient records to unauthorized personnel
- Strictly follow local protocols for requests for patients' records from people you do not know. This includes telephone and email requests

Principles of good record keeping

Records should:
- Be factual, consistent and accurate

Exercise

- Read the policy and procedures for record keeping within your Trust.
- Identify potential barriers to good record keeping.
- Decide how you would overcome these barriers.

- Be written as soon as possible after an event has occurred, providing current information on the care and condition of the patient
- Be written clearly, in such a way that the text cannot be erased or altered
- Ensure that any alterations or additions are dated and signed
- Be readable on photocopies (use black ink)
- Be dated, timed and signed, with the name of the author being alongside the first entry
- Be clear, unambiguous, concise and jargon- and abbreviation-free
- Not include meaningless phrases, irrelevant speculation, offensive statements, or irrelevant personal opinions regarding the patient
- Be consecutive
- Be written in terms the patient can understand
- Where possible, be written with the involvement of the patient or carer
- Provide evidence of the care planned, the decisions made, the care delivered and the information shared
- Provide evidence of actions agreed with the patient

Summary

- Good record keeping helps protect the welfare of patients by promoting high standards of care, continuity of care, improved communication and an ability to detect problems at an early stage
- All information recorded about a patient's care can be called upon by a court as evidence and can be used as evidence in an

investigation or complaints procedure

- The Access to Health Records Act 1990 gives patients the right to access manual records made about them after 1 November 1991. The Data Protection Act 1998 gives patients the right of access to their computer-held records and also regulates the storage and protection of such information

References

Access to Health Records Act 1990

Data Protection Act 1998

Department of Health (1997c). *The Caldicott Committee: Report on the Review of Patient-Identifiable Information.* London: HMSO.

Department of Health (1999c). *The Health Service Circular: Using Electronic Patient Records in Hospitals: Legal Requirements and Good Practice.* HSC 1998/153. London: HMSO.

Nursing and Midwifery Council (2002). *Guidelines for records and record keeping.* London: Nursing and Midwifery Council.

Tingle, J. (1998). Nurses must improve their record keeping skills. *British Journal of Nursing,* 7, 5, 245.

Young, A. (1995). Law Series 3: Record Keeping. *British Journal of Nursing,* 4, 3, 179.

Useful website

www.nmc-uk.org/aFrameDisplay.aspx?DocumentID= 516 (Nursing and Midwifery Council)

Test yourself

 To check your progress, locate this section on CD-ROM 1 and work through the interactive questions at the end.

Section 4: Clinical supervision

Clinical supervision forms an integral part of practice, as it seeks to enable mental health workers to develop skills and maintain high standards of patient care. It links to the clinical governance agenda outlined in Section 1.

Regular clinical supervision is seen as an 'integral part of a framework of activities that are designed to manage, enhance and monitor delivery of high-quality services' (Butterworth & Woods, 1998).

Clinical supervision is defined as:

'A formal process of professional support and learning which enables individual practitioners to develop knowledge and competence, assume responsibility for their own practice and enhance consumer protection and safety in complex situations.'

Department of Health, 1993

Models of clinical supervision

Several models of supervision have evolved over the last decade, with three being the most commonly recognized:

1 Growth and Support Model (Faugier, 1992)
2 Integrative Approach (Hawkins & Shohet, 1989)
3 Three Function Integrative Model (Inskipp & Proctor, 1993)

The most commonly adopted model is the Three Function Integrative Model, which details the key functions of clinical supervision as:

- **Formative**: the part of supervision concerned with the educational development of the practitioner through the maintenance and expansion of skills and knowledge
- **Restorative**: the aspect of supervision that addresses the practitioner's need for support through the management and minimization of occupational stressors
- **Normative**: seen as the managerial component of supervision, concerned with the practitioner delivering efficient and effective healthcare; a quality assurance and quality control process

In order to benefit from clinical supervision, learners will need to recognize the importance of structured reflection on their current knowledge and skills and their competence to apply these to practice. Schön (1987)

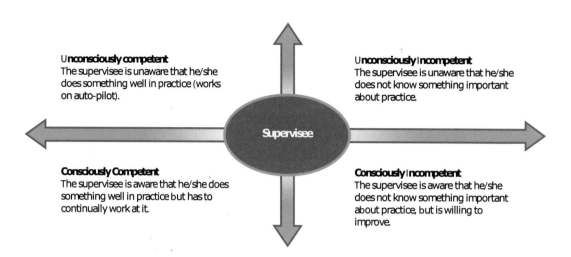

Figure 2: Four stages of learning (Driscoll, 2000)

differentiates between two types of reflection:

- **Reflection-in-action**: thinking about something whilst doing it
- **Reflection-on-action**: looking back at something after the event

Driscoll's (2000) model (Figure 2) demonstrates how, through the use of supervision, learners can move from a position of knowing something important now, to knowing something well and applying it automatically.

Where on the diagram would you place yourself? As a novice practitioner, it is likely that this will be within the consciously incompetent quadrant. Knowing your limitations is the first step towards overcoming them.

Exercise

- Where on the diagram in Figure 2 would you place yourself at this present time in relation to your role as a mental health worker?
- Where are you on the diagram in relation to your level of competence, working with patients with depression?
- Where are you on the diagram in relation to your level of competence, working with patients with anxiety?

Through a process of supervision and parallel course work, with time you will move towards the consciously competent quadrant. The danger zone is the unconscious incompetent quadrant, as it is those things that we do not realize we are not yet good at that pose the greatest threat (Race, 2001).

Knowledge gained through education and reading, etc., is known as 'declarative knowledge', which consists of theories, concepts, principles and facts that can be stated by the supervisee (Inskipp & Scaife, 2001). Knowledge that is applied in practice is known as 'procedural knowledge' and is believed to be automatic in nature.

Effective supervision encourages structured reflection upon your knowledge and explores how emerging skills are applied in practice. It offers an opportunity to identify gaps in knowledge and prompts health workers to examine their own strengths and weaknesses.

Greenwood (1993) identifies three stages in the reflective process:

Stage One: Triggered by uncomfortable feelings arising from the realization that the knowledge one is applying is not sufficient

Stage Two: Critical analysis of the situation

Stage Three: Development of a new perspective on the situation

Johns (2000) refined a model for structured

reflection (Figure 3), to enable practitioners to gain maximum benefit from the process of reflection. In short, it poses an ordered series of brief questions to aid personal reflection. It may be helpful to enhance your reflective skills in individual clinical supervision. Ensure that both you and your supervisor have copies of the prompt questions to help structure the reflection session.

Types of supervision

Clinical supervision can be offered in a variety of different ways. As a supervisee you can receive supervision from one other person known as 'individual supervision'. This is often with a line manager or more experienced practitioner. When individual supervision is offered with a peer and you take it in turns in the role as supervisor and as supervisee, this is known as 'co-supervision'. Clinical supervision can also be offered in a small group with peers from the same discipline and level of experience. This is known as 'peer group supervision' (Scaife, 2001). Alternatively, clinical supervision can be offered in a team involving different disciplines with different levels of experience, which is known as 'team supervision' (Carroll & Holloway, 1999). Recently, more flexible supervision arrangements have become popular; particularly where supervi-

Exercise

- Write down brief notes about a recent patient encounter. Tell the story of what happened. Select an everyday situation you feel you can learn from.
- Now revisit this story and take your time to reflect on your involvement and write down your responses to each of the questions in Johns's Model (Figure 3).
- What have you learnt from this reflective process?

Aesthetics

- What was I trying to achieve?
- Why did I respond as I did?
- What are the consequences of that for:
  ○ the patient?
  ○ others?
  ○ myself?
- How was this person feeling?
- How did I know this?

Personal

- How did I feel in this situation?
- What internal factors were influencing me?

Ethics

- How did my actions match my beliefs?
- What factors made me act in incongruent ways?

Empirics

- What knowledge did or should have informed me?

Reflexivity

- How does this connect with previous experiences?
- Could I handle this better in similar situations?
- What would the consequences be of alternative actions for:
  ○ the patient?
  ○ others?
  ○ myself?
- How do I NOW feel about this experience?
- Can I support myself and others better as a consequence?
- Has this changed my way of knowing?

Figure 3: Johns's model for reflection

sors and supervisees are geographically distant from one another as often occurs in primary care. Telephone and email supervision can be offered on their own or to complement any of the above supervision arrangements. All of the above include retrospective accounts of practice experience.

An alternative is concurrent, live supervision whereby the supervisor directly observes the supervisee in their work, with consent of the patient. This approach offers a more immediate feedback to the supervisee. In such arrangements, careful consideration is needed so that the supervisor is positioned so that the supervisee's relationship with the patient is not compromised.

There is no right or wrong method for delivering clinical supervision. The advantages and disadvantages of each type will depend on whether the type of supervision is viewed from a supervisor or supervisee perspective, or from a team or organizational perspective. It is important that, whatever type of supervision is used, all participants consider its strengths and limitations and make efforts to overcome any obstacles. To facilitate this, the supervisor and supervisee should regularly review the supervisory process.

The contracting process in supervision

An important component of successful supervision is the contracting process, through which the supervisor and supervisee negotiate and reach an agreement upon such matters as the timing and frequency of contacts and the role relationships (Inskipp & Scaife, 2001). The topics that might be included in a supervisory contract are as follows:
*   Ground rules
*   What is to be learned and how
*   Supervisory relationship/roles
*   Dealing with problems such as a busy supervisor, differences of opinion and ethical dilemmas

Contracting is an ongoing process and should be reviewed regularly.

Exercise

List the advantages and disadvantages of each of the different types of supervision listed below:
*   Individual
*   Group
*   Team
*   Telephone/email
*   Concurrent/live

Overcoming barriers to successful supervision

It is vital to identify potential barriers to successful supervision at the outset. A useful first step is to agree ground rules with your supervisor. One of the most commonly cited reasons for not accessing supervision is lack of available time (Duarri & Kendrick, 1999; McKeown & Thompson, 2001). It is important that you discuss this openly with your supervisor and choose the least busy times of the week.

Environment also plays an important part in ensuring successful supervision. Ensure the phone is off the hook and mobile phones are turned off, and (where appropriate) indicate that you are not to be disturbed.

Supervision is not an opportunity to catch up on gossip; remember to prepare your supervision agenda in advance and to agree on it at the start of the session. This will prevent the session losing focus. It is good practice for the supervisee to prepare for a supervision session by focusing on a question, developed from a recent experience, to take to supervision. Supervision can then be structured to problem-solve and develop solutions focused on improving clinical practice. A supervisee can then be given work to undertake between supervision sessions.

There may be occasions where a clash of personality occurs between supervisor and supervisee. It is important that this is discussed, openly, honestly and professionally, to determine the way forward. On occasions, it may be appropriate to agree that a new supervisor must be sought. CD-ROM 1 includes a video clip which shows an inappropriate referral for Samantha, a primary care mental health worker, and an audio clip of a supervision session in which she voices her concerns. Transcripts of both sessions are given below.

Video: Inappropriate referral – referral discussion

Dr Lindley: I would like you to see Mr Jones. He has a long history of chronic depression with three previous admissions to the psychiatric unit. He is starting to dip in his mood again, he is not eating, his sleep pattern is very disturbed, and he has started to have some suicidal thoughts. He has no plans as yet to act on these thoughts, but I am extremely worried about him. He was made redundant a few months ago, and this happened shortly after his wife walked out on him for another man, so naturally he is very angry and upset. I'd like you to see him as a matter of great urgency as the waiting list at the community mental health team is several weeks – unless, of course, you know they are a great danger to themselves. He also has a long history of drinking heavily, and has been waiting to be seen by the drug and alcohol team for assessment and treatment. Last week he was arrested for drunk and disorderly behaviour, and unfortunately he hit the arresting officer.

Mental health worker (Samantha): I feel a bit confused about this to be honest. I'm not really supposed to see people with such complex problems.

Dr Lindley: I'm very concerned about the long waiting time before Mr Jones can be seen by the drug and alcohol service. You're based here, and you can see him next week in our practice. It will be much easier for you to liaise with me after you have assessed him.

Samantha: The problem is that my training doesn't really prepare me to see people with such complex difficulties. I can see, from what you say, that he is depressed and that's

fine, but my concern is about his alcohol problems, and also the level of violence. I think he sounds more appropriate for secondary care.

Dr Lindley: I agree. However, the waiting time is too long as I've already said, and I think it would be good experience for you.

Samantha: I'm feeling under a lot of pressure to see this man, and I do appreciate he does need to be seen very soon. Is there no way you can put a bit of pressure on the drug and alcohol team to see him a bit quicker?

Dr Lindley: What about helping out just this once? I'll get on to the drug and alcohol team, but if you'd just agree to see him for a few weeks I'd really appreciate it.

Samantha: I can see that, but Dr Lindley I just feel really uncomfortable about this. I just don't think he is an appropriate case for me. I feel like I've got to talk about this to my supervisor. I will get back to you as soon as possible, but I really feel that I've got to do that.

Dr Lindley: Well, if you can let me know as soon as you can whether you can see him, and in the meantime I'll get on to the drug and alcohol team and see if they can speed up the referral.

Audio: Supervision – inappropriate referral

Supervisor: Okay Samantha, let me just check that I've got this right. You left it with Dr Lindley that she is chasing up for this person to be seen by the drug and alcohol team, and you agreed to come back to her as to whether it is appropriate for you to undertake some face-to-face work with him. So your question is, 'Do I see this man for Dr Lindley as requested?'

Mental health worker (Samantha): Yes, that pretty much sums it up.

Supervisor: So what do you think?

Samantha: Well, I'm not really sure to be honest. I was pretty sure at first, when I was discussing the referral, that it was completely inappropriate because of the complexity of the patient's presenting problems, but I'm also aware that I do work with people with depression and provide short-term guided self-help. The other thing is that I'm also aware that this man might need to wait a while to be seen, and Dr Lindley is really busy, and she did just ask me to do this as a one-off favour.

Supervisor: So are you saying that the reason for seeing this patient is because of the long waiting time to be seen by the drug and alcohol team, and you wanting to help Dr Lindley out of a difficult situation?

Samantha: Well, when you put it like that, it doesn't sound appropriate.

Supervisor: So what would be the reasons for you offering face-to-face and telephone contact to this patient?

Samantha: If Mr Jones's main problem was depression, and after assessment it was still considered that he could benefit from low-intensity interventions, then I'd feel much happier about seeing him.

Supervisor: And is this the case?

Samantha: Well no, he has complex needs.

Supervisor: So is it appropriate that you see him?

Samantha: Well no, I suppose not.

Supervisor: So what do you need to do next?

Samantha: I think I need to speak to Dr Lindley about it and just tell her that, after reflecting on it, and also talking to you as my supervisor, this case is just not appropriate for me to see. I could also suggest that she try to push the referral through a bit quicker by telling the drug and alcohol team about his recent arrest.

Supervisor: It sounds like you've worked this out for yourself and reached a decision that hasn't been an easy one to make. I'm impressed with how you've been able to come to a decision based on the facts, and separated this out from the pressures that you were feeling under.

Samantha: Thank you. It's not been easy, to be honest, but I do feel a lot better having talked it through.

Supervisor: I'll be interested to hear how you get on. Now, I know that we're meeting up next week at our health centre for our next supervision session, so let's put it on the agenda for that session.

Samantha: Okay. Thanks. I'll see you next week.

Exercise

Find out if your Trust has a policy guide on the implementation of clinical supervision.
- Is there a preferred model of supervision to support clinical practice?
- What type of supervision is encouraged?
- Does the policy guide offer advice or illustrative materials on the writing-up of clinical supervision sessions?

Summary

- Clinical supervision is a formal process of professional support and learning, which enables practitioners to develop knowledge and competence, and protects patients
- Clinical supervision enables a formal process of reflection
- Contracting is an important component of successful supervision
- Establishing ground rules on the timing and frequency of meetings is a useful starting point
- There are a number of different types and models of clinical supervision, each with their own advantages and disadvantages

References

Butterworth, T. & Woods, D. (1998). *Clinical Governance and Clinical Supervision Working Together to Ensure Safe and Accountable Practice.* Manchester: School of Nursing, Midwifery and Health Visiting, University of Manchester.

Carroll, M. & Holloway, E. (1999). *Counselling Supervision in Context.* London: Sage.

Department of Health (1993). *A Vision for the Future: The Nursing, Midwifery and Health Visiting Contribution to Health and Health Care.* London: HMSO.

Driscoll, J. (2000). *Practising Clinical Supervision: A Reflective Approach.* London: Balliere Tindall.

Duarri, W. & Kendrick, K. (1999). Implementing Clinical Supervision. *Professional Nurse*, 14, 12, 849–852.

Faugier, J. (1992). The supervisory relationship. In Butterworth, T. & Faugier, J. (eds) *Clinical Supervision and Mentorship in Nursing*. London: Chapman & Hall.

Greenwood, J. (1993). Reflective Practice: a critique of work of Argyris & Schön. *Journal of Advanced Nursing*, 18, 8, 1183–1187.

Hawkins, P. & Shohet, R. (1989). *Supervision in the helping professions*. Milton Keynes: Open University Press.

Inskipp, F. & Proctor, B. (1993). *The art, craft and tasks of supervision: making the most of supervision*. London: Cascade.

Inskipp, F. & Scaife, J. (2001). *Supervision in the Mental Health Professions: A Practitioner's Guide*. Hove: Philadelphia Taylor Francis.

Johns, C. (2000). *Becoming a reflective practitioner. A reflective and holistic approach to clinical nursing practice development and clinical supervision*. London: Blackwell Science.

McKeown, C. & Thompson, J. (2001). Implementing Clinical Supervision. *Nursing Management*, 8, 6, 10–13.

Race, P. (2001). *The Lecturer's Toolkit* (second edition). London: Routledge Falmer.

Scaife, J. (2001). *Supervision in the Mental Health Professions: A Practitioner's Guide*. Hove: Brunner-

Exercise

Before you start the next section, try to think of all the 'legal' words that relate to healthcare practice. Your list will probably look something like this:

Law	Crime/Criminal
Ethics	Act of Parliament
Competence	Inquiry
Capacity	Civil law
Practice	Statute
Liability	Sentence
Negligence	Restraint
Common Law	Consent
Duty of Care	Tort
Solicitor	Judge
Barrister	Jury
Court	Plaintiff
Confidentiality	Appellant
Defence	Prosecution

Next, try to list the Acts of Parliament that you think relate to healthcare practice. Once again, this is the sort of list you're likely to have made:

Abortion Act, 1967	Mental Health Act, 1983
Access to Health Records Act, 1990	NHS Reform & Health Care Professions Act, 2002
Care Standards Act, 2000	
Children Act, 1989	NHS and Community Care Act, 1990
Data Protection Act, 1998	Nurses, Midwives and Health Visitors Act, 1997
Disability Discrimination Act, 1995	
Health Act, 1999	Police and Criminal Evidence Act, 1984
Health and Safety at Work Act, 1974	Race Relations Act, 1976
Human Fertilisation & Embryology Act, 1990	Sex Discrimination Act, 1967
Medicines Act, 1967	Suicide Act, 1961

Routledge.

Schön, D. (1987). *Educating the Reflective Practitioner: How Professionals Think In Action.* New York: Basic Books.

Test yourself

 To check your progress, locate this section on CD-ROM 1 and work through the interactive questions at the end.

Section 5: English law

Defining Terms and Acts of Parliament

In England and Wales, our laws are constituted as formally enacted laws and customary law. Formally enacted laws are called 'statutes', legislated by Parliament. Customary law in this context means 'common law'.

Although Acts of Parliament can affect Scotland, much of Scottish law is different to English law, due to historical differences in practice.

Context of Law

Many people think law is absolute, merely a question of right or wrong. However, common law requires the interpretation of previous legal precedents to consider the implications of the issue at stake. On many occasions, the appropriate statute law may not be as clear as first intended, and may require further interpretation. Laws tend to reflect the society in which they are made, and, as society changes and other laws are introduced, older laws need updating to reflect the changes. A good example of when this has occurred has been with the incorporation of the Human Rights Act 1998 into English law, which now means that all future laws must be considered with the Human Rights Act in mind.

Summary

- Law is: the body of rules, whether formally enacted or customary, which a state or community recognizes as binding on its members or subjects
- Statute law is made by Parliament
- Laws can be customary – known as common law in England and Wales
- Laws change as society changes

References

Abortion Act 1967
Access to Health Records Act 1990
Care Standards Act 2000
Children Act 1989
Crime and Disorder Act 1998
Data Protection Act 1998
Disability Discrimination Act 1995
Health and Safety at Work Act 1974
Human Fertilisation & Embryology Act 1990
Medicines Act 1967
Mental Health Act 1983
NHS Reform & Health Care Professions Act 2002
NHS and Community Care Act 1990
Nurses, Midwives and Health Visitors Act 1997
Police and Criminal Evidence Act 1984
Race Relations Act 1976
Sex Discrimination Act 1967
Suicide Act 1961

Useful websites

www.hmso.go.uk/acts or www.legislation. hmso.gov.uk/acts/acts2003/20030043.htm (Her Majesty's Stationery Office (Acts))

Test yourself

 To check your progress, locate this section on CD-ROM 1 and work through the interactive questions at the end.

Section 6: Common law

Common law was developed after the Norman Conquest of 1066 as the law common to the whole of England. As the court system developed, and judges' decisions became recorded in law reports (both known as precedents), the English system of common law by precedent began to develop. This means that, when deciding a particular case, the court and judge must have regard to legal principles laid down in earlier cases on similar points of law.

Because it consists of using what has gone before as a guide, common law places great emphasis on precedents. The essence of common law is that it is made by judges sitting in courts, applying their common sense and knowledge of legal precedent to the facts before them.

Patients who believe they have been wronged during healthcare treatment may seek recourse through common law. Usually an individual (or a group of people) takes action against another person (or group of people or organization). Such a case is known as a tort.

Tort

A tort is a wrongful act that causes injury or damage. Tort is a branch of civil law that covers duties towards other people, where the responsibility to take action lies with the individual, and not with the state – unlike, for example, criminal proceedings, which involve the police and Crown Prosecution Service.

Negligence

Negligence is perhaps the most well-known, and possibly most notorious, aspect of healthcare law. In legal terms, negligence has been defined as:

> '...the omission to do something, which a reasonable man, guided upon those considerations, which ordinarily regulate the conduct of human affairs, would do, or doing something, which a prudent and reasonable man would not do.'
>
> *Blyth v Birmingham [1856]*

Negligence can also occur when people fail to do something that could have prevented harm occurring. For instance, in healthcare this could be a failure to tell a patient about the full risks of a particular treatment, or failure to pass on important information regarding a patient's care. This is known as an 'act of omission'.

People turn to the courts for redress for negligence, using the branch of law known as 'tort', because they want some compensation. The purpose of compensation is to put the injured person in the place of where they would have been had the harm not occurred.

In order for a negligence case to be brought, harm (or damage) must have occurred. But this alone is not enough. There also has to be:

- A duty of care
- The duty of care has to be breached by the defendant
- The harm caused must not be too remote a consequence of the breach

This can be simplified as damage, breach of duty, and a link between the two. A further important aspect is that the damage must have been foreseeable and could have been prevented, and be reasonably closely linked to the duty (proximity; see the ruling by Lord Atkins, below).

Duty of care

According to common law we all have a duty of care under certain circumstances. In healthcare there is a well-established principle that duty exists once treatment has started. In general circumstances, this is referred to as the 'neighbour principle'. Lord Atkins's speech, considered by some to be the most important words ever spoken by a judge, helps define this, and also explains the principles of 'foreseeability' and 'proximity':

> 'The rule that you are to love your neighbour becomes in law, you must not injure your neighbour and the lawyer's question, who is my neighbour? receives a restricted reply. You must take reasonable care to avoid acts or omissions which you can reasonably foresee would be likely to injure your neighbour. Who, then, in law is my neighbour? The answer seems to be – persons who are so closely and directly affected by my act (Proximity) that I ought reasonably to have them in contemplation as being so affected when I am directing my mind to the acts or omissions which are called in question.'
>
> *Lord Atkins, in Donoghue v Stevenson (1932)*

Legally speaking, there is no obligation on an individual to assist others, unless:

- They have undertaken a task, when they have a duty to perform it carefully
- They have a personal relationship with the other person
- When harm occurred caused by a third party that the defendant should control. Acts of third parties are not the responsibility of a defendant, unless there is a common law duty to prevent the third party from causing injury or other harm

If there is such a duty, then proximity may be found to exist.

Examples of duty of care relationships

- Employers and their employees
- Manufacturers and consumers
- Teachers and their pupils
- Home occupiers and their visitors
- Motorists and other road users
- Doctors, nurses and their patients

Vicarious liability

In the NHS, most claims for negligence are brought in tort, as they are 'non-contractual civil wrongs'. This is because there is no contract between the two parties concerned. In such a claim, it is the employing NHS organization that has the action brought against them, not the individual. This is because of 'vicarious liability'.

An employer is vicariously liable for negligent acts or omissions by their employee in the course of employment, whether or not such act or omission was specifically authorized by the employer. To avoid vicarious liability, an employer must demonstrate either that the employee was not negligent, in that they were reasonably careful, or that the employee was acting in his own right rather than on the employer's business. Employers are not normally legally responsible for the criminal acts of employees, although this has happened (see Lister and Others v. Hesley Hall Limited [2001]).

There is a term often inserted into contracts of employment that 'an employee will exercise all reasonable care and skill during the course of employment'. An employee who is negligent can be found to be in breach of the terms of their employment. The employer who has been held vicariously liable could seek an indemnity from the employee to make good the loss.

As claims for medical negligence have risen significantly lately, NHS Trusts are covered by a type of insurance scheme, called the 'Clinical Negligence Scheme for Trusts'. Employees of a Primary Care Trust are covered by this scheme.

The Bolam Test and best interests

There is, under common law, a requirement that doctors (and all healthcare professionals should act in accordance with professional standards set by the medical profession ('The Bolam Test') when determining 'Best Interests'.

This gives rise to the question of at what standard we expect doctors (and by extension, other healthcare professionals) to perform. As we discussed earlier, negligence is 'the omission to do something which a reasonable man would do'.

In general terms, the reasonable man has been described as 'the man on the street' or 'the man on the Clapham omnibus'.

Clearly, there is a different expectation for the standards of the reasonable doctor (or other healthcare practitioner). Again, the precedent set by the Bolam case is helpful:

> 'The test is the standard of the ordinary skilled man exercising and professing to have that special skill. A man need not possess the highest expert skill, at the risk of being found negligent. It is a well-established law that it is sufficient if he exercises the ordinary skill of an ordinary man exercising that particular art.'
>
> *Bolam v. Friern Hospital [1957]*

Healthcare professionals' standards of conduct are governed by the terms of their employment, by common and statute law, and by the standards of their professional body. Good examples of 'codes of conduct' you may choose to look at are the Nursing and Midwifery Council Code of Professional Conduct (NMC, 2004), the British Psychological Society (1993)

The Bolam Test

Bolam v Friern Hospital [1957] All ER 118 QBD

In this case, the plaintiff was given electro-convulsive treatment (ECT) without a muscle relaxant, causing him to suffer fractures. At the time, there were two schools of thought on the use of muscle relaxants in ECT, one view being that it was necessary, the other that this only increased the risk. Whilst there is a duty of care on the doctor to 'act in accordance with the practice accepted by a body of medical men skilled in that particular art', negligence and failure to act in the 'best interests' cannot be inferred, merely because there was a body of opinion which took contrary views.

As well as having a common law duty of care, doctors have a further duty to act in the 'best interests' of a mentally incapacitated patient. The convenience of those caring for the patient is not a consideration when determining the 'best interests' of the patient.

Recent judgements have further explained this, so that now it is not enough that there is a reasonable body of medical opinion; this opinion must also have a logical basis (see Bolitho v. City & Hackney Health Authority, [1997]).

Code of Conduct, Ethical Principles & Guidelines and the Health Professions Council, Standards of Conduct, Performance and Ethics (HPC, 2003).

Case references

Donoghue v. Stevenson [1932]

Donoghue found a snail in a bottle of ginger beer bought from a café. Being unable to sue the proprietor, Donoghue successfully sued the manufacturers.

Lister and Others v. Hesley Hall Limited [2001] UKHL 22 (3 May 2001)

Hesley Hall Ltd employed Mr Grain as warden

Exercise

- Read one of the professional codes of conduct mentioned in the previous paragraph (see list of useful websites).
- Write down some of the key themes that seem to apply generally to the codes of conduct and professional standards that you have read.

of a home for maladjusted children. Over the course of several years, Mr Grain sexually abused the children under his ward. As employers, Hesley Hall were found vicariously liable.

Bolam v Friern Hospital [1957] All ER 118 QBD

See box 'The Bolam Test' (box).

Schloendorff v. Society of New York Hospital [1914] 211 NY 125

In this case, brought by the plaintiff against the Society of New York Hospital, the plaintiff entered the hospital in 1908 with a stomach disorder. After some weeks of treatment as an inpatient the house physician discovered a lump, thought to be a fibroid tumour. The visiting surgeon advised an operation. The plaintiff testified that she was told the character of the lump could not be determined without an examination. The plaintiff consented to the examination, but stated that she told the physician that there must be no operation. She received the examination, but whilst under anaesthesia the tumour was removed. Following the operation, and according to witness testimony, gangrene developed in her left arm causing intense suffering and requiring amputation of some fingers.

This case was heard as an appeal from the plaintiff, following an earlier hearing in which the judgement had been found in favour of the defendant. The case had been brought against the hospital for negligence. In this appeal, the previous judgement was affirmed, deciding that the physicians/surgeons performing the operation had committed the wrong, but the defendant was not liable for their actions, as they themselves had not acted negligently.

Gillick v. West Norfolk & Wisbech Health Authority [1985] 3 All ER 402, HL

A mother of five daughters sought a declaration that a doctor would be acting unlawfully if he gave contraceptive treatment for any of her daughters without the mother's consent. The House of Lords said a child under 16 who has sufficient intelligence to understand fully the implications of the proposed treatment (a 'Gillick competent' child) can give her own consent to medical treatment. The fact that her parents have not consented, or even that they have expressly refused the treatment, is then irrelevant.

Re C (Adult: Refusal of Treatment) [1994] 1 All ER 819

A 68-year-old man suffering from paranoid schizophrenia developed gangrene in his foot. Doctors advised amputation, and put C's chance of survival at only 15 per cent if the leg was not amputated soon. C refused to consent, and his decision was upheld by the court. Granting an appropriate declaration, Judge Thorpe said C had sufficient understanding to take in and consider the information given him and to make a decision. The presumption of his right of self-determination was not changed.

Sidaway v. Bethlem Royal Hospital [1985] 1 All ER 643, HL

S agreed to have an operation on her spine, but Dr F did not warn her of a risk (about 1 per cent) of paralysis resulting from the operation, which, it was conceded, had been competently performed. S claimed F's failure to warn her was itself a breach of duty, but the House of Lords disagreed. Lord Scarman felt the American rule of 'informed consent' should apply, and that there should generally be full disclosure, unless 'therapeutic privilege' could be invoked. But the

majority said the Maynard test should apply, to vindicate any course supported by a substantial body of responsible medical opinion, subject to a duty to answer any direct questions truthfully and fully. Given the low level of risk, a substantial body of neuro-surgical opinion was for non-disclosure, and that was sufficient.

Bolitho v. City & Hackney Health Authority [1997] 4 All ER 771, HL

A two-year-old boy, B, suffered serious brain damage following respiratory failure, and his parents alleged medical negligence. The doctor's treatment decisions were supported by several expert witnesses, and, on that basis, the judge found that the doctor had not been negligent. B's appeal failed. Lord Browne-Wilkinson said [...] that a judge is not bound to find that a doctor is not negligent merely because there is a body of medical opinion in his favour: he must also be able to show that this opinion has a logical basis. But only very rarely would a judge decide that the opinions of a number of otherwise competent doctors were not reasonably held, and this was not such a case.

St George's Healthcare Trust v. S [1998] Times 3/8/98, CA

S was 36 weeks pregnant, and doctors advised a Caesarian delivery because of complications that threatened the lives of both S and the unborn child. S wanted the baby born naturally and (while understanding the advice) refused to follow it. A social worker then arranged for S to be admitted to hospital as a compulsory patient under the Mental Health Act 1983, and the doctors were authorised in a hearing to perform the operation without S's consent. The baby was successfully delivered, but S then appealed against the judge's order. Allowing the appeal, Judge LJ said the 1983 Act cannot be used to detain an individual against her will, merely because her thinking is unusual, bizarre, irrational or contrary to the views of the community at large. Even a patient properly detained cannot be forced into medical procedures unconnected with her mental condition, unless her capacity to consent is in some way diminished. While pregnancy may increase a woman's personal responsibilities, it does not diminish her entitlement to decide whether or not to undergo medical treatment, and a foetus's need for medical treatment cannot prevail over its mother's rights.

Appleton v Garrett [1996] PIQR 1, Dyson J

A dentist, G, deliberately over-treated a number of patients for financial reasons, supposedly obtaining their consent by giving the impression that the treatment was medically necessary. The court said a surgeon who performs an operation without his patient's consent commits an assault for which he is liable to damages. Here there was no real consent, and the trespass was of such a nature as to justify an award of aggravated, as well as compensatory damages. D was struck off the dental register for serious professional misconduct, but was reinstated two years later after retraining.

Blyth v. Birmingham Water Works Co.Court of Exchequer [1856]11 Exch. 781, 156 Eng.Rep. 1047.Prosser, pp. 132–133

The defendants installed a fire hydrant near the plaintiff's house that leaked during a severe frost, causing water damage. The jury found the defendant negligent, and the defendant appealed. The court they appealed to found that the extreme frost that caused the damage in this case was 'not within the contemplation' of the defendants and that the result of the frost was an accident. The court entered a verdict for the defendants.

Re S [1992] 4 All ER 671, Brown P

A 30-year-old woman S was six days overdue to give birth, and examination showed the baby was in a breach position and could not be born naturally. S, supported by her husband, refused to consent to a Caesarean section on religious grounds, in spite of doctors' clear advice that it was the only way in which her life and the baby's could be saved. The doctors applied to the court for permission to proceed with the operation without her consent, and the judge authorized the doctors to perform the operation in the hope of saving the baby. In the event, the operation was unsuccessful and the baby died.

Summary

- Common law is based on judges' interpretations and understanding of previous cases (known as precedents). These are written down and form Case Law
- Tort is a branch of common law that people use when they think they have been wronged, and there is no statutory duty on the part of the state or the police to act
- Compensation is used to put someone in the position they would have been in if the wrong (negligence) had not occurred
- For negligence to be proven, there must be:
  - Harm or damage
  - A duty of care
  - A breach of the duty of care
  - A link between the duty of care and the harm
- Doctors, and other healthcare professionals, have a duty of care to their patients, especially towards mentally incapacitated patients
- Under vicarious liability, employers are liable for the actions of their employees
- Healthcare professional standards are governed by employment terms and conditions, common and statute law, and the standards of professional bodies

References

British Psychological Society (1993). *Code of Conduct, Ethical Principles & Guidelines.* The British Psychological Society. Leicester.

Health Professions Council (2003). *Standards of Conduct, Performance and Ethics. Your Duties as a Registrant.* London: Health Professions Council.

Nursing and Midwifery Council (2004). *The NMC Code of Professional Conduct I: Standards for Conduct, Performance and Ethics.* London: Nursing and Midwifery Council.

Law report references

Blyth v Birmingham Waterworks [1856] 156 ER 1047

Donoghue v Stevenson, [1932] All ER Rep 1; [1932] AC 562; HL

Lister and Others v. Hesley Hall Limited [2001] UKHL 22 (3rd May, 2001)

Bolitho v City & Hackney Health Authority [1997] 4 All ER 771, HL

Bolam v Friern Hospital [1957] QBD All ER 118

Test yourself

 To check your progress, locate this section on CD-ROM 1 and work through the interactive questions at the end.

Section 7: Consent

It has long been a common law principle in English law that every person has a right to have their body protected against 'invasion' by other people, as part of a right to self-determination. This has been further defined in case law. One case, which is often used as a reference for 'consent', helps define the principle underpinning consent for healthcare.

> '...every person being of adult years and sound mind has a right to determine what shall be done with his own body and a surgeon who performs an operation without his patient's consent commits an assault.'
>
> *Schloendorff v. Society of New York Hospital [1914]*

Recent cases in English courts have supported this principle. In Appleton v. Garrett [1996], it was reported that the court said 'a surgeon who performs an operation without his patient's consent commits an assault for which he is liable in damages'.

Bearing in mind the duty of care principle to act in the patient's best interests, doctors may want to treat somebody (a) against their wishes or (b) when consent is unobtainable.

In (a), this is sometimes referred to as a 'paternalistic' view of healthcare. The argument can be constructed along the following lines: 'Good health is preferable to ill health; therefore, a patient will be better off if treated, whether they consent or not.' This can be put simply as: 'doctor knows best'.

In (b), treatment is only justified in limited circumstances. Emergency treatment to save an unconscious patient's life can be justified by the rationale that treatment is needed to restore the patient to a position where they can make up their own mind; or the patient would wish it, were they able to express consent. In the case of an unconscious adult, no other person, including the next of kin, is able to give consent on their behalf, although it is recommended good practice to discuss interventions with relatives or close friends as close to the event as practical.

The law on consent is subject to intense debate and lobbying by special interest groups. The 'doctrine of necessity' attracts particular controversy, as it is also possible for a court to overrule a patient's refusal to consent. Using the 'sanctity of life' principle, it can be necessary to intervene, even when a patient refuses on religious grounds (see *Re S [1992]*).

Consent and mental health

Generally, the only other times when somebody can be treated against their wishes are when they lack the capacity to consent to treatment due to mental impairment or age. The first instance may refer to a psychiatric emergency (where the common law principle of the duty of care could apply) or to more formal, longer-term treatment when the patient is treated under the Mental Health Act 1983, and there is a risk to the patient's or other people's life.

Children and consent

Under the Family Law Reform Act 1969 s.8(1), children between 16 and 18 have a right to consent to some medical and dental treatments; but their refusal to consent could be overruled.

Parents generally have a right to determine whether or not their child under the age of 16 has medical treatment. However, some children under the age of 16 can be given contraceptive

The Fraser Guidelines

1 The young person understands the advice being given.
2 The young person cannot be convinced to involve parents/carers or allow the medical practitioner to do so on their behalf.
3 It is likely that the young person will begin or continue having intercourse with or without treatment.
4 Unless he or she receives treatment/contraception their physical or mental health (or both) is likely to suffer.
5 The young person's best interests require contraceptive advice, treatment or supplies to be given without parental consent.

Department of Health (2004d)

advice and treatment without parental consent, provided they fulfill a set of criteria. These criteria are assessed against the Fraser Guidelines. These guidelines were formerly known as Gillick Competence, referring to a landmark case when a mother went to court because her daughter, who was under 16, had been given contraceptives against the mother's wishes (Gillick v. West Norfolk and Wisbech Area Health Authority [1984]).

However, sometimes the wishes expressed by parents to start or stop treatment can be overruled, in order to act in the child's best interests. An example may be parents refusing to allow their child a life-saving blood transfusion on religious grounds. Section 1(1) of the Children Act 1989 places a requirement that the child's welfare be the paramount consideration when determining interventions. This is an important principle to bear in mind when dealing with all issues relating to children.

Where consent is necessary, it can be expressed (such as saying 'Yes'), or implied (such as visiting a GP). However, any consent only refers to a specific action/intervention at a defined time, and should not usually be extended into other areas or taken as a licence for 'carte blanche' intervention. It can also be withdrawn, by the patient, at any time.

Failure to obtain consent for treatment in any other situation could be construed as assault and provoke civil and criminal proceedings. It may also be actionable under the Human Rights Act 1998.

Capacity and lawful consent

Consent is only lawful if it can be shown to be 'real consent' or 'true consent'. This is a legal term that requires a patient to have been informed in broad terms of the treatment or procedure, and has indicated their acceptance of it.

Patients also have a right to information about their treatment under the NHS Charter. Healthcare professionals are under an obligation to disclose information to the patient about the nature and possible risks of a likely course of treatment, and must also act as advocates for the patient (act in their best interests). Although of unproven legal standing, the term 'informed consent', introduced from the United States, has now been adopted into common healthcare practice.

Whilst consent can be implied, written or verbally expressed, all are of equal legal standing. However, proving consent has been given is clearly easier if it has been written down. It is against the law to consent to an unlawful act. Even if consent has been given, if this was under undue influence or coercion it is not lawful. Consent by a minor or someone who 'lacks capacity' or 'competence' is also unlawful.

Exercise

- Read your Trust's policy on obtaining consent from patients, including the consent to share information policy.
- Go to the Department of Health website, download the guidelines on consent (www.dh.gov.uk/assetRoot/04/ 01/91/86/ 04019186.pdf), and read them.

Summary

- Consent means 'to give permission', 'to allow'
- Everyone has a right to determine what is done to their bodies
- Failure to obtain consent could be seen as assault
- Sometimes it is necessary to treat people without or against their consent. This might be to save the life of an unconscious person, or to treat someone who is at risk of harming themselves or other people because of a mental illness, and are unable or will not give their consent
- Some children under 16 can consent to some healthcare interventions, provided they are able to understand the consequences. This is called 'Gillick competence'
- Children's needs must be paramount when making any decisions that will affect them
- In order to consent, a person must be able to:
  ◦ Understand the information
  ◦ Retain and believe it
  ◦ Weigh it up in the balance, and make a choice
  ◦ And communicate their decision
- Consent can be expressed, written down, or implied, but it only refers to the intervention in question, cannot be extended to mean any other intervention, and must always be sought
- Consent can be withdrawn at any stage

References

Children Act 1989
Family Law Reform Act 1969 s.8(1).
Mental Health Act 1983
Department of Health (2004d). *Best practice guidance for doctors and other health professionals on the provision of advice and treatment to young people under 16 on contraception, sexual and reproductive health*. London: Department of Health.

Law report references

Gillick v West Norfolk and Wisbech Area Health Authority [1984] QB 581
Schloendorff v Society of New York Hospital [1914] 211 NY 125
Appleton v Garrett [1996] PIQR
Re S [1992] 4 All ER 671

Test yourself

 To check your progress, locate this section on CD-ROM 1 and work through the interactive questions at the end.

Section 8: Capacity

In order for an adult to be able to give consent, they must be mentally competent (now called having mental capacity). There is now a widely accepted three-stage test for assessing competence, known as the 'Re C' test after Re C (Adult: Refusal of Treatment, 1994). According to the 'Re C' test, a patient is competent to give consent if they are able to:
- Comprehend and retain treatment information
- Believe it
- Weigh it in the balance to arrive at choice

The Mental Capacity Bill (2003) adds a fourth test, that the patient is able to:
- Communicate that decision

This is also known as 'capacity to consent'. Recent cases have shown that less weight is now being given to the 'belief' aspect of consent.

The Mental Capacity Bill (2003) also adds that everyone should be given as much help as possible to help them make their own decision, before they can be treated as unable to make the decision. This will include interpreter services, and any other aids for communication. This will affect people whose command of English is not sufficient to enable them to understand and

Exercise

Find out how you can access interpreter services within your Trust, including sign language and Makaton (see www.makaton.org/about about.htm).

retain information, unless it is in a language they can understand (including sign language, etc.).

The Mental Capacity Bill

We have been discussing case law and statute laws that have been enacted. Statute laws that are proposed are called 'bills' before they become Acts of Parliament. The Mental Capacity Bill (2003) came before Parliament in the 2004/5 session. It makes provisions for people who are unable to make decisions for themselves (and are over the age of 16). There are some key points we need to be aware of.

What the Bill is about

The starting point is always that everyone has capacity (even if they have a learning disability). The Bill goes on to say:

Key principles

- Everyone should be given as much help as possible to assist them in making their own decision, before they can be treated as not able to make the decision
- No one should be thought of as lacking capacity just because they make an unwise decision
- Everything done for someone who lacks capacity must be in their best interests
- Everyone must be very careful with the person's rights and freedom of action
- A person lacks capacity if they are unable to make a decision for themselves, due to impairment or disturbance in the functioning of the mind or brain. This can be permanent or temporary
- Because a person may lack capacity in one aspect of their life, it does not mean they lack capacity in every aspect
- The Bill refers to all areas of decision making, not just healthcare
- The Bill allows a person to appoint someone to look after their affairs if they lose capacity (Lasting Power of Attorney)
- The Bill allows a person to decide what medical treatment they would not want in the future. This is called an advance deci-

sion to refuse treatment (also known as 'advance directives')
- The Bill will appoint a Court of Protection to help make very difficult decisions. If someone does not have a Lasting Power of Attorney, the Court of Protection will appoint a Deputy
- The Public Guardians Office will be created to ensure that people with authority to make decisions for people who lack capacity do not abuse the power
- It will be a criminal offence to abuse, treat badly or neglect people who lack capacity

Summary

- Everyone must be presumed to have capacity to make decisions
- The Mental Capacity Bill (2003) refers to a person's ability to make decisions about all their affairs
- A person may lack capacity in one area of their life but still retain it in other areas
- People will need to be given as much help and time as possible to make a decision
- Because people make unwise decisions, it does not mean they lack capacity

References

The Mental Capacity Bill (2003). London: TSO.
Re C (Adult: Refusal of Treatment) [1994] 1 OER 819

Test yourself

 To check your progress, locate this section on CD-ROM 1 and work through the interactive questions at the end.

Section 9: Confidentiality

Confidentiality related to practice

Confidential information is information entrusted by one individual to another in confidence, and where there is a legitimate expectation that it will remain in confidence unless consent is sought and given.

Consent must be explicit, and not given under duress or through coercion. In order to consent, a person must be able to:

- Understand the information
- Believe it
- Use it to reach a rational decision
- Communicate that decision

It is important that a person is also informed of the consequences of not sharing information when they reach a decision. Consent to share information can be withdrawn at any time, and a person may limit whom they consent to share their information with (such as different members of the healthcare team). Where decisions have been made by an adult with capacity, and the consequences of the decision have been fully explained, they must be respected.

Confidential information can include personal details and personally sensitive information (such as race, sexuality, religion, politics, criminal and health records). It can be stored in any format, including on paper, electronically and on video- or audio-tape. Any such information that could identify a person is, therefore, seen as confidential.

Confidentiality is possibly the most common source of moral and ethical dilemmas for healthcare professionals. All NHS employees have a common law duty of confidentiality, which has now become a statutory duty under the Data Protection Act 1998. Confidentiality is a key requirement of codes of conduct for healthcare professionals. The law protects the privacy rights of individuals in respect of their personal data. The right to respect for privacy in private life, family, home and correspondence is a right under Article 8 of the Human Rights Act 1998.

Any disclosure of information or breach of confidentiality would be in breach of this article, unless other legislation exists, or it was necessary for:

- The interests of national security
- Public safety
- Prevention of a crime
- Protection of health or morals
- Protection of rights and freedom of others

In some situations, healthcare professionals may be required by statute or common law to break confidentiality. Some information may also be disclosed in certain situations if it is 'in the public interest' to do so; or, if by disclosing the information, you are acting in the patient's best interest. Such an example may be when there is serious risk to the patient or to others. This could also be covered by provision under the Children Act 1989, or the Mental Health Act 1983. The Police and Criminal Evidence Act 1984 allows a constable to apply to a circuit judge for a warrant to have access to certain categories of information, which may well breach confidentiality. The Crime and Disorder Act 1998 gives power to any person to disclose information lawfully to the police, probation service, local and health authorities, when it is expedient or necessary for the purposes of any provision under the Act. However, it is not a statutory duty to disclose, nor does the Act contain any power to demand disclosure.

Other statute laws, such as the Freedom of Information Act 2000, and the Access to Health Records Act 1990, give people the right to see some information, about themselves, that is held by healthcare organizations.

Data protection

The Data Protection Act 1998 covers the holding, using, retaining and destruction of all personally identifiable data. The Act applies to all personal data, either stored manually or electronically in any media (such as on computer, but also video- and audiotape). It is an offence to process information, except in accordance with the principles of data protection.

Because confidentiality is such a sensitive area, the Chief Medical Officer of England commissioned the *Report on the Review of Patient-Identifiable Information* (1997c), a review of how patient-identifiable information is used within the NHS. Known as the Caldicott Review, this was in response to increasing concern about the ways in which patient information was being used in the NHS and the need to ensure that confidentiality is not undermined.

It introduced the notion of data custodians and outlined principles for data collection and use.

Since then, the NHS has issued updated guidance, encompassing the latest legal advice and guidance, *The NHS Confidentiality Code of Practice* (2003a), which covers holding, obtaining, recording (including record keeping), using and sharing information.

The key principles of Data Protection state that information should be:

- Shared on a 'need to know basis'
- Used on a 'need to know basis'
- Processed fairly and lawfully
- Obtained only for one or more specific purposes
- Adequate, relevant and not excessive
- Accurate and up-to-date
- Processed in accordance with rights of subjects under the Act
- Protected against unauthorized/unlawful processing, accidental or technical loss

Information shall not be:

- kept for longer than necessary
- transferred outside the European Union (unless measures are in place to ensure protection)

This has been simplified into *The NHS Model of Data Protection*, known as HORUS (NHSIA Information Governance Toolkit, 2003), which states that information shall be:

- **H**eld securely and confidentially
- **O**btained fairly and efficiently
- **R**ecorded accurately and reliably
- **U**sed effectively and ethically
- **S**hared appropriately and lawfully

 CD-ROM 1 includes a video clip of a supervision session discussing confidentiality. A transcript of the clip is shown below.

Video: Confidentiality discussion in supervision

Mental health worker (Waseem): I've been thinking a little bit about issues of confidentiality, and the question I would like to ask you for supervision is, how do I know who I can and can't talk to about patients?

Supervisor (Barbara): Mmmmm, that's a really important thing to talk about. Is there a particular patient that has made you bring this up today?

Waseem: Yes, there is actually. I saw a patient last week called Ed, and after he had left the practice, one of the receptionists, Emma, asked me what his problem was, and to be honest with you, I didn't really know what to say.

Barbara: So, what did you say?

Waseem: Well, to be honest with you, I didn't. I just made an excuse that I was busy, and left it there. The only thing is, I don't know what I'll say next time I see her. I've also since found out that Ed and Emma actually live on the same street. I really don't know how to tackle it.

Barbara: So what are your concerns for Ed?

Waseem: I'm mostly concerned that he probably doesn't want his neighbours knowing his business, so I wouldn't like to be talking about him to people who weren't involved in his care.

Barbara: So, what do you think you might say to Emma the next time that you see her?

Waseem: I think I'd probably say to Emma that I couldn't talk to her about a patient, or couldn't talk to anybody who wasn't directly involved with the patient about that patient's issues.

Barbara: Okay. So, what about if Emma wasn't Ed's neighbour; would it be different then?

Waseem: I don't think it should be any different, no. They are not directly involved in his care after all.

Barbara: And that includes anybody that you might see, your family and friends, people that you might talk to after work.

Waseem: Yes, we did this on the course.

Barbara: Okay. Let's look at this from a different angle now. What would you do if you phoned Ed at home and someone else answered the phone?

Waseem: I would ask to speak to Ed.

Barbara: And what if he wasn't there; what would you say?

Waseem: I'd find out when Ed was due back, and, perhaps, make a time when I could ring him when it was convenient.

Barbara: That's right. It is important not to assume that he has told his family that he is coming to see somebody about a mental health problem. It's something that you should talk about really early on with your patients, when you first see them. Let's move on. When is it alright to talk to other people about a patient's problems? Do you think there are times when a patient might tell you something that you feel you really need to disclose to somebody else?

Waseem: You mean if, say, Ed for example, told me that he was having violent thoughts, or feeling suicidal perhaps?

Barbara: Yes. There are a number of Trust policies on how best to deal with situations like this. Have you seen the Trust policy on child protection?

Waseem: I've seen it, but I haven't had a chance to read it just yet, but I am going on the Child Protection Study Day next week.

Barbara: I think it would be a good idea for you to read the policy before you go on the study day. Do you know where you can get hold of a copy?

Waseem: The Practice Manager, Angela has a copy. I'll take hers.

Barbara: Okay. Something else related; what do you think you would do if somebody phoned you up, and asked you for information about a patient that you were seeing?

Waseem: That's not really going to happen, is it?

Barbara: It might do. Somebody might ring up and say they were from Social Services, and say that a patient had been referred to their service, and they wanted information about him.

Waseem: Right. Thinking about it, I think that would be alright. They're involved in his care, so yes, I'll give them the information.

Barbara: So you're saying that somebody that you don't know, whose voice you don't recognize, rings up, and you would give them that information?

Waseem: Yes, well if you put it like that, it does sound a little bit risky, doesn't it?

Barbara: So what might you do to check out that they are who they say they are, and that your patient has consented for them to have that information about them?

Waseem: I see what you are getting at. I think what I'd do is, I'd take their number and I could check them out, and then call them back. It also gives me a chance to check with the patient to see whether he has consented.

Barbara: Sure, that's absolutely right. Okay, something slightly different. How would you respond if a patient asked you if they could read their notes?

Waseem: I haven't really thought about that.

Barbara: There is another Trust policy on this and that might be useful for you to read. Shall we talk about that in supervision next time?

Waseem: Okay, let's do that.

Exercise

- Read your employing Trust's policy on confidentiality.
- How would you handle a phone call from somebody you didn't know, who is asking for personal information about a patient?

Summary

- Confidential information is private information given by a person to another, where they expect it to remain private unless consent is given
- Confidential information is personally sensitive information (such as religion, sexual history, criminal record, healthcare history) that could also identify a person
- You must ask for a person's consent before their private information is shared with other people. The need for consent can only be overridden if: there is a risk of harm to the person concerned or other people; it is in the interests of national security, public safety, prevention of a crime, protection of health or morals, or

protection of rights and freedom of others
- Healthcare professionals have a duty to maintain confidentiality under common law, their employment terms and conditions, and their professional code of conduct
- The right to respect for privacy in private life, family, home and correspondence is a right under Article 8 of the Human Rights Act 1998
- The Data Protection Act 1998 applies to all forms of information that is stored. It applies to information on paper, computer, video- or audio-tape. Healthcare professionals have a duty to store information safely

References

Department of Health (1997c). *The Caldicott Committee: Report on the Review of Patient-Identifiable Information*. London: HMSO.

Department of Health (2003a). *The NHS Confidentiality Code of Practice; Guidelines on the use and protection of patient information*. London: HMSO.

NHS Information Authority (2003). *The NHS Model of Data Protection. Information Governance Toolkit*. NHSIA.

Access to Health Records Act 1990

Children Act 1989

Crime and Disorder Act 1998

Data Protection Act 1998

Freedom of Information Act 2000

Human Rights Act 1998

Mental Health Act 1983

Police and Criminal Evidence Act 1984

Test yourself

 To check your progress, locate this section on CD-ROM 1 and work through the interactive questions at the end.

Section 10: The Human Rights Act 1998

Based on the 1950 European Convention on Human Rights, the Human Rights Act 1998 has now passed into English law. It now allows British citizens to enforce their rights in UK courts.

The act came into force on 2nd October 2000 and incorporates into UK law certain rights and freedoms set out in the European Convention on Human Rights. These are numbered as listed below (note that there is no article number 1 or number 13):

Article 2: The Right to Life

Article 3: Freedom from Torture or Inhuman or Degrading Treatment

Article 4: Freedom from Slavery or Forced Labour

Article 5: Personal Freedom

Article 6: Right to a Fair Trial

Article 7: No Punishment without Law

Article 8: Private Life and Family

Article 9: Freedom of Belief

Article 10: Free Expression

Article 11: Free Assembly and Association

Article 12: Marriage

Article 14: Freedom from Discrimination

There are also four Protocols within the Act:
1. The right to property
2. The right to education
3. The right to free and fair elections
4. The abolition of the death penalty in peacetime

The new law does three simple things:
1. It makes it unlawful for a public authority, like a government department, a local authority or the police, to breach the convention rights, unless an Act of Parliament meant it couldn't have acted differently
2. It means that cases can be dealt with in a UK court or tribunal, without plaintiffs having to go to Strasbourg to enforce their rights
3. All UK legislation must be given a meaning that fits with the convention rights, if that is possible. If a court says that this is not possible, it will be up to Parliament to decide what to do

According to the Human Rights Act 1998, you, and the patients you see in your role as a mental health worker, have the same rights. At times you may find yourself acting as an advocate for patients with mental health problems, communicating and acting on their behalf. The role of advocacy is explored in Chapter 2.2, Section 2.

Exercise

- Why do you think the Human Rights Act is important in relation to health-care law?
- What implications does the Human Rights Act have for you and your role as a mental health worker in primary care?

Summary

- The Human Rights Act has passed into law rights that had previously only been accessible through the European Convention of Human Rights
- All new UK legislation has to be given a meaning that fits with convention rights

Reference

Human Rights Act 1998

Test yourself

 To check your progress, locate this section on CD-ROM 1 and work through the interactive questions at the end.

Chapter 1.3
Managing the patient's journey through primary care and the role of mental health workers in primary care

Aims

- To provide an opportunity to critically examine the role of the mental health worker in primary care
- To facilitate critical evaluation of the epidemiology of mental health in primary care
- To provide an opportunity to critically appraise the concept of healthcare inequalities and the approach to care and treatment in primary care

Learning outcomes

At the end of Chapter 1.3 the reader will be able to critically:
- Evaluate the epidemiology of mental heath in primary care
- Appraise the use of self-help materials available in primary care
- Evaluate the roles and responsibilities of the mental health worker in primary care
- Appraise the stepped care approach and case management model
- Examine the use of antidepressant medication in primary care
- Examine the needs of patients with serious mental health problems

Part 1.3 content is as follows:

1 Mental health in primary care: epidemiology
2 The role of mental health workers in primary care
   ◦ Face-to-face work
   ◦ Telephone support
   ◦ Liaison and networking
3 A Stepped Care approach
4 Guided self help
   ◦ Interactive/computerized assisted help
   ◦ A guide to self help materials
5 Case management
6 Pharmacological management of depression: antidepressants
   ◦ Basic principles
   ◦ Antidepressants
   ◦ Tricyclic antidepressants
   ◦ Selective serotonin re-uptake inhibitors (SSRIs)
   ◦ Monoamine oxidase inhibitors (MAOIs)
   ◦ Principles of stopping treatment
7 Mental health indicators in primary care:
   ◦ Serious mental health problems
      – Schizophrenia
      – Bipolar affective disorder
      – Antipsychotic medication
8 Addressing health inequalities
   ◦ Mental illness registers
   ◦ Audit

Section 1: Mental health in primary care: epidemiology

Most of us experience stresses and strains at some time in our lives; if not ourselves directly, then friends, family or work colleagues. Most people who seek help from the health service turn to primary care. Approximately 90% of people with mental health problems in the UK are treated solely in primary care (Goldberg & Huxley, 1992).

The World Health Organisation in 2001 estimated 121 million people worldwide currently live with depression, and around 24 million people have a diagnosis of schizophrenia. An estimated 23% of the total burden of disease in developed countries is due to mental illness (www.who.int/mediacentre/factsheets: go to the alphabetic list, click 'M' and scroll down to 'mental and neurological disorders' for further information).

The undefined burden of mental health problems refers to the economic and social burden on families, communities and countries. Although substantial, this burden has not been efficiently measured. This is because of the lack of quantitative data and difficulties in measuring and evaluating.

The hidden burden refers to the burden associated with stigma and violations of human rights and freedom. Again, this burden is difficult to quantify. This is a major problem throughout the world, as many cases remain concealed and unreported (www.who.int/mediacentre/factsheets: go to the alphabetic list, click 'M' and scroll down to 'mental health problems' for further discussion of these concepts).

Further discussion of the economic impact of mental ill health can be found in the Layard Report, *Mental Health: Britain's Biggest Social Problem* (2004), which addresses the issue of the interface between the NHS and work and the role of psychological approaches in the journey from welfare to work.

The NHS Plan recognizes that most mental health problems are managed in primary care. As many as one in four GP consultations touches upon a mental health issue, second only to consultations for respiratory infections. The NHS Plan aims to improve primary care resources in order to improve the mental health and well-being of the population (Department of Health, 2000d).

While most people will experience mild conditions and recover quickly, a significant number of people with serious mental health problems are cared for by general practitioners (Department of Health, 2001). The main aims of the survey were to estimate the prevalence of adult mental health problems according to diagnostic category; to identify the extent of disability and availability of mental health services.

The results (see Table 1) highlighted that 1 in 6 adults (164 cases per 1000) were assessed as having experienced a 'neurotic' disorder, often described as common mental health problems. Approximately 25% were receiving treatment of some kind for a mental or emotional problem. Twenty percent were prescribed medication, 9% were receiving therapy of some description, with only 4% receiving both. This is in contrast to suffering from a psychotic disorder, of whom 85% were in receipt of treatment, 84% being on medication and 40% receiving therapy.

A number of personal characteristics are associated with a higher prevalence of anxiety

Table 1: Prevalence of mental disorders in men and women (Department of Health, 2001d)

	Rates per 1000		
	Men	**Women**	**Total**
All neurosis	135	194	164
Mixed anxiety and depression	68	108	88
Generalized anxiety	43	46	44
Depression	23	28	26
Phobias	13	22	18
Obsessive-compulsive disorder	9	13	11
Panic Disorder	7	7	7
Personality disorder	54	34	44
Probable psychosis	6	5	5

and depression. They include the following:

- have female gender
- are aged between 35 and 54
- are separated or divorced
- are living as a one-person family unit or as a lone parent
- have no formal educational qualifications
- have a predicted IQ of <90
- come from social class V
- are economically inactive
- are tenants of Local Authorities and Housing Associations
- have moved two to three times in last 2 years
- are living in an urban area
- are also suffering from a physical complaint

The World Health Organisation Collaborating Centre for Research and Training for Mental Health (2000) published a useful guide to Mental Health in Primary Care including an overview of prevalence of mental disorders in primary care and criteria for assessment of mental disorder and learning disability based on the International Classification of Diseases. The text also includes disks for printing assessment tools and resources that can be used by mental health practitioners in primary care.

A document discussing psychiatric morbidity among adults who live in private households has been published by the Office for National Statistics (Department of Health, 2001d), and is available online at www.statistics. gov.uk/downloads/theme_health/psychmorb.pdf.

Summary

- Common mental health problems are very prevalent in primary care
- The statistics may not reveal the true extent of mental health difficulties in primary care as detection rates are poor; the figures could actually be far greater
- Approximately 450 million people worldwide are affected with various mental health problems

References

Department of Health (2000). *The NHS Plan: a Plan for Investment, a Plan for Reform*. London: HMSO.

Department of Health (2001d). *Office of National Statistics: Psychiatric Morbidity Among Adults Living in Private Households*, 2000. London: HMSO.

Goldberg, D. & Huxley, P. (1992). *Common Mental Disorders: A biosocial module*. London: Routledge.

Layard, R. (2004) *Mental Health: Britain's Biggest Social Problem?* Paper presented at a seminar hosted by the Prime Minister's Strategy Unit. Available online at www.strategy.gov

World Health Organisation Collaborating Centre for Research and Training for Mental Health (2000). *WHO Guide to Mental Health in Primary Care*. London: Royal Society of Medicine Press.

Useful websites

www.statistics.gov.uk/downloads/theme_health/ psychmorb.pdf (Department of Health)

www.who.int/mediacentre/factsheets (World Health Organisation)

Test yourself

 To check your progress, locate this section on CD-ROM 1 and work through the interactive questions at the end.

Section 2: The role of mental health workers in primary care

With the publication and implementation of *Shifting the Balance of Power* (Department of Health, 2001b), Primary Care Trusts (PCTs) are now at the cornerstone of the NHS as both commissioners and providers of mental health services. They are charged with delivering the targets set out within the National Service Framework for Mental Health (Department of Health, 1999a).

One of the strategies within the NHS Plan has been to enable these targets to be met through the recruitment, training and

Meet Nigel

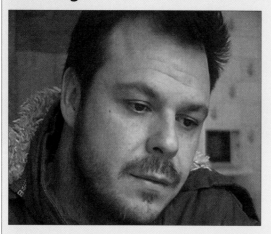

Nigel is a 45-year-old man, recently separated from his wife. He presents with low mood and reduced energy. He used to be very sporty, but he has given up these activities as he gets no pleasure from them any more. He has early morning wakening and difficulty concentrating. He was always a self-confident person, but has experienced a loss of confidence of late. He blames himself for the breakdown of his marriage. He has occasional suicidal thoughts, but dismisses these and has no plans to take his life. He became depressed four months ago after his wife left him for another man. His GP has recommended that he commence anti-depressant medication, but Nigel is reluctant to do so as he believes that 'taking tablets means that I am weak and a failure'.

Although he and his wife Jenny appeared to have a stable relationship, it turned out that she had been having an affair for the past five years. Nigel was unaware of this, and her leaving came as a complete shock. Nigel has not told her of his diagnosis of depression, as he feels that she would not understand and he would lose her respect, thereby reducing his chances of winning her back. They have two grown-up children who no longer live at home. His son David is training to be an accountant. His daughter Patricia is currently doing well at university. Nigel usually enjoys his job as a clerical officer at the local county council, but has been struggling more recently. He has been on sick leave for the past three weeks and is anxious about his return to work.

 CD-ROM 1 includes video clips which show Nigel as he talks of how he feels, and then as he meets with Waseem, a mental health worker assigned to Nigel's case. Transcripts of the videos follow.

deployment within PCTs of 1000 new graduate mental health workers in primary care (Department of Health, 2000). The date for this target to be achieved was December 2004. These workers are a new resource for primary care. In practice, mental health work within primary care can be undertaken by a range of different disciplines, with appropriate education and training.

A useful resource for further information is the Knowledge Community at the Care Services Improvement Partnership (CSIP) website: kc.csip.org.uk.

Face-to-face work

The NIMHE publication *Improving Access to Psychological Therapies* (2004) acknowldges that people with depression and anxiety have for too long been offered little more than medication which, for some, is not enough to help them recover, and that waiting times for psychological therapies are long, despite the mass of evidence to demonstrate this.

There is now developing evidence of improved patient outcomes in the treatment of anxiety and depression using low-intensity interventions such as problem solving (Mynors-Wallis et al, 2000) and facilitated patient self-management (Bower et al, 2001). These interventions are based on cognitive behavioural therapy (CBT). Training does not require a professional qualification (Richards et al, 2002).

Face-to-face sessions may not need to be restricted to the traditional timing of therapy sessions, offering an hour to each patient, and to accommodate a high volume of patients they can be brief – as short as twenty minutes. Behavioural techniques are designed to alleviate symptoms of anxiety and depression, such as increasing pleasurable activities by reducing fear responses to situations and facilitating a change in a person's lifestyle. Cognitive techniques are designed to reduce negative and/or anxiety-provoking thoughts. The emphasis of patient contact is on developing a collaborative relationship between the mental health worker and the patient, and empowering them to make changes between sessions.

When undertaking face-to-face work with patients it is important to create a suitable working environment that is conducive to you, as a mental health worker, engaging with a patient and working therapeutically. It is important to prepare the room and take control of the environment that you have booked for face-to-face work. Points you should consider include the following:

- Is there a quiet room available at a regular designated time?
- Is this accessible for patients with physical disabilities?
- Is the room isolated from the clinical area?
- Is there a panic button?
- How would you deal with telephone disturbances (e.g. calls being put through to you)?
- Are mobile phones switched off?
- Is there an 'engaged' sign on the door?
- Are there two similar chairs?
- Are there noises outside (e.g. a busy waiting room)?
- Is there adequate sound proofing?
- Are other staff likely to need equipment from the room?

Video: Introducing Nigel (Depression)

Nigel: I haven't been feeling very good since Jenny, my wife, left me for another man. I think I caused all that, I never took her out or anything. I never told her how nice she looked, and she did look nice. No wonder someone else fancied her, and she went off at the first opportunity. They were together for years and I didn't even notice. Now I can't stop thinking about it, I can't get it out of my head. I know it's all my fault, what I deserved, but now I can't eat or sleep properly. I haven't been able to concentrate at work, so I've been on the sick now for the past three weeks. That's bothering me too, because I'm never off, and I'm worried about what my colleagues think of me, but to be honest I just can't face it right now. I'm waking up about 4 o'clock every morning and I find it impossible to get back to sleep. I'm so exhausted during the day that I can't be bothered to do anything, never mind drag myself into work. When I was there, I didn't seem to be able to do very much anyway. I sometimes wonder whether I'd be better off dead to be honest, but I wouldn't do anything, I couldn't do it to the kids. I should be able to handle this. I can't even tell Jenny I've been diagnosed with depression. What would she think of me? She'd see me as pathetic and weak for sure. I'm going to see Dr Rushforth today. She's really nice but I just can't imagine why she wants to bother with me.

Video: Nigel in a session with his mental health worker, Waseem

Waseem: So you say that you have been having some time off work recently and this isn't like you?

Nigel: Yes I've been off work for the last three weeks. I just can't face it.

Waseem: What do you think is stopping you going to work?

Nigel: Well, since Jenny left me I haven't felt like doing anything. I've just had no energy to do anything.

Waseem: So how are you feeling now?

Nigel: Not good.

Waseem: If you had to try and say what kind of feeling this was, what would it be?

Nigel: I'd say I was miserable and depressed.

Waseem: I'd be interested to know how it is affecting other areas of your life Nigel. Have you had any other symptoms?

Nigel: Well it's taking me ages to get to sleep at night. I'm mulling things over in my head all the time. I'm not sleeping until 2am and then in the morning I'm shattered and want to stay in bed.

Waseem: You know you've said you haven't been working, when you've stayed off work; have you been staying in bed?

Nigel: Yes, I've been staying in bed until tea-time. That's really not like me.

Waseem: How does that you make you feel?

Nigel: It makes me feel angry at myself; I feel pathetic. I can't really explain how I feel.

Waseem: I think you're actually doing okay in explaining how you are feeling, Nigel. It must be very distressing and frustrating for you to feel this way about yourself. So you have said that you have stayed in bed a lot on days that you haven't gone to work. Can you tell me how it is affecting you with day-to-day things? How are you spending the rest of your time at home?

Nigel: I can't concentrate on anything. I'm forgetting things, I just can't remember things.

Waseem: What about your appetite, how's your appetite been recently?

Nigel: Normally it's good but I've not been eating in the day at all, then I've just been eating a sandwich at night.

Waseem: What do you normally do to relax?

Nigel: Normally I play badminton with a group of friends once a week and go to the pub afterwards, but I've not done that for the last few weeks.

Waseem: What do you think stopped you?

Nigel: I don't want to bring everyone down, I don't want to depress people.

Waseem: Nigel, it certainly sounds like things have changed a lot for you since Jenny left, and you've experienced a lot of quite distressing symptoms. I am keen to listen to this and to work out the best way we can help you. Have you an idea what you think you need help with?

Nigel: Yes, I just want to get myself back to normal, back to the way I usually feel, but it seems impossible.

Waseem: Okay. Well, from what you've said to me and the information that your GP

Exercise

- When you next arrange a face-to-face meeting with a patient, take time to prepare your environment, considering the factors in the list on page 37.
- After the session, reflect on the changes made that were within your control.
- What factors were you unable to control?
- Few people will have a perfect working environment. Some improvements can often be made. If the environment still remains unsatisfactory, discuss it with your line manager to explore alternative solutions.

passed on to me, it seems like you've experienced several symptoms: low mood; lack of energy; poor sleep; poor concentration; and lack of motivation. We find that if a person experiences several of these symptoms for a period of time it can be signs of depression.

Nigel: Yes, the doctor said I was depressed.

Waseem: Depression is a recognized illness, but it can be treated. What I can offer is some information to read in a workbook, with follow-up support and help from me. Would you be interested in that?

Nigel: How would that work?

Waseem: Well, I'll give you the workbook and we'll agree how much you would need to take in, and we'll arrange to meet up occasionally at the health centre. I could arrange regular telephone conversations with you as well. How does that sound?

Nigel: How long would the sessions be?

Waseem: Not long, 20 minutes to half an hour, and telephone conversations would last round about 10 minutes. How does that sound?

Nigel: Yes, that sounds good.

Waseem: Okay. I'm also going to give you this booklet on depression. If you get a chance to have a read of this, maybe we can talk about the main points in there next time we meet up.

Nigel: My reading has been a bit off since I can't really concentrate so well, but I'll give it a go.

Waseem: Okay. I appreciate that your concentration might be reduced, but perhaps if you can highlight the important bits or read it in little chunks, then we can discuss it next time.

Telephone support

Telephone support is a low-intensity intervention which aims to improve the care and outcomes for people living with depression. Primary care mental health workers are ideally placed to deliver this intervention. When patients are newly prescribed antidepressant medication by their GP, follow-up structured telephone support has proved an effective intervention in improving compliance with medication and discussions on side-effects and emerging difficulties (NHS Centre for Reviews and Dissemination, 2002). Medication management using scheduled telephone contact is covered in depth in Part 3.4, Section 3.

There is increasing interest in simple and cost-effective health technologies, for example self-help manuals, information handouts and assistance with computerized Cognitive Behaviour Therapy programmes that have proved effective in reducing symptoms (NIMHE North West Development Centre, 2004b).

Checklist for managing telephone work with patients

- It is important to check that you have the right telephone number
- Are you telephoning from an environment that is not too disruptive?

> ## Exercise
>
> What are the potential problems associated with telephone contacts? Read the checklist and then make notes. Identify actions to address these problems. You may want to discuss some of the issues with your supervisor.

- Check if patients have changed their telephone number: they may not have informed the surgery
- If your patient's partner answers the telephone, be familiar with the local policy on how you would explain who you are and why you are telephoning
- Respect confidentiality of patients at all times
- Always ask a patient if it is acceptable to them for you to leave a message
- Be aware of any financial considerations in the place of work restricting use of telephones. Many people now have a mobile telephone
- Remember that booking scheduled times for regular telephone conversations with patients is more likely to be effective
- Be clear on what contact telephone number you leave with a patient, particularly if you have more than one base
- Be clear on how you could arrange a telephone message system in your place of work
- Locate and read local policy and guidelines on actions to follow if the person you call appears much worse than usual and you think they might be at risk
- Having the telephone number of your clinical supervisor available for ad hoc supervision is helpful for support and guidance

> ## Exercise
>
> Examine the feasibility of starting a telephone support service in your workplace. Think particularly about these questions:
> - Where?
> - When?
> - What changes can be made?
> - Are there any restrictions?

Liaison and networking

Liaison is a key role for the mental health worker in primary care, especially with other members of the primary care team. It is important for all primary care staff to understand each others' roles so that appropriate referrals can be made and expertise be utilized. Liaison may also involve networking with external agencies outside of the PCT, including other providers of mental health services such as Mental Health Trusts and Social Services. It may also involve contact with specialist services such as the police and criminal justice liaison service. A fundamental part of this role will require contact with the Council for Voluntary Services and various local voluntary sector and charitable organizations. Visits to these organizations would be very beneficial to enable a mental health worker to understand the scope of their work and how they are funded. Liaison also involves making contact with patients, their family and carers, depending on each patient's individual need. Consequently, liaison involves many varied activities including Mental Health Promotion (for more information see Part 2.2, Section 3).

The benefits of liaison

- Leads to improved communication for medication management
- Improves a patient's mental health
- Helps others understand your role
- Helps you understand the role of other health and social care professionals
- Establishes and encourages positive working relationships with voluntary sector organizations
- Provides an opportunity to challenge stigma related to patients with mental health problems
- Provides an opportunity to act as a positive advocate for mental health services
- Provides an opportunity for mental health promotion

Summary

- The environment for both face-to-face work and telephone support needs careful consideration
- Liaison with many professional disciplines and non-medical staff will be an important component of the work

References

Bower, P., Richards, D. & Lovell, K. (2001). The clinical and cost-effectiveness of self-help treatments for anxiety and depressive disorders in primary care: a systematic review. *British Journal of General Practice*, 51, 838–845.

Department of Health (1999a). *A National Service Framework for Mental Health*. London: HMSO.

Department of Health (2000). *The NHS Plan: a Plan for Investment, a Plan for Reform*. London: HMSO.

Department of Health (2001b). *Shifting the Balance of Power within the NHS: Securing Delivery*. London: HMSO.

Mynors-Wallis, L.M., Gath, D.H., Day, A. & Baker, F. (2000). Randomized controlled trial of problem solving treatment, antidepressant medication, and combined treatment for major depression in primary care. *British Medical Journal*, 320, 26–30.

National Institute for Mental Health in England (2004). *Improving Access to Psychological Therapies*. London: NIMHE.

National Institute for Mental Health in England North West Development Centre (2004b). *Primary Care Graduate Mental Health Workers – a practical guide*. Hyde: NIMHE North West.

NHS Centre for Reviews and Dissemination (2002). Improving the recognition and management of depression in primary care. *Effective Health Care Bulletin*, 7, 5.

Richards, D.A., Richards, A., Barkham, M., Williams, C. & Cahill, J. (2002). PHASE: a health technology approach to psychological treatment in primary mental health care. *Primary Health Care Research and Development*, 3, 159–168.

Useful website

kc.csip.org.uk (Knowledge Community at the Care Services Improvement Partnership (CSIP))

Test yourself

 To check your progress, locate this section on CD-ROM 1 and work through the interactive questions at the end.

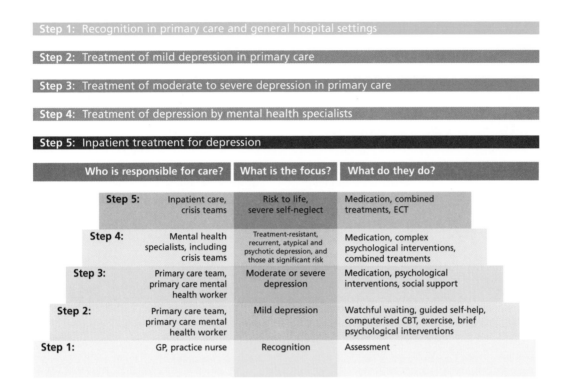

Figure 4: The Stepped Care model for depression, taken from the NICE guidelines

Section 3: The Stepped Care approach

The Stepped Care approach for the treatment of depression and anxiety proposes that low-intensity interventions are given initially to patients with depression and anxiety, before the introduction of more complex treatments for those patients who fail to respond (Hegel et al, 2002).

The Stepped Care Approach acknowledges that primary care is at the forefront of treatment of depression and anxiety. Patients with depression have up to three times more primary care consultations than the general population (Katon et al, 1997), and treatment of depression accounts for 7% of primary care expenditure in pharmacotherapy (Peveler et al, 1999).

Mental health services have conflicting priorities in meeting the needs of patients with common mental health problems in primary care. The National Service Framework for Mental Health sets out a clear agenda for investment and priorities for services providing treatment and care of patients with mental health problems (Department of Health, 1999a).

Guidelines have been developed for the management of depression and anxiety summarizing key research findings and recommendations for the implementation of management of depression in primary and secondary care, and the management of anxiety in adults in primary, secondary and community care.

The NICE guidelines on managing depression (NICE 2004a) and anxiety (NICE 2004b) are available in PDF format on CD-ROM 1. They are also available online at www.nice.org.uk/guidance/CG22/niceguidance/pdf/English (anxiety) and www.nice.org.uk/guidance/CG23/niceguidance/pdf/English (depression). Figure 4 shows the stepped care model for depression taken from the NICE guidelines.

The Stepped Care approach is covered in greater depth in Part 3.4, Section 1.

Summary

- The Stepped Care approach for the treatment of depression and anxiety advocates that low-intensity interventions are given initially to patients with depression and anxiety, before the introduction of more complex treatments for those patients who fail to respond
- The *Enhanced Services for Depression under the new GP Contracts* emphasizes the importance of patients having access to assessment, defined pathways, monitoring and choice of treatment

References

Department of Health (1999a). *A National Service Framework for Mental Health*. London: HMSO.

Hegel, M., Imming, J., Cyr-Provost, M., Noel, P., Arean, P. & Unutzer, J. (2002). Role of Behavioural Health Professionals in a Collaborative Stepped Care Treatment Model for Depression in Primary Care: Project IMPACT. *Families, Systems and Health*, 20, 3, 265–277.

Katon, W., Korff, M., Lin, E., Unutzer, J., Simon, G., Walker, E., Ludman, T. & Bush, T. (1997). Population Based Care of Depression: Effective Disease Management Strategies to Decrease Prevalence. *General Hospital Psychiatry*, 19, 169–178.

National Institute for Mental Health in England, North West Development Centre (2004a). *Enhanced Services Specification for Depression under the new GP Contract: A Commissioning Guidebook*. Hyde: NIHME, North West Development Centre.

National Institute for Mental Health in England, North West Development Centre (2004b). *Enhanced Services Specification for Anxiety under the new GP Contract: A Commissioning Guidebook*. Hyde: NIHME, North West Development Centre.

Peveler, R., George, C., Kinmonth, A., Campbell, M. & Thompson, C. (1999). Effect of antidepressant drug counselling and information leaflets on adherence to drug treatment in primary care: randomised controlled trial. *British Medical Journal*, 319, 612–615.

Useful website

www.nice.org.uk (National Institute for Clinical Excellence)

Test yourself

 To check your progress, locate this section on CD-ROM 1 and work through the interactive questions at the end.

Section 4: Guided self-help

Despite research indicating both the popularity and clinical effectiveness of psychological therapies, most general practitioners have significant challenges in accessing the right treatment at the right time (Lovell & Richards, 2000).

There are only limited numbers of mental health workers who have completed education and training courses relevant to providing services in primary care, and they often have long waiting lists. A major improvement of recent years has been the development of self-help interventions. These forms of treatment are often based on the principles and practice of cognitive behavioural therapy (CBT).

The following methods can be used to deliver self-help:

- Bibliotherapy
- Book prescription
- Interactive computerized programmes for depression and anxiety
- Web-based interactive sites

In 2001, the Department of Health Policy Research Programme commissioned a major review of research evidence about self-help interventions for people with mental health problems. The report (Department of Health, 2003b) acknowledged that most studies reported a significant benefit from self-help materials, based on CBT approaches, for depression, anxiety, bulimia and binge eating disorder. It suggested that the use of self-help materials was 'probably safer' if their use was supported by a healthcare professional, and suggested that self-help interventions could be a very useful first step in a Stepped Care approach.

The majority of books highlighted in the above report employ a structured CBT approach and present complete step-by-step treatment programmes with exercises, self-assessments, diary sheets, etc. Many are self-help adaptations of well-established clinical treatments of proven effectiveness. Furthermore, several of the books have been subjected to clinical trial (Department of Health, 2003b).

The effectiveness of bibliotherapy depends on the motivation and application (as well as the literacy) of the person using the text. Those who actively read self-help material and enthusiastically engage with it are much more likely to benefit than those who pay little attention to reading in their day-to-day activities. However, total adherence to a complete programme is not necessary for the person to gain some significant beneficial effect (Frude, 2004a). 'Bibliotherapy' is highly acceptable to patients, with a high adherence (Frude 2004b). Frude (2004a), from Cardiff and Vale NHS Trust, devised the idea for the Cardiff Book Prescription Scheme.

These treatments are not dependent on specialist psychological training, and provide real choice to patients, especially in areas where there are scant specialist resources to support primary care mental health services. Self-help is often best delivered with a watchful eye. Mental health workers are ideally placed to deliver such an approach, often termed 'facilitated' or 'guided self-help', to patients with common mental health problems.

Gloucestershire's Primary Mental Health Service have developed, and is using to positive effect, an eight-week self-help workbook for anxiety, 'Gaining Control of your Life', which was specifically designed to be supported by telephone contact. For more information and self-help leaflets, contact www.pmhsglos.org.uk.

The Department of Health (2001e) has produced an informative leaflet on psychological therapies, 'Choosing Talking Therapies', available in PDF format on CD-ROM 1, or online at www.dh.gov.uk/assetRoot/04/08/27/09/04082709.pdf.

A useful source of information is *Organising and Delivery of Psychological Therapies* at the NIMHE website, www.nimhe.org.uk.

Guided self-help is the foundation of a Stepped Care approach, offered as a first-step treatment for patients with common mental health problems. Ways of using guided self-help are covered in Part 3.4, Section 4.

Research into the use of CBT in addressing the needs of patients with common mental health problems, such as depression, has established its effectiveness. Certainly CBT has been found to be effective in the treatment of negative cognitions associated with depression, such as hopelessness and poor self-esteem (Hollon et al, 1987). Patients with depression who have undergone CBT are said to have less of a need to seek social approval, are more optimistic about the future, less likely to avoid perceived stressful situations, have less of a negative evaluation of self, and are less likely to hold irrational beliefs and cognitive biases (Robins & Hayes, 1993).

Despite the effectiveness of CBT for anxiety and depression, access is poor (Lovell & Richards, 2000), with a limited number of accredited CBT therapists being available for patients to access (www.babcp.com). Moreover, as 30% of patients who present at primary care have mental health problems as their main issue (Kendrick et al, 1994), this underlines the need for us to promote the availability of more accessible, less clinician-intensive methods of delivering psychological support (Lovell & Richards, 2000).

CBT adopts a collaborative approach to the delivery of psychological management, the aim being that the patient learns to adopt strategies that they can effectively use in their daily lives. Completing tasks between sessions is seen as fundamental to the process of learning new skills. For this purpose, an array of material has been produced to assist the patient in addressing their needs outside the clinical session. This material is often referred to as self-help material (NIMHE, 2003).

The use of between-session activities, sometimes referred to as homework assignments, has been a major part of psychotherapy since as far back as the 1930s (Burns & Spangler, 2000). Homework assignments are present in a number of treatment manuals for a variety of disorders, such as alcohol misuse, anxiety and psychotic disorders (Kazantzis, 2000).

Within CBT, there is evidence that patients who participate in between-sessions activities have better therapeutic outcome than those who do not. Kazantzis et al (2000) conducted a meta-analysis of research focusing on the impact of between-sessions activity. The authors explored the impact of the differing types of activity engaged in as part of therapy on therapeutic outcome. They concluded that compliance in the between-sessions activity appears to impact directly on the improvement of the patient in therapy, as well as being a predictor of positive therapeutic outcome. In particular, the effect size was larger for those patients who utilized a range of between-sessions activities, than for those who completed one type of between-sessions activity.

A range of issues has led to an interest in developing the effectiveness of patients engaging in therapy outside the confines of a clinical session. Certainly, the volume of psychological morbidity in primary care, together with the concerns held by patients about the use of medication to address their needs, has stressed the need for effective accessible psychological management initiatives being available for patients experiencing difficulties such as depression and anxiety, with guided self-help advocated as a first line treatment.

Guided self-help is seen as a means of

Exercise

- Identify which members of your primary care team currently use guided self-help.
- How might you use guided self-help in your role as a mental health worker?

delivering CBT and building on what we know about the effectiveness of engaging in between-sessions tasks. It promotes the availability of more accessible, less clinician-intensive methods of delivering psychological support that could help to address the morbidity of common mental health problems in primary care.

The National Service Framework (NSF) (Department of Health 1999a) stresses how important it is that accessible mental health treatment is provided within primary care. The 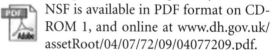 NSF is available in PDF format on CD-ROM 1, and online at www.dh.gov.uk/assetRoot/04/07/72/09/04077209.pdf.

In summary, self-help provides a flexible approach to address mental health distress in patients, an approach which is more accessible than traditional models of delivering therapy, with a focus on empowering patients to address their current and future difficulties. It also reduces some of the potential barriers to patients actively accessing support for their mental health distress, by being based in primary care; patients will not feel the stigma associated with having contact with secondary mental health services. The Department of Health's publication *Self-help interventions for mental health problems* (DOH, 2003b) is available in PDF format on CD-ROM 1, and online at www.dh.gov.uk/assetRoot/04/12/57/94/04125794.pdf.

The use of self-help materials across a variety of mental health disorders has demonstrated its effectiveness (Fritzler et al, 1997; Bowman et al, 1996; Evans et al, 1999; and Bower et al, 2001). With guided self-help, the patient receives brief input from a facilitator who guides them in the use of appropriate evidence-based self-help material to meet their assessed need. There is growing evidence for the effectiveness of this model of delivering self-help (Barkham et al, 1996).

There is evidence that the approach can be successfully taught to non-mental health professionals (Richards et al, 2002).

Interactive/computerized-assisted help

Current research suggests that the delivery of cognitive behavioural therapy (CBT) via a computer interface (CCBT) may be of value in the management of anxiety and depressive disorders. An effectiveness review by the National Institute for Health and Clinical Excellence (2002) advised caution and counselled against the general introduction of this technology into the NHS. To establish the contribution and place of CCBT in the management of common mental health problems, including its role in Stepped Care approaches, the NHS should consider supporting an independent programme of research into CCBT, including carefully monitored pilot implementation projects. The research should include investigations into user preferences, suitability, needs and educational/cultural characteristics (NICE, 2002).

NICE (2002) has issued guidance on the clinical and cost effectiveness of CCBT. There appears to be a role for CCBT within Stepped Care approaches, with primary care mental health workers being in a prime position for the facilitated delivery. Processes for appropriate screening and referral will need to be fully established and implemented before mental health workers use this treatment mode. Several CCBT packages are currently available. These have been developed for a specific target group or groups and use different CBT algorithms. Variations between the individual packages include computer requirements, content, interactivity, amount of between-session activity, requirement for facilitator time and input, and cost. Specific programmes/ training will be dependent on funding from each individual PCT.

NICE (2002) has produced the document *Guidance on the use of Computerised Cognitive* *Behavioural Therapy for depression and anxiety*, which is available in PDF format on CD-ROM 1, and online at www.nice.org.uk/download.aspx?o=ta097 guidance&template=download.aspx.

Exercise

- Look on the website www.mind. org.uk. to access factsheets on self-help. Identify which ones might be appropriate for your patient group.
- Also visit www.depression-primarycare. org.
- Now access the website www.nhsdirect. nhs.uk. Imagine you were experiencing problems with depression and/or anxiety and accessed this site yourself.
- What are the strengths and limitations of the NHS Direct site?

Summary

- During guided self-help, a patient receives brief input from a facilitator who guides them in the use of appropriate evidence-based self-help material, to meet their assessed needs
- Self-help promotes the availability of more accessible, less clinician-intensive methods of delivering psychological support that could help to address the extensive morbidity of common mental health problems in primary care
- There is a range of methods for delivering guided self-help, including the use of leaflets, workbooks, video/audio cassettes, CD-ROMs and interactive computerized packages

References

Barkham, M., Rees, A., Stiles, W., Shapiro, D., Hardy, G. & Reynolds, S. (1996). Dose-effect relations in time-limited psychotherapy for depression. *Journal of Consulting and Clinical Psychology*, 64, 927–935.

Bower, P., Richards, D. & Lovell, K. (2001). The clinical and cost-effectiveness of self-help treatments for anxiety and depressive disorders in primary care: a systematic review. *British Journal of General Practice*, 51, 838–845.

Bowman, D., Scogin, F. & Brenda, L. (1996). The efficacy of self-examination and cognitive biblio-therapy in the treatment of moderate depression. *Psychotherapy Research*, 5, 131–140.

Burns, D.D. & Spangler, D.L. (2000). Does psychotherapy homework lead to improvements in depression in CBT or does improvement lead to increased homework concordance? *Journal of Consulting and Clinical Psychology*, 68, 1, 46–56.

Department of Health (1999a). *A National Service Framework for Mental Health*. London: HMSO.

Department of Health (2001d) *Choosing Talking Therapies?* London: Department of Health.

Department of Health (2003b). *Self-Help Interventions for Mental Health Problems*. London: Department of Health.

Evans, K., Tyrer, P., Catalan, J., Schmidt, U., Davidson, K., Dent, J., Tata, P., Thornton, S., Barber, J. & Thompson, S. (1999). Manual-assisted cognitive behaviour therapy (MACT): a randomized controlled trial of a brief intervention with bibliotherapy in the treatment of self-harm. *Psychological Medicine*, 29, 19–25.

Fritzler, B., Hecker, J. & Loose, M. (1997). Self-directed treatment with minimal therapist contact: preliminary findings for obsessive-compulsive disorder. *Behavioural Research and Therapy*, 35, 627–631.

Frude, N.J. (2004a) A book prescription scheme in primary care. *Clinical Psychology*, 39. 11–14.

Frude, N.J. (2004b). Bibliotherapy as a means of delivering psychological therapy. *Clinical Psychology*, 39, 8–10.

Hollon, S., DeRubeis, R. & Evans, M.D. (1987). Casual mediation of change in treatment for depression: Discriminating between nonspecificity and noncausality. *Psychological Bulletin*, 102, 1, 139–149.

Kazantzis, N. (2000). Power to detect homework effects in psychotherapy outcome research. *Journal of Consulting and Clinical Psychology*, 68, 1, 166–170.

Kazantzis, N., Deane, F.P. & Ronan, K.R. (2000). Homework assignments in cognitive and behavioural therapy: A Meta-Analysis. *Clinical Psychology: Science and Practice*, 7, 2, 189–202.

Kendrick, T., Burns, T., Freeling, P. & Sibbard, B. (1994). Provision of care to General Practice patients with a disabling long term illness: a survey in 16 practices. *British Journal of General Practice*, 44: 301–309.

Lovell, K. & Richards, D.A. (2000). Multiple access points and levels of entry (MAPLE): ensuring choice, accessibility and equity for CBT services. *Behavioural and Cognitive Psychotherapy*, 28, 4, 379–392.

National Institute for Health and Clinical Excellence (2002). *Guidance on the use of computerised cognitive behavioural therapy for anxiety and depression*. London: National Institute for Clinical Excellence. www.nice.org.uk/pdf/ 51_CCBT_Full_guidance.pdf.

National Institute for Mental Health in England (2003). *Self-help interventions for mental health problems*. London: National Institute for Mental Health in England.

Richards, D., Richards, A., Barkham, M., Williams, C. & Cahill, J. (2002). PHASE: a health technology approach to psychological treatment in primary mental health care. *Primary Health Care Research and Developments*, 3: 159–168.

Robins, C.J. & Hayes, A.M. (1993). An appraisal of cognitive therapy. *Journal of Consulting and Clinical Psychology*, 61, 2, 205–214.

Useful websites

www.babcp.com (British Association for Behavioural and Cognitive Psychotherapy)

www.depression-primarycare.org (The Macarthur Foundation Initiative on Depression in Primary Care)

www.dh.gov.uk/assetRoot/04/07/72/09/04077209.pdf (Department of Health)

www.nhsdirect.nhs.uk (NHS Direct On line)

www.mind.org.uk (MIND for Better Mental Health)

www.pmhsglos.org.uk (Primary Mental Health Service Gloucestershire Health and Social Care Community)

Test yourself

 To check your progress, locate this section on CD-ROM 1 and work through the interactive questions at the end.

Section 5: Case management

Where guided self-help has had limited effect, a more proactive approach is required, which extends the support offered to patients within primary care in the treatment of their mental health difficulties.

Despite the volume of common mental health problems in primary care, the treatment offered for patients with depression and anxiety has been criticised for being of poor quality and for doing little in helping them overcome their problems (Rost et al, 2000).

Primary care practitioners are criticised on several counts: for being inadequate in their detection of depression, with up to 50% of patients attending GP consultations with a depressive disorder not being diagnosed; for being inadequate in its treatment once identified; and for prescribing antidepressants with little advice or support, with subsequent non-concordance with treatment (NHS Centre for Reviews and Dissemination, 2002).

The most successful interventions are those that are provided by a primary care mental health worker, with the skills to deal with the needs of patients with mental health problems. When patients with depression receive such treatment, depression is treated as effectively as within mental health services (Rost et al, 2000).

Interest is growing in models of chronic disease management in the management of depression. These recommend the allocation of a worker who actively engages in a proactive collaborative relationship with the patient experiencing a period of depression, supporting the general practitioner (GP) in their treatment of the patient.

At this point, you are advised to access information on chronic disease management principles (available online at www.improving chroniccare.org) and consider the philosophy being advocated within the case management model for mental health workers in primary care.

Antidepressant medication is acknowledged to be an effective treatment for depression, when compared to a placebo (Furukawa et al,

Exercise

What are the issues that need to be considered in the recognition and management of depression in primary care?

The bulletin *Improving the recognition and management of depression* (NHS Centre for Reviews & Dissemination, 2002), available in PDF format on CD-ROM 1, and online at www.york.ac.uk/ inst/crd/ehc75.pdf, will assist you in developing your answer.

Exercise

Read The Cochrane Review *Interventions for Helping Patients to follow Prescriptions for Medication* (Haynes 2004), available in PDF format on CD-ROM 1.
* What interventions can be used to improve patients' concordance with prescribed medicines?

Exercise

Read *Improving Quality in Primary Care: A Practical Guide to the National Service Framework for Mental Health*, second edition, Autumn 2003 (available online at www.npcrdc.man.ac.uk).
* What does the document advocate for the provision of effective primary care services and the Collaborative Care Models?
* What role does the mental health worker have in primary care in supporting the use of antidepressant medication?

2002). For depression to be treated effectively in primary care, it is not enough to prescribe antidepressant medication in isolation, for patients often fail to improve without the simultaneous support of a member of the healthcare team who assists the patient in taking their medication as prescribed. Evidence indicates that between 30% and 68% of depressed patients fail to continue with their prescription in the first month of it being prescribed (Korff & Goldberg, 2001). It would therefore appear useful for a mental health worker to follow up such patients to offer information, advice and support and to problem-solve any difficulties. See Part 3.4, Sections 2 and 3.

A number of factors are suggested as being associated with non-concordance: for example, the patient's experience of adverse side-effects, or their perception that they no longer need to take medication because they feel better. There is also some evidence that patients who see stigma associated with depression and treatment with antidepressants are less likely to comply with taking medication (Demyttenaere, 2003).

Exercise

Recall an occasion when a patient did not fully comply with antidepressant treatment.
- What were the reasons?

These are some of the general issues related to non-concordance that you might want to consider:
1 Non-intentional – due to forgetfulness, complex drug regimen, lifestyle restrictions, confusion, lack of understanding
2 Habitual minimization – under-medication due to health beliefs despite presence of symptoms, may decrease dose, frequency or reduce days taking
3 Deliberate – due to drug (e.g. side-effects, taste of medication, lack of efficacy)

Compliance versus concordance

The pursuit of compliance suggests that the aim of prescribing is to encourage patients to follow doctors' orders.

> 'There is an assumption that the patient's role was to be passive and that the prescriber's view was rational and evidence-based.'
>
> *Royal Society, 1997, p3*

These assumptions are challenged by an alternative model of engagement with patients. Concordance is based on the notion that prescribers and supporting primary care workers negotiate with the patient, where both parties are equals and the aim is to build a therapeutic alliance. Its strength lies in an assumption of respect and openness in the relationship, and both can proceed together on the basis of the reality of the patients' circumstances.

Exercise

Write down what ideas you have on improving concordance with antidepressant medication.

You might want to consider some of the following measures to improve concordance:
1 Monitoring whether the patient's depression is responding to the prescribed medication
2 Asking whether they are taking the medication as prescribed. Remember to ask non-judgemental questions, such as 'I've had trouble remembering to take medicines at times. How are you doing?'
3 Making it clear you are listening and responding to the patient's concerns and goals
4 Building reminders into the treatment plan. The leading reason most people fail to take their medication is simple: they forget. Use of coloured stickers on calendars or bleepers on watches can help. For a sample list of what is available, see online at www.epill.com/ind.html.
5 Empathizing with any difficulties and side-effects experienced by the patient
6 Feeding back information on the patient's progress and adherence to the responsible primary care physician

Summary

- A clear written protocol which details the scope of primary care worker involvement in monitoring antidepressant and other pharmacological treatments needs to be fully signed-up-to by the primary care team and employer

- The chronic disease management principle advocates the allocation of a worker who actively engages in a proactive collaborative relationship with the patient suffering from depression

References

Demyttenaere, K. (2003). Risk factors and predictors of concordance in depression. *European Neuropsychopharmacology*, 13, 69–75.

Furukawa, T., McGuire, H. & Barbui, C. (2002). Meta-analysis of effects and side-effects of low dosage tricyclic antidepressants in depression: systematic review. *British Medical Journal*, 325, 991–1001.

Haynes, R.B, McDonald, H, Gang, A.X. & Montague, P. (2004). *Interventions for helping patients to follow prescriptions for medications.* Chichester: Cochrane Database of Systematic Reviews.

Korff, M. & Golberg, D. (2001). Improving outcomes in depression: the whole process of care needs to be enhanced. *British Medical Journal*, 323, 948–949.

NHS Centre for Reviews and Dissemination (2002). Improving the recognition and management of depression. *Effective Health Care*, 7, 5, 1–12.

Rost, K., Nutting, P., Smith, J. & Werner, M. (2000). Designing and implementing a primary care intervention trial to improve the quality and outcome of care for major depression. *General Hospital Psychiatry*, 22, 66–77.

Royal Society of Great Britain (1997). *From compliance to concordance: achieving shared goals in taking medication.* London: The Royal Society.

Useful websites

www.improvingchroniccare.org (Improving Chronic Illness Care)

www.npcrdc.man.ac.uk (National Primary Care Research and Development Centre)

Test yourself

 To check your progress, locate this section on CD-ROM 1 and work through the interactive questions at the end.

Section 6: Pharmacological management of depression: antidepressants

It is important to adhere to the local PCT protocols/guidelines on medication management (see Part 3.4, Section 3, for information on medication management). Training will be required in advance for primary mental health workers to monitor medicines prescribed by the general practitioner. Primary care mental health workers should not be offering advice or negotiating changes to medication, unless the written protocol expressly allows this, and only if all the conditions detailed in the protocol are met.

Meet Sarah

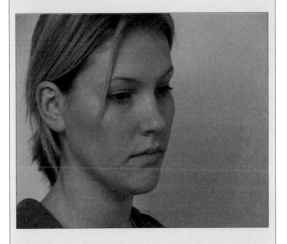

Sarah is a 24-year-old single woman who lives with a female flatmate of similar age. Sarah has been feeling increasingly depressed over the last three months since she lost her job as a secretary at a local building firm when it went into liquidation. Her mood is low and she is tearful a good deal of the time. She has done little to find another job and tends to spend her days moping around the house, doing very little. Her flatmate takes care of the shopping and housework, as Sarah feels unable to get started to do anything. She rarely goes out and, despite her flatmate's encouragement, her social life is now non-existent. Her appetite is

Meet Sarah (*continued*)

poor and she has lost weight, but not to a degree that would cause concern for her physical health. She has lost her self-confidence, and her self-esteem is very low. She is very negative about the future, finding it difficult to see herself getting another job. She has recently started having thoughts of suicide but has dismissed these so far.

 CD-ROM 1 includes a video clip in which Sarah introduces herself, and an audio clip of a telephone support session between Sarah and Katie, a practice mental health worker, in which they discuss side-effects Sarah has experienced as she begins to take her prescription medication.

Video: Introducing Sarah (Depression)

Sarah: I've been feeling more and more down over the past three months or so. It all started when I lost my job at Myles and Kelly Builders. I really liked my job, it was a good laugh and the work was easy. I know it probably sounds stupid, but I can't stop crying about it. Sometimes I just start crying and don't even know why. I haven't done anything about getting another job just yet, I haven't been able to face it. Now I just sit around all day doing nothing apart from drinking tea and watching telly. I just don't feel up to doing anything. I feel really guilty about it. I'm just so tired though, I think that's why I can't be bothered. I'm not sleeping well either. I'm waking up really early, and I just can't get back to sleep. Karen, my flatmate, she's been really great about it, but it's not fair that she's having to do everything. She tried to drag me out the other night, she's always doing that, but I can't face going out any more. God, I can't even face eating half the time, never mind going on a night out. I can't see how things are

going to get any better. Dr Mehra has put me on some tablets which he reckons might help. I'm going to give them a go. Let's hope they help. He's also asked me to see a mental health worker at the practice. I think he thinks I could do with someone to talk to. I think I might find that helpful.

Audio: Medication Management - Side effects

Sarah: Hello.

Mental Health Worker (Katie): Hello, is that Sarah Goodfellow?

Sarah: Yes, speaking.

Katie: Hi Sarah, it's Katie Walsh here, the mental health worker from Cochrane Park Health Centre. I arranged to telephone you to discuss how you've been getting on with taking your antidepressants since you were prescribed them just over a week ago by Dr Mehra.

Sarah: I'm pleased you've called because I've been having a few problems.

Katie: Okay, is that what you'd like to talk about for the 10 minutes we have today?

Sarah: Yes, I'm a bit concerned about it.

Katie: What type of problems have you been experiencing, Sarah?

Sarah: I've had a dry mouth and been feeling a bit sick.

Katie: And when did this start?

Sarah: It's been in the last three days or so.

Katie: How severe is the dry mouth?

Sarah: It's making me drink more, but I never feel like I quench the thirst.

Katie: Is it there all the time?

Sarah: Pretty much so.

Katie: Okay, what about the nausea, how severe has that been?

Sarah: I've felt pretty sick at times but I haven't actually been sick.

Katie: You say at times, are there times when you don't feel sick?

Sarah: Yes. I suppose the nausea is worse in the morning, but after lunch it's not as bad.

Katie: Are there any other problems you're experiencing?

Sarah: No, that's it.

Katie: Okay. What you've described is completely normal. It's very common for people to experience some minor difficulties within the first couple of weeks of starting antidepressants. It sounds like what you're experiencing is a bit unpleasant, but most people find that these symptoms subside after a few days. This is the tough part at the moment, because you're getting the side-effects but not getting the benefits yet. Considering this, are you happy to continue to take the medication as prescribed, and for us to review how you're getting on in a week's time?

Sarah: Yes, it's not unbearable.

Katie: What you may find helpful is to suck a boiled sweet when you've got the dry mouth, and sipping drinks can also help too.

Sarah: That's useful to know. I'll try that.

Katie: You might also find it helpful to take the medication just before food, as this can help with nausea.

Sarah: Oh, that's useful to know, as I've been taking them several hours before food.

Katie: Okay, good. Now, have you read the leaflet explaining about your antidepressants?

Sarah: No, I didn't get round to it.

Katie: Could that be something that you could do between now and the next time we speak in a week's time?

Sarah: Yes, I'll do that. I haven't started the diary either, yet, that you asked me to complete, on what I'm doing on an hour-by-hour basis. Maybe I could fill that in too.

Katie: Good. That would be really helpful. So, we've acknowledged how this can be a particularly difficult time when you start to experience some side-effects, but I'm really pleased to hear that it's not too unbearable, and that you are willing to stick with it. Is there anything else about side-effects that you want to talk about today?

Sarah: No, I think I'll read the leaflet.

Katie: Okay, that's good. Well we seem to have covered everything we set out to cover. Can I just check with you that we're both clear about what you plan to do until we speak again next week?

Antidepressant drugs are effective in the treatment of moderate to severe depression; however, they are not seen as particularly effective in milder forms of depression. The major classes of antidepressants include the Tricyclics and related antidepressants, the Selective Serotonin Re-uptake Inhibitors (SSRIs) and the Monoamine Oxidase Inhibitors (MAOIs). The choice of antidepressants will be based on the individual patient's requirements, including suicide risk, and previous response to antidepressant therapy (Bazire, 2003–4; British Medical Association and Royal Pharmaceutical Society of Great Britain, 2004; The National Prescribing Centre, 2000).

Exercise

Familiarize yourself with the most commonly prescribed antidepressants in your GP practice. It may well be worth asking a GP about their preferred choice of medication.

Antidepressants are not generally recommended for patients in steps 1–2 of the Stepped Care model because the risk–benefit ratio is poor. However, due to past custom and practice, many people with mild depression will still be prescribed antidepressants.

Medication is more commonly prescribed in steps 3–5. Exceptions may be made when patients have failed to benefit from other interventions at lower steps, or where patients have a previous history of moderate to severe depression. Please refer to the NICE Guidelines for Depression (2004a) and the *Enhanced Services Specification for depression under the new GP contract*, a commissioning guide (National Institute for Mental Health in England North West Development Centre 2004a). The basic principles of the *Enhanced Services Specification* that relate to the prescription of antidepressant medication are as follows:

- Prescription is in accordance with NICE guidelines
- Antidepressants are not recommended in the initial treatment of mild depression

- Maintenance prescribing is monitored regularly
- Information is given to the patients

Other useful considerations

- Carers should be provided with appropriate information on the nature, course and treatment of depression, including the use and likely side-effects of medication
- Antidepressants may affect driving and other skilled tasks
- Great caution is necessary for pregnant and nursing mothers. Antidepressants are not recommended for children under 16
- Alcohol interacts with most antidepressants
- Antidepressants work by increasing levels of noradrenaline, serotonin or dopamine, or a combination of these
- Antidepressants do not work immediately
- Antidepressants can take up to six weeks before benefit is felt (longer in the elderly)
- Treatment should continue for at least 6 months after resolution of symptoms

Anon., 1999; Bazire, 2003–4; The National Prescribing Centre, 2000

Tricyclic antidepressants

This group of drugs was developed in the 1960s and is still used today, although the number of new prescriptions is declining, with preference given to new-generation SSRI antidepressants. Tricyclic antidepressants improve mood by blocking the reuptake of serotonin and noradreniline, and, to a lesser degree, of dopamine (Wilbourn & Prosser, 2003). These drugs are most effective for treating moderate to severe depression associated with physiological changes – for example, sleep disturbances or loss of appetite (British Medical Association and Royal Pharmaceutical Society of Great Britain, 2004; The National Prescribing Centre, 2000).

Contraindications
- Recent myocardial infarction, arrhythmias, severe liver disease

Cautions
- Cardiac disease, epilepsy, hepatic impairment, thyroid disease, phaeo-chromocytoma, history of mania, psychosis, closed angle glaucoma, history of urinary retention

Side-effects
- Common: dry mouth, blurred vision, urinary retention, constipation, drowsiness, weight gain
- Uncommon: headache, nausea, palpitations, postural hypotension, sexual dysfunction, sweating
- Rare: tremor

Discontinuation reactions
- Cholinergic rebound, headache, restlessness, diarrhoea, nausea, vomiting, flu-like symptoms, lethargy, abdominal cramps, sleep disturbance, movement disorders

Selective serotonin re-uptake inhibitors (SSRIs)

SSRIs work by increasing serotonin and are often the first line of treatment in routine care. They tend to be tolerated better than tricyclic antidepressants and have fewer anti-cholinergic and cardiovascular side-effects, and they are safer in overdose than tricyclic antidepressants. They are preferred where there is a significant risk of deliberate overdose (Bazire, 2003–4; British Medical Association and Royal Pharmaceutical Society of Great Britain, 2004; The National Prescribing Centre, 2000).

Contraindications
- Less pro-convulsive, but still some risk in epilepsy

Cautions
- In-patients with renal and hepatic impairment

Side-effects
- Common: gastric disturbance, loss of appetite, nausea, vomiting, anxiety,

restlessness, diarrhoea, insomnia
- Fairly common: sexual dysfunction
- Uncommon: dizziness, drowsiness, headache
- Rare: dry mouth, rashes, hyponatraemia, tremor

Discontinuation reactions

- Dizziness, vertigo/light-headedness, nausea, fatigue, headache, a sensation like electric shocks in the head, insomnia, abdominal cramps, chills, flu-like symptoms, increased dreaming, anxiety, agitation and volatility

Monoamine oxidase inhibitors (MAOIs)

MAOIs work by blocking the breakdown of the central nervous system stimulatory neurotransmitters, adrenaline, noradrenaline and dopamine (Wilbourn & Prosser, 2003). They also prevent breakdown of naturally occurring monoamines, particularly tyramine. MAOIs are used much less frequently than tricyclics or SSRIs, because of the dangers of dietary and drug interactions (Bazire, 2003–4; British Medical Association and Royal Pharmaceutical Society of Great Britain, 2004; The National Prescribing Centre, 2000).

Contraindications
- Liver disease, blood dyscrasias, congestive heart failure, cerebrovascular disease, phaeochromocytoma, hyperthyroidism
- Numerous drug interactions with prescribed and over-the-counter medicines (e.g. ephedrine, pseudoephedrine, and many cough and cold remedies)

Cautions
- Elderly patients
- Epilepsy
- Ingestion of tyramine can result in hypertensive crisis
- Food and drink to be avoided: cheese, Bovril, OXO, meat extracts, broad bean pods, banana skins, Marmite, yeast extract, pickled herrings, textured vegetable protein, stale food, Chianti wine, home brew, real ales
- Need to be particularly careful when swapping to and from other antidepressants. Washout periods needed

Side-effects
- Common: postural hypotension
- Uncommon: constipation, drowsiness, dry mouth, fatigue, headache, insomnia
- Rare: blurred vision, oedema, skin rashes, sweating, urine retention

Discontinuation reactions
- Psychosis, hallucinations, disorientation, catatonia, irritability, hypomania, nausea, sweating, palpitations, nightmares, delirium

Reactions to the discontinuation of MAOIs

- Usually start 1–2 days after stopping
- Resolve within 24 hours of restarting
- More common with longer courses or high doses
- Can occur with missed doses
- Symptoms will be consistent with the antidepressant groups

Principles of stopping antidepressant treatment

The basic principles when discontinuing antidepressant medication is to withdraw the medication gradually over a 1–2-week period in patients who have received less than 8 weeks of continuous medication. For patients who have received 6–8 months of treatment, the antidepressant should be tapered off over 6–8 weeks. Where patients have been maintained on antidepressants for a longer period of time, the dose is usually reduced by 25% every 4–6 weeks.

Patients should be clearly advised to discuss with their GP their intention to stop antidepressant treatment.

Questions that may arise

Patients prescribed antidepressant medication often have concerns and questions about their medication. Typical of such questions are the following:

- Are they addictive?
- How long will I need to take them?
- What are the side effects?
- Can I drink whilst taking them?
- Will they make me put on weight?
- Will they affect my contraception or other medication I am taking?
- Can I drive while taking them?

Exercise

As a mental health worker, it is useful for you to be able to respond to the questions listed above. Read the following publications (downloadable from www.mind.org.uk) in order to familiarize yourself with patient issues related to this treatment::

- *Making Sense of Antipsychotics*: www.mind.org.uk/Information/Booklets/ Making+sense/antip.htm.
- *Getting the Best from your Pharmacist*: www.mind.org.uk/Information/Factsheets/ Treatments+and+drugs/GETTING+ THE+BEST+FROM+YOUR+ PHARMACIST.htm.
- *Mind Rights Guide 3: Consent to treatment*: www.mind.org.uk/Information/Booklets/ Rights+guide/RG3.htm.
- *Making Sense of Antidepressants*: www.mind.org.uk/Information/Booklets/ Making+sense/Making+sense+of+ antidepressants.htm.

Summary

- Antidepressants are used for moderate to severe depression
- There are two main groups of commonly prescribed antidepressants, the Selective Serotonin Re-uptake Inhibitors and Tricyclic antidepressants
- There are certain difficulties associated with the side-effects of this group of medication

- The primary care mental worker can facilitate aspects of medication management

References

Anon. (1999). Withdrawing Patients from Antidepressants. *Drugs and Therapeutics Bulletin.* 37, 49–52.

Bazire, S. (2003–4). *Psychotropic Drug Directory*. Wiltshire: Quay Books.

British Medical Association and Royal Pharmaceutical Society of Great Britain (2004). *British National Formulary*. London: British Medical Association and Royal Pharmaceutical Society of Great Britain.

National Institute for Mental Health in England North West Development Centre (2004a). *Enhanced Services Specification for Depression under the new GP Contract: A Commissioning Guidebook.* Hyde: NIHME, North West Development Centre.

The National Prescribing Centre (2000). The drug treatment of depression in primary care. *MeRec Bulletin*, 11, 9, 33–36.

Wilbourn, M. & Prosser, S. (2003). *The pathology and pharmacology of mental illness*. Cheltenham: Nelson Thornes Ltd.

Useful websites

www.bnf.org (British National Formulary)
www.mind.org.uk (MIND for Better Mental Health)

Test yourself

 To check your progress, locate this section on CD-ROM 1 and work through the interactive questions at the end.

Section 7: Mental health indicators within primary care: serious mental health problems

This section focuses on the needs of patients with serious mental health problems. Most people with mental health problems are managed in primary care. A small minority of patients have regular contact with secondary care mental health services. While many mental health workers in primary care will work for the majority of their time with patients with common mental health problems, there may be occasions when it is appropriate that someone with schizophrenia or bipolar affective disorder is seen in a primary care setting. Such patients will contact their GP with physical health problems, and it may be appropriate for them to be seen by a mental health worker if they present with anxiety and/or depression and the schizophrenia or bipolar affective disorder is well controlled. It is not uncommon for some practice nurses to provide such patients with their regular depot injections.

As a minimum standard, it is important that primary care staff enhance their knowledge and understanding of serious mental illness and assist in the screening process and referral to the appropriate services (Department of Health, 1999a; Department of Health, 2000). Before patients with serious mental health problems can be referred to Mental Health Trusts for assessment and treatment, primary care mental health workers and other primary care staff need to be able to screen and detect serious mental illness.

Traditional classifications of serious mental health problems tend to describe mental illness as a group of symptoms leading to a diagnosis and subsequent treatment. Terms such as schizophrenia or bipolar affective disorder are used to classify a group of symptoms which, primarily, characterize the patient groups referred to as patients with serious mental health problems (The British Psychological Society, 2000).

Schizophrenia

The core symptoms of schizophrenia are:
- Hallucinations, such as hearing voices when no one is around; hallucinations may be via any of the senses
- Delusional ideation (i.e. strange beliefs or fears which are not in keeping with the person's culture)
- Thought disorder, shown by disorganized or strange speech patterns
- Affective symptoms (extreme or labile emotional state)
- Agitation or bizarre behaviour

These symptoms are often referred to as positive or overt symptoms. However, people suffering from schizophrenia also identify other symptoms characterized by a reduction in activity, referred to as negative symptoms, such as apathy and reduced emotional response, that affect their quality of life.

More information on schizophrenia – how widespread a problem it is, more detail on the symptoms experienced by patients and the prognosis – is available online at:
- www.rcpsych.ac.uk/campaigns/cminds/ schizophrenia.htm
- www.mind.org.uk/Information/Booklets/ Understanding/Understanding+schizophrenia. htm

The most common hallucinations experienced by patients diagnosed with schizophrenia are auditory hallucinations, and the consensus view is that people who hear voices have difficulty distinguishing their own thoughts or inner speech from voices with an external origin (Morrison & Haddock, 1997). The voices tend to be worse when people are anxious or distressed (Margo et al, 1981). Beliefs and explanations about voices also appear to be highly significant, as they appear to affect the amount of distress experienced by the patient (Chadwick & Birchwood, 1994).

A delusion is characterized by an irrational belief that defies normal reasoning. Delusions are often related to the patient's hallucinations, and strengthen the conviction with which they are held. Delusions can take many forms; for example, the individual may be plagued by the belief that someone is plotting against them and out to harm them, or that there is something physically wrong with them (Maxmen & Nicholas, 1995).

Our current understanding of the aetiology of severe mental health problems is as follows: patients who experience severe forms of mental illness have a biological vulnerability to developing the illness; these vulnerable patients experience symptoms when they have been under high levels of stress (e.g. acute stress following a bereavement, or chronic stress resulting from situations such as unhappy relationships, not having enough money, etc.). This model of understanding schizophrenia is referred to as the 'stress vulnerability' model.

For more details of the stress vulnerability model, see www.npi.ucla.edu/ssg/stress.htm and www.psychosissucks.ca/epi/index.cfm?action= whatcauses.

You should also read the report by the British Psychological Society (2000), *Recent Advances in Understanding Mental Illness*, available in PDF format on CD-ROM 1, and online at www. mentalhealthcare.org.uk/download/ psychosis/Understanding_Mental_ Illness. pdf.

Bipolar affective disorder

Bipolar affective disorder is also known as manic depression. Patients diagnosed as suffering from bipolar affective disorder experience marked mood swings which are beyond what most people experience, more extreme and more prolonged than the common, everyday ups and downs. Emotions may vary from depression and hopelessness through to feeling overly elated or 'high'. People usually go through periods of normal mood between episodes of illness and do not necessarily experience highs and lows alternately.

The typical symptoms of mania are feeling euphoric, with increased levels of energy. Patients are, therefore, very active, restless and distractible. Patients, when experiencing mania, have a reduced need for sleep and can have an increased sex drive; their thoughts tend to race and to be grandiose in nature; they can, therefore, be full of new and exciting ideas and have unrealistic beliefs about their abilities and powers (Lam et al, 1999).

When patients are depressed they feel sad, lack any interest or pleasure, and they typically have no energy and feel tired. They often appear "slowed down", and have poor concentration and find it difficult to remember things. They will often express feelings of low self-esteem, despair and hopelessness, worthlessness and/or guilt, with ideas of suicide and/or actual self-harm.

For more information on bipolar affective

disorder see www.yorkmind.org.uk/inf_manic. htm and www. makingspace.co.uk/pdfs/ manic_depression.pdf.

Dementia

For information on what is meant by the term dementia, how the diagnosis is made, and the current evidence base related to aetiology and care, visit: www.alzheimers.org.uk. For services available to patients with dementia, visit: www.fordementia. org.uk and www.dh.gov.uk /assetRoot/04/07/12/83/ 04071283.pdf.

The *National Service Framework for Older People: Modern Standards and Service Models* (Department of Health 2001f) is available in PDF format on CD-ROM 1, and online at www.dh.gov. uk/assetRoot/04/07/12/83/04071283.pdf.

Antipsychotic medication

A brief summary of antipsychotic medication is given below.
* Older drugs (typical), e.g. Chlorpromazine, Haloperidol. Some are available as long-acting depot injections
* Newer drugs (atypical), e.g. Olanzapine, Risperidone
* All drugs are effective at treating positive symptoms
* Atypicals may help negative symptoms and are less likely to cause some of the troublesome side-effects of the older ones

How do they work?

* Dopamine hypothesis: over-activity of dopamine receptors in limbic system
* Antipsychotic drugs block dopamine receptors
* Atypical antipsychotic drugs block serotonin receptors. Important in treatment of negative symptoms
* Blockade of these and other receptors explains side-effects

Uses of antipsychotic drugs

* Schizophrenia

- Mania
- Other psychotic illnesses
- Rapid tranquilization
- Agitation and anxiety
- Behavioural control in dementia
- Sleep disturbances
- Antiemetic
- Hiccups

Summary

- While many mental health workers in primary care will work for the majority of their time with patients with common mental health problems, there may be occasions when it is appropriate that someone with schizophrenia or bipolar affective disorder is seen in a primary care setting
- Patients with schizophrenia can experience hallucinations via any of the senses, strange beliefs or fears which are not in keeping with the person's culture, disorganized or strange speech patterns, and/or a reduction in activity
- These patients have a biological vulnerability to developing these symptoms when they have been under high levels of stress
- Patients diagnosed as suffering from bipolar affective disorder experience marked mood swings, which are beyond what most people experience, more extreme, and more prolonged than the common, everyday ups and downs

References

British Psychological Society (2000). *Recent advances in understanding mental illness and psychotic experiences*. Leicester: The British Psychological Society.

Chadwick, P.D.J. & Birchwood, M. (1994). The omnipotence of voices: A cognitive approach to auditory hallucinations. *British Journal of Psychiatry*, 164, 190–201.

Department of Health (1999a). *A National Service Framework for Mental Health*. London: HMSO.

Department of Health (2000). *The NHS Plan: a Plan for Investment, a Plan for Reform*. London: HMSO.

Department of Health (2001f). *National Service Framework for Older People: Modern Standards and Service Models*. London: Department of Health.

Lam, H.L., Jones, S.H., Hayward, P. & Bright, J.A. (1999). *Cognitive Therapy for Bipolar Disorder*. Chichester: Wiley.

Margo, A., Hemsley, D. & Slade, P. (1981). The effects of varying auditory input on schizophrenic hallucinations. *British Journal of Psychiatry*, 139, 122–127.

Maxmen, J. & Nicholas, G. (1995). *Essential Psychopathology and Its Treatment* (second edition). New York: W.W. Norton.

Morrison, A. & Haddock, G. (1997). Cognitive factors in source monitoring and auditory hallucinations. *Psychological Medicine*, 27, 3, 669–679.

Useful websites

www.alzheimers.org.uk (Alzheimer's Society: Dementia Care and Research)

www.dh.gov.uk/assetRoot/04/07/12/83/04071283.pdf (Department of Health)

www.fordementia.org.uk (For Dementia)

www.makingspace.co.uk/pdfs/manic_depression.pdf (Making Space)

www.mind.org.uk/Information/Booklets/Understanding/Understanding+schizophrenia.htm (MIND for better mental health)

www.npi.ucla.edu/ssg/stress.htm (Family Social Support Project)

www.psychosissucks.ca/epi/index.cfm?action= whatcauses (Early Psychosis Intervention Program Fraser Health Authority)

www.rcpsych.ac.uk/campaigns/cminds/schizophrenia.htm (The Royal College of Psychiatrists)

www.rcpsych.ac.uk/info/mhgu/pdfs/Sheet21.pdf (The Royal College of Psychiatrists)

www.yorkmind.org.uk/inf_manic.htm (York and District MIND)

Test yourself

 To check your progress, locate this section on CD-ROM 1 and work through the interactive questions at the end.

Section 8: Addressing health inequalities

An improvement in healthcare and lifestyle has led to great advances in the life expectancy and health status of many. However, despite a general increase in prosperity and access to healthcare, many groups within our community experience premature death and increased infant mortality relative to the average. The social circumstances experienced by an individual, as well as their ability to access healthcare have a major impact upon their health and mortality. Issues such as gender, race, educational achievement, and disability are seen as impacting on our personal behaviour, which in turn might influence our health.

At this point it would be useful to read more information on the health inequalities encountered by many disadvantaged groups. The *Tackling Health Inequalities Programme* (2003c) was launched by the Department of Health, and is available in PDF format on CD-ROM 1, and online at www.dh. gov.uk/assetRoot/04/01/93/62/04019362. pdf. It advocates that Primary Care Trusts and local authorities target disadvantaged groups and areas, and proactively seek out the views of local people of the services that affect their health.

Serious mental illness has a major impact upon an individual's social circumstances. Patients with serious mental illness are more likely to experience a number of disadvantages, such as unemployment, reduced income, stigma and social exclusion (International Council of Nurses, 2001). As with other disadvantaged groups, these inequalities impact significantly on the behaviour of the patient. Patients with serious mental illness have a higher incidence of smoking than the general population (Kelly & McCreadie, 1999) and tend to have diets high in fat and low in fibre, as well as taking less exercise (Brown, 1997; Bradshaw, 2005). Patients with schizophrenia also have the added burden upon their physical health of the adverse consequences of their treatment, with weight gain, diabetes mellitus and cardio-

---

Exercise

Find out:
- How disadvantaged groups are identified by your Primary Care Trust.
- How the views of local people about mental health in primary care are obtained.

More information is available on the Programme for Action and Health Inequalities at: www. dh.gov.uk/PolicyAnd Guidance/HealthAndSocialCareTopics/ HealthInequalities/fs/en; and on Health Action Zones at www.haznet. org.uk. In particular, focus on any local initiatives and how they might impact on the social exclusion and discrimination experienced by patients with serious mental health problems.

---

toxic side-effects recorded as side-effects of antipsychotic drugs (Sim, 1987).

Patients with schizophrenia are four times more likely than the general population to die of coronary heart disease and to be more vulnerable to respiratory disease (Murie, 2004). The average life expectancy is reduced by 10 years for men with schizophrenia, and by nine years for women (Allebeck, 1989). Herrman et al (1983), in their study of 592 patients with schizophrenia, found that ischaemic heart disease was the commonest cause of death.

Exercise

Find out what specialist services are available within your work setting to help meet the physical health needs of people with mental health problems.

Most health centres, GP practices and surgeries have access to specialist clinics either on site or at a neighbouring practice, providing screening and management of asthma, diabetes, hypertension, smoking cessation and many others. These clinics are organized and managed by practice nurses and nurse practitioners. The input received by patients with serious mental health problems, in monitoring and addressing their physical healthcare needs, has been heavily criticised. Patients generally fail to recognize physical health difficulties themselves (Brown et al, 2000). However, despite this, mental health professionals tend to overlook the physical needs of their patients, particularly if they experience high levels of positive symptoms. Primary care services are said to be equally

---

Exercise

Find out what clinics are provided by primary care staff in your work setting for people with physical health problems.

- Are all high-risk patients informed about these clinics?
- Are there other ways of accessing hard-to-reach people with serious mental health problems to address hidden physical illness?

---

inactive in providing an accessible service for this patient group (Felker et al, 1996).

The government has called for a major cultural shift in attitudes towards people with mental health problems. A report by the Social Exclusion Unit (2004), *Action on Mental Health: A Guide to promoting Social Inclusion* sets out a programme to foster greater social inclusion. It details strategies for the delivery of services in a non-stigmatizing manner. The guide is available in PDF format on CD-ROM 1, or online at www. socialexclusion.gov.uk/downloaddoc. asp?id=300.

MIND has produced a guide for what it sees are the priorities in addressing mental health and social exclusion. This is available online at www.mind.org.uk/News+policy+and+campaigns/ Policy/SEUP.htm.

Mental illness registers

Primary care providers are given direction on the implementation of services to include the improved mental health quality indicators. Services involve the registration of the personal details of patients with serious mental health problems, and a reduction of the adverse health outcomes experienced by this and other patient groups. For more information, please access and read the PDF file *Delivering Investment in* 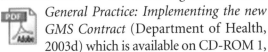 *General Practice: Implementing the new GMS Contract* (Department of Health, 2003d) which is available on CD-ROM 1, or online at 195.33.102.76/assetRoot/04/07/02/ 31/ 04070231.pdf.

The NSF for Mental Health (Department of Health, 1999a) calls upon primary and mental health services to work closely, within agreed protocols, in order to implement a strategy that ensures that the comprehensive needs of patients with serious mental illness are met. These principles are outlined in Standards Four and Five, which detail how addressing the physical healthcare needs of patients is fundamental to the process of providing effective services for this patient group. Primary care services are given the responsibility to take a lead in meeting the physical needs of this patient group.

In order to provide better services, Primary Care Trusts will have to produce registers of the prevalence of serious mental health problems in patients on their lists, in order to monitor their clinical progress, compliance with medication and, in particular, to review and manage their physical healthcare needs (Murie, 2004). The *Enhanced Services Specification for Depression* recommends that there should be a separate register for patients with depression to those with severe mental health problems (NIMHE North West Development Centre, 2004a).

Audit

Primary Care Trusts are also being asked to identify patients on their practice lists with depression, and develop protocols to: screen vulnerable groups, offer effective interventions and support, meet identified needs, and monitor the efficiency of what they offer (NIMHE North West Development Centre, 2004a).

The *Enhanced Services Specification for Depression under the new GP Contract* (NIMHE North West Development Centre, 2004a) recommends auditing of the following within PCTs, to demonstrate that enhanced services for depression are evident:

- Protocols are in place and adhered to for screening high-risk groups
- Screening tools are used to aid diagnosis
- Standard questionnaires are used to monitor progress
- Patients are offered an appropriate number of monitoring and review appointments
- Medication is prescribed appropriately and monitored regularly
- Appropriate psychological therapies are available and offered to patients
- Patient satisfaction is monitored using standardized questionnaires

Summary

- Patients with serious mental illness experience health inequalities that adversely affect their life expectancy and health status
- Primary and mental health services are asked to work closely, within agreed protocols, in order to implement a strategy that ensures that the comprehensive needs of patients with serious mental illness are met
- Patients with mental health problems will present in primary care for management of physical health problems, and will benefit from attending clinics offering specialist screening and monitoring
- It is important for primary care staff to screen all patients for possible mental health problems, liaise with mental health workers, and refer to appropriate support through the GP

References

Allebeck, P. (1989). Schizophrenia: A Life Shortening Disease. *Schizophrenia Bulletin*, 15, 1, 81–89.

Bradshaw, T. (2005). A systematic review of the efficacy of healthy living interventions for adult with a diagnosis of schizophrenia, a schizo-affective disorder. *Journal of Advanced Nursing*, 49, 6, 634–654.

Brown, S. (1997). Excess mortality of schizophrenia: A meta-analysis. *British Journal of Psychiatry*, 171, 12, 502–508.

Brown, S., Inskip, H. & Barrowclough, B. (2000). Causes of the excess mortality of schizophrenia. *British Journal of Psychiatry*, 177, 212–217.

Department of Health (1999a). *A National Service Framework for Mental Health*. London: HMSO.

Department of Health (2003c). *Tackling Health Inequalities: A Programme for Action*. London: HMSO.

Department of Health (2003d). *Delivering Investment in General Practice: Implementing the new GMS Contract*. London: HMSO.

Felker, B., Yazel, J.J. & Short, D. (1996). Mortality and medical co-morbidity among psychiatric patients: A review. *Psychiatric Services*, 47, 12, 1356–1363.

Herrman, H.E., Baldwin, J.A. & Christie, D. (1983). A record-linkage study of mortality and general hospital discharge in patients diagnosed as schizophrenic. *Psychological Medicine*, 13, 581–593.

International Council of Nurses (2001). Mental Health: Stop exclusion – Dare to care. Nursing matters, www.icn.ch/matters_mentalhealth.htm.

Kelly, C. & McCreadie, R.G. (1999). Smoking habits, current symptoms and premorbid characteristics of schizophrenic patients in Nithsdale, Scotland. *American Journal of Psychiatry*, 156, 11, 1751–1757.

Murie, J. (2004). Contract will address needs of patients with severe mental illness. *Guidelines in Practice*, 7(3), 35–42.

National Institute for Mental Health in England North West Development Centre (2004a). *Enhanced Services Specification for Depression under the new GP Contract: A Commissioning Guidebook*. Hyde: NIHME North West Development Centre.

Sim, A. (1987). Why the excess mortality from psychiatric illness? *British Medical Journal*, 294, 986–987.

Social Exclusion Unit (2004). *Action on Mental Health: A guide to promoting social inclusion*. London: SEU.

Useful websites

www.dh.gov.uk/PolicyAndGuidance/HealthAnd
SocialCareTopics/HealthInequalities/fs/en
(Department of Health)
www.haznet.org.uk (Health Action Zone)
www.icn.ch (International Council of Nurses)
www.mind.org.uk (MIND for better Mental Health)

Test yourself

 To check your progress, locate this section on CD-ROM 1 and work through the interactive questions at the end.

Part 2
Practice-based working with users, carers and support agencies

Authors: Julie Attenborough, Barbara Goodfellow and Ian Light

Chapter 2.1

The Modernization Agenda and social inclusion

Aim

To provide in-depth knowledge and a critical understanding of the NHS Modernization Agenda (specifically as it applies to mental health and primary care); exploring the concept of social inclusion/ exclusion as it applies to mental health (focusing on groups where social exclusion has been demonstrated).

Learning outcomes

By the end of this Chapter, the reader will be able to:
*   Critically reflect on the policy documents that drive the modernization of the NHS
*   Discuss the proposed changes to the law as they relate to mental healthcare, taking into account the views of service user organizations
*   Describe and discuss the structural changes being made nationally to the NHS
*   Critically discuss the locally-based organizations which have been created to assess quality and promote user and carer involvement
*   Discuss and evaluate the concepts of social exclusion and social inclusion as applied to users of mental health services
*   Critically consider the subject of social exclusion/inclusion as it relates to ethnicity, gender and disability in the fields of mental health and primary care

Introduction

Throughout this Chapter (and the programme as a whole), ideas such as 'health', 'mental health', 'well-being' and 'illness' will constantly come into play; before you start, it is worth thinking about what you mean by these terms, and why. The act of promoting health and well-being is always value-laden; definitions of health may raise the possibility for individuals subjectively to 'feel' personally healthy, despite the experience of 'symptoms' that others would view as indicative of poor health (e.g. hearing voices).

Reference

World Health Organisation (WHO) (1998). *Health Promotion Glossary*. Geneva: WHO.

Chapter 2.1 content is as follows:

1   The Modernization Agenda, including the National Service Framework and mental health targets
2   Social inclusion and mental health

Section 1: The Modernization Agenda, including the National Service Framework and mental health targets

This section is divided into six parts:
1   Introduction: the policy context
2   The National Service Frameworks (NSFs)
3   The NHS Plan: a Plan for Investment, a Plan for Reform
4   The specific targets proposed for mental health and primary care
5   Structural changes at the national level
6   Organizational changes at the local level

'The long-term goal of the modernisation programme is a radical re-shaping of services around the experience of service users and carers.'

Readhead & Briel, 2001

'The people who use mental health services will be involved, as equal partners and at every level, to ensure the new services make sense.'

Department of Health, 2001a

Introduction: the policy context

When the Labour government came to power in 1997, it undertook a major review of the National Health Service and, during its first years in office, produced several major policy documents – including:

- *The New NHS: Modern, Dependable* (1997)
- *Modernising Mental Health Services* (1998a)
- *The Future Organisation of Prison Health Care* (1999a)
- *Managing Dangerous People with Severe Personality Disorder* (1999b)
- *The National Service Framework for Mental Health* (1999c)
- *Saving Lives: Our Healthier Nation* (1999d)
- *The NHS Plan: a Plan for Investment, a Plan for Reform* (2000a)
- *The Expert Patient: A New Approach to Chronic Disease Management for the 21st Century* (2001b)

Of these, two of the most important for our purposes are the *National Service Framework for Mental Health* (1999c) and *The NHS Plan* (2000a).

Both the National Service Framework for Mental Health and the NHS Plan are included in PDF format on CD-ROM 2, and are available online at www.dh.gov.uk/ assetRoot/04/07/72/09/04077209.pdf (the NSF) and www.dh.gov.uk/assetRoot/04/05/57/83/ 04055783.pdf (the NHS Plan).

You may find it helpful to access these documents as you complete the exercises, or research the full text of the documents on which this programme draws.

The principles that were first mooted in the white paper *Modernising Mental Health Services* (1998a) act as the guiding principles behind the *National Service Framework for Mental Health* (1999c). These propose that a modernized system of mental healthcare should:

- involve users and their carers in the planning and delivery of care
- deliver high-quality treatment and care, which is known to be effective and acceptable
- be well suited to those who use it and be non-discriminatory
- be accessible, so that help can be obtained when and where it is needed
- promote patient safety and that of their carers, staff and the wider public
- offer choices which promote independence
- be well coordinated between all staff and agencies
- deliver continuity of care for as long as it is needed
- empower and support staff
- be properly accountable to the public, users and carers
- reduce suicides

The document from which this summary of principles is taken is *The Journey to Recovery: The Government's Vision for Mental Health Care* (2001a). It is included on CD-ROM 2 in PDF format, and is available online at www.dh.gov.uk/assetRoot/04/05/89/00/ 0405 8900.pdf.

As a preliminary, you might wish to consider to what extent you think these principles have been achieved – or are even achievable. For example, you might pinpoint interagency coordination as a problem; or consider the potential conflicts that may occur between service users and clinicians.

At present, the legal document that governs the treatment of people with mental illness is the *Mental Health Act* (1983), which provides (among other things) the framework for 'sectioning' patients. The mental health charity MIND has produced an outline guide to the Act which can be accessed on www.mind.org.uk/ Information/Legal/OGMHA.htm.

The government is proposing changes to this, as detailed in *Reforming the Mental Health Act, Part I and II* (2000b and 2000c): a summary of these documents is included on CD-ROM 2, and the complete documents are available online at www. dh.gov.uk/assetRoot/04/05/89/ 14/04058914.pdf (Part 1) and www.dh.gov.uk/ assetRoot/04/05/89/15/ 04058915.pdf (Part 2).

Exercise

Read the above documents and consider:
- Where do you stand on the issue of compulsory treatment in the community?
- What are your views on the breadth of the inclusion criteria for admittance to compulsion under the act?
- The proposed reforms highlight proposals for a right to independent advocacy for people subject to compulsion – do you think this is feasible, desirable or practicable?
- You may find it useful to read the response from the Mental Health Foundation (2002), available in PDF format on CD-ROM2.

National Service Frameworks (NSFs)

Mental health, along with coronary heart disease and cancer, was one of the first three National Service Frameworks to be created – as mental health issues were felt to be a pressing health concern:

> 'Depression is the third most common reason for consultation in UK general practice. In the UK, suicide is now the commonest cause of death amongst the under 35s and stress is the most common cause of sickness absence. Mental health problems are now implicated in possibly as many as one in four primary care consultations.'
>
> *National Institute for Mental Health in England and Department of Health, 2003a*

The previous passage is taken from *Fast-Forwarding Primary Care Mental Health*, which is available in PDF format on CD-ROM 2, and online at www.dh.gov.uk/assetRoot/ 04/07/02/02/04070202.pdf.
The ten-year strategy contained in the NSF

The seven standards of the NSF for Mental Health

Mental health promotion (standard 1) Ensure health and social services promote mental health and reduce the discrimination and social exclusion associated with mental health problems.

Primary care and access to services (standards 2 and 3) Deliver better primary mental healthcare, and ensure consistent advice and help for people with mental health needs, including primary care services for individuals with severe mental illness.

Effective services for people with severe mental illness (standards 4 and 5) Ensure that each person with severe mental illness receives the range of mental health services they need; that crises are anticipated or prevented where possible; ensure prompt and effective help if a crisis does occur, and timely access to an appropriate and safe mental health place or hospital bed, as close to home as possible.

Caring about carers (standard 6) Ensure health and social services assess the needs of carers who provide regular and substantial care for those with severe mental illness, and provide care to meet their needs.

Preventing suicide (standard 7) Ensure that health and social services play their full part in reducing the suicide rate.

---

sets out the kind of care that adults of working age with mental health problems should expect. It proposes to do this by:
- setting national standards and identifying key interventions
- putting in place strategies to support implementation
- establishing ways to ensure progress within an agreed timescale

The mental health needs of older people, children and adolescents are considered in the National Service Frameworks for those age groups. The development of each NSF includes an external reference group (ERG) that seeks to bring together health professionals, service users and carers, health service managers, partner agencies, and other advocates. All the various NSFs are available on the Department of Health website (www.dh.gov.uk/ Home/fs/en): enter 'NSF' into the website's search engine. The NSF for Mental Health is available in PDF format on CD-ROM 2.

The seven standards of the mental health NSF are grouped under five headings (see Box).

The NSF cites that 4,000 suicides committed each year in England are attributed to depression, and, while most people who are depressed seek help from primary care, only about 30–50% of depression is recognized by GPs. Depression in people from the African-Caribbean, Asian, refugees and asylum seekers communities is said to be 'frequently overlooked' (Department of Health, 1999c).

The NSF highlights standards two and three as being directly related to primary care.

As examples of good practice, the government mentions the following telephone helplines:

'The telephone service offered by the Samaritans receives around 4.5 million calls each year. SANEline takes around 70,000 calls per year; the National Schizophrenia Fellowship has a large network of local helplines.'

Department of Health, 1999c

In addition, standard four mentions GP services specifically, in that the Care Programme Approach (CPA) should give them guidance on how to respond if the service user needs additional help.

Standard six proposes that the needs of carers are formally assessed by health and social services.

Meet Deborah

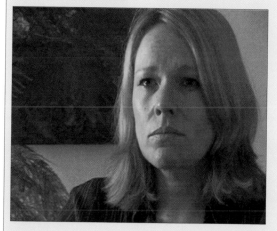

Deborah is a 42-year-old married woman who lives with her husband and 19-year-old son. She has difficulty leaving home unaccompanied for fear that she will faint, despite having no history of fainting. Her problem started a year ago when she was hospitalized following a severe blood virus. She spent several weeks recuperating at home and found that when it came to leaving the house she had lost her confidence. She has made a full recovery from her physical illness,

which is not relevant to her current problem with agoraphobia, apart from the need to recuperate which resulted in her loss of confidence in going out. Deborah's husband had already taken over the shopping while she was in hospital, and continues to do so. She will go out accompanied but will only go as far as the local shop alone.

The anticipation of going out alone makes her feel extremely anxious and leads to lightheadedness, dizziness, palpitations and trembling. She is worried that her problem is deteriorating as she now finds that even going to the local shop is causing some anxiety, and she would like some help to regain her confidence in going out alone.

The relationship between Deborah and her husband Paul is not straightforward, as we shall see.

 CD-ROM 2 includes two video clips in which Deborah introduces herself, and, with her husband Paul, meets Waseem, her primary care mental health worker. Notice how Waseem works towards ensuring the terms of standard six are met. Transcripts of the clips follow.

Exercise

Do you think that the needs of carers are always formally assessed by health and social services?

Video: Introducing Deborah (Agoraphobia)

Deborah: I suppose my problems started a few months ago when I was in hospital. I had this funny virus, anyway I was in hospital for a while, and when I came home, when I came out of hospital, I couldn't go anywhere, I couldn't go out and then when I could go out it seemed like I couldn't. Well, whenever I went out, I'd get this really, really dry mouth and felt that I couldn't swallow. My heart was beating so loud, it was almost like I thought people could hear it, and I just felt like I couldn't swallow, I had to hang onto things. I sometimes felt I was going to be sick or I'd faint. It was just awful and it was much, much worse when I went into crowded places. If I went on the bus, or if I went on the tube and it was crowded, it just made me feel like I would faint at any moment. It just was awful, and then I found that I couldn't even go into the supermarket, which meant that Paul, my husband, had to do all the shopping and everything outside of the house because I just haven't been able to go out at all really. I just can't see it getting any better.

It's like, whenever I even think about going out, I start to feel really nervous and it's like a feeling of having lost all your confidence, having no confidence at all. If it hadn't been for Paul, I just don't know what I'd have done because he's been so fantastic. He's really done everything for me and everything that I have to do inside the house is fine but anything to do with going out, he's doing all of it and I just don't know how long he can carry on doing that, because it

must be really difficult for him, and that worries me a lot.

I've been seeing my GP, and he referred me to a mental health worker at the practice and that's actually been quite helpful I think, but now the mental health worker wants to see Paul and I together today and that's what we're going to do. I do hope it goes okay.

Video: Assessing and supporting carers

Mental health worker (Waseem): I'm glad you're both here. I wanted you both to come in, to see how the treatment is working, and to see if there are any ways in which we can support you, Paul.

Paul: Well, I think you're getting a little bit better, aren't you?

Deborah: Yes, I have been out a bit. It's been good actually, I think I am a bit better. I suppose one thing to say is that obviously, if it hadn't been for Paul, I don't think I would have got better so quickly. I've had a lot of help from you, obviously, but he's just been fantastic, he's done everything really. You've done such a lot of the things that I used to do, haven't you? You're still doing all the shopping and things that involve going into busy, crowded places.

Paul: I don't really mind doing the shopping to be honest, I mean, if that helps. You couldn't really do it on your own, could you?

Deborah: Well, I don't know. I think I'm getting back to the stage where I probably could.

Paul: Yes, well it's just that Deborah used to complain about feeling very giddy, and that she was close to collapse. At first we thought it was women's problems but it seemed to go on a bit, didn't it? And we couldn't get to the bottom of it, and I don't know what we would have done if it wasn't for the help that we've had. I just don't want us to rush it and suddenly find we're back to square one. I would just like us to take our time, because the last thing I want is to have you ringing me at work saying 'I don't feel well,

I can't get to the shop, I'm feeling faint'. I'm quite happy doing the shopping.

Deborah: But I really do want to start doing those things again.

Waseem: Okay, it seems like it might have been quite a difficult time for you for the last couple of weeks. You seem to be coping.

Deborah: I think it's been going okay.

Paul: It's been quite hard for me. To be honest I don't think you really felt sometimes how difficult it has been for me, because I didn't know how ill you were. At one point, I thought you were dying and then you were really ill and then, and now it's this and I'm not really quite sure how much attention to pay now, and I sometimes feel that maybe you don't need my help at this point, and that I'm in some way interfering. What do you think?

Waseem: It sounds like it's been quite a tough time for you. Paul, as Deborah's situation changes, then I think of course your role is changing. I think maybe you are having one or two difficulties in, perhaps, finding out what the best ways are for you to support her. We'll talk more about it a little bit later on. I wonder whether, at this point, if you would be interested in attending a relatives' support group?

Paul: I don't know about that.

Waseem: Well, it's run here at the practice, and it is fully confidential. There's nobody from the practice who will attend. It's people who have been in similar situations who can discuss the stresses, and I think it might help you. A lot of the relatives who attend find it very useful indeed.

Deborah: That sounds really good, love. Why don't you go along and give it a go?

Paul: Well I suppose I could. Would you be alright if I did that?

Deborah: Yes, of course I would.

Waseem: It's fully confidential, Paul, there's nobody from the practice here, so you get the chance to talk to other people with similar problems and maybe that will help you.

Paul: Okay.

Waseem: Well, I'll tell you more about it: it runs on a Tuesday between 8 o'clock and 9 o'clock and, as I said, it's run here. In fact, Paul, it might be worthwhile for you to meet one of the relatives who goes to this group, before you attend. I'm sure I could arrange that for you. It gives you a chance to think about it a little bit more before you attend. What do you think?

Paul: Sounds alright.

Waseem: Shall we get that sorted?

Deborah: Sounds good.

Waseem: Okay. I'll make a note of that and we'll get that sorted out.

The NHS Plan

Published in July 2000, *The NHS Plan* made a number of proposals for change in mental healthcare, which included:

- changes to primary care (including new staff)
- additional early intervention to reduce the period of untreated psychosis
- new crisis resolution teams
- more assertive outreach services
- redesign of services for women
- improved support for carers
- further investment in secure psychiatric and prison services

If you are unfamiliar with some of the terminology used above (e.g. crisis resolution teams, assertive outreach), you will find explanations in *The NHS Plan*.

The government also proposed establishing a small number of taskforces to drive forward the NHS Plan. The proposed taskforces will look at waiting times, heart disease, cancer, mental health, older people, children, inequalities and public health, the workforce, quality, and the capital and information systems infrastructure.

Targets for mental health and primary care

In the appendices of its 2002 document *Improvement, Expansion and Reform: The Next Three Years* (2002a) (included on CD-ROM 2 in PDF format, and available online at www.dh.gov.uk/assetRoot/

04/05/98/31/04059831.pdf), the Department of Health sets out its public service agreement. Some proposals in this document included that, by December 2004:

- a single phone call to NHS Direct would be a one-stop gateway to out-of-hours health-care
- up to 3,000 family doctors' premises would be substantially refurbished or replaced
- 500 'one-stop' centres would have been established

The document sets out five key dimensions for a 'good patient experience'. These are:
1 improved access and shorter waiting time
2 more information and more choice
3 the building of closer relationships
4 safe, high-quality, coordinated care
5 a clean, comfortable, friendly environment

The NHS Plan set other targets specific to the provision of mental health services. These include the provision of:
- 50 early intervention teams
- 335 crisis resolution teams
- 220 assertive outreach teams
- 700 extra staff to work with carers
- 1000 graduate primary care mental health workers

National structural changes

Alongside these frameworks, plans and targets, the organization of healthcare has been undergoing a thoroughgoing restructuring. For example, since The Health Act (1999), local councils and the NHS have been encouraged to work together more closely, making use of:
- pooled budgets
- lead commissioning (i.e. either the local authority or the Primary Care Trust can take the lead in commissioning services)
- integrated provision (local authorities and Trusts merge their services to deliver a one-stop package of care)

Workforce and manpower changes have also been proposed. With respect to primary care, the government is creating new posts – which include graduate primary care mental health workers and community mental health staff (now known as Gateway Workers), and 'Support, Time and Recovery' (STR) workers (Department of Health, 2003). There is an additional proposal to employ 300 extra prison in-reach staff, 500 community development workers for black and minority ethnic communities, 200 staff, and 6 outreach teams for personality disorder (Department of Health, 2002a).

The policy document *Shifting the Balance of Power* (2001c) has changed how care is managed. Locally-based Primary Care Trusts (PCTs) have been given the role of day-to-day running of the NHS – assessing need, planning and securing all health services, and improving health. Strategic Health Authorities (SHAs) have been established to manage the performance of PCTs, NHS Trusts and Workforce Development Directorates (previously known as Workforce Development Confederations), among other functions. *Shifting the Balance of Power* is included in PDF format on CD-ROM 2, and available online at www.dh.gov.uk/assetRoot/04/07/35/54/04073554.pdf.

At the national level, the proposed changes are being overseen by a Mental Health Taskforce. It includes representatives of government, the NHS and social services, service users and voluntary groups, and explicitly aims to develop mental health services planned and delivered around the needs and aspirations of service users. It is one of the ten national taskforces that support the NHS Modernisation Board, which is responsible for the implementation of *The NHS Plan*.

The following organizations also have an important role in the national Modernization Agenda:

The Modernisation Agency (MA) Acts as a resource of current thinking and practical advice for improvement for everyone involved in improving patient care.

The National Institute for Mental Health in England (NIMHE) Seeks to reshape services and practice in line with the evidence-base and to communicate best practice.

The National Institute for Health and Clinical Excellence (NICE) Provides guidance on new and existing technologies and develops clinical guidelines and clinical audit.

The Social Care Institute for Excellence (SCIE) Reviews information about what works in social care and produces guidelines on best practice.

Healthcare Commission: Commission for Healthcare Audit and Inspection (CHAI) Replaced the Commission for Health Improvement (CHI), the healthcare component of the National Care Standards Commission (NCSC) and the NHS value for money components of the Audit Commission's remit.

The Commission for Patient and Public Involvement in Health (CPPIH) Carries out national reviews of services from the patient perspective and makes recommendations.

Locally-based organizations

At the local level, there is a Local Implementation Team (LIT) to plan and deliver change. It also comprises the statutory services (such as health, social services and housing) for the area, together with service users, carers and local voluntary groups. Each Local Implementation Team is charged with producing a Local Implementation Plan (LIP) setting out how the NSF standards, *The NHS Plan*, and other changes will be translated into new local services.

The system of Patient and Public Involvement (PPI) that was put before parliament on 1 September 2003 requires that the patient should be at the centre of the NHS. With a view to this, further bodies have been created, which include:

- Patient Advice and Liaison Service (PALS)
- Independent Complaints Advocacy Service (ICAS)
- Patient and Public Involvement Forums (PPIFs)

- Overview and Scrutiny Committee (OSC)

You might wish to look at the summaries of their roles found in the Glossary, or by searching for the relevant terms on the Department of Health website (www.dh.gov.uk/Home/fs/en).

Exercise

There may be problems inherent in this network of organizations that you may wish to consider. For example, do they constitute too complex a bureaucracy? How will they relate to each other in practice? Are they an example of transparency or 'joined-up thinking'?

It is important to remember that advocacy (in a more general sense, i.e. not solely associated with complaints) and service user groups exist outside the NHS. Most advocacy provision is located in the voluntary sector (as we shall examine in Chapter 2.2, Section 2, 'Challenges of advocacy'), as are a variety of organized service user groups (including national and local forums). All of these groupings are subject to the vicissitudes and insecurities of funding in the voluntary sector; nevertheless, they provide much in the way of valued support and contributions to various consultations and networks.

Section summary

- The modernization of the NHS and provision of mental healthcare is driven by a number of crucial policy documents, including the *National Service Framework for Mental Health* (1999c) and *The NHS Plan* (2000a)
- Service user organizations are poised to play a role in this process, from shaping services to commenting on proposed changes to mental health legislation
- The needs of carers should be assessed and addressed
- Primary care is specifically targeted by the Modernization Agenda
- Local and national organizations have been created to drive the agenda forward,

and structural changes to health and social care provision have been made

References

Department of Health (1997). *The New NHS: Modern, Dependable*. London: HMSO.

Department of Health (1998a). *Modernising Mental Health Services*. London: HMSO.

Department of Health (1999a). *The Future Organis-ation of Prison Health Care*. London: HMSO.

Department of Health (1999b). *Managing Dangerous People with Severe Personality Disorder*. London: HMSO.

Department of Health (1999c). *The National Service Framework for Mental Health*. London: HMSO.

Department of Health (1999d). *Saving Lives: Our Healthier Nation*. London: HMSO.

Department of Health (2000a). *The NHS Plan: a Plan for Investment, a Plan for Reform*. London: HMSO.

Department of Health (2000b). *Reforming the Mental Health Act, Part I, The New Legal Framework*. London: HMSO.

Department of Health (2000c). *Reforming the Mental Health Act, Part II, High Risk Patients*. London: HMSO.

Department of Health (2001a). *The Journey to Recovery: The Government's Vision for Mental Health Care*. London: HMSO.

Department of Health (2001b). *The Expert Patient: A New Approach to Chronic Disease Management for the 21st Century*. London: HMSO.

Department of Health (2001c). *Shifting the Balance of Power within the NHS: Securing Delivery*. London: HMSO.

Department of Health (2002a). *Improvement, Expansion and Reform: The Next Three Years*. London: HMSO.

Department of Health (2003). *Mental Health Policy Implementation Guide: Support, Time and Recovery (STR) Workers*. London: HMSO.

National Institute for Mental Health in England (NIHME) and Department of Health (2003a). *Fast-Forwarding Primary Mental Health: Graduate Primary Care Mental Health Workers – Best Practice Guidance*. London: HMSO.

Readhead, E. and Briel, R. (2001). *Review of the Mental Health Training Process*. Durham: Northern Centre for Mental Health.

Test yourself

 To check your progress, locate this section on CD-ROM 2 and work through the interactive questions at the end.

Section 2: Social inclusion and mental health

This section is divided into five parts:
1 The concepts of social exclusion and social inclusion
2 Mental health and social exclusion
3 Minority ethnic communities
4 Physical disability: the example of deaf people
5 Women

'**NSF Standard 1**: "Ensure health and social services … reduce the discrimination and social exclusion associated with mental health problems." '

Department of Health, 1999c

The concepts of social exclusion and social inclusion

In some senses, social exclusion and inclusion can be defined as opposites of each other. The following details conditions that might promote one or the other.

When Labour came to power in 1997, it was felt that social exclusion in this country was at unacceptable levels as compared to other countries in Europe (Social Exclusion Unit, 2001), and a governmental unit was set up to try and move from social exclusion and towards social inclusion. Emphasis was placed on the 'joined-up' nature of the social problems involved:

'Social exclusion includes low income, but is broader and focuses on the link between problems such as, for example, unemployment, poor skills, high crime, poor housing and family breakdown. Only when these links are properly understood and addressed will policies really be effective.'

Social Exclusion Unit, 2001

The government proposed three broad

Social Exclusion

Social exclusion is a shorthand term for what can happen when people or areas suffer from a combination of linked problems such as unemployment, poor skills, low incomes, poor housing, high crime environments, bad health and family breakdown.

Social Exclusion Unit (SEU)
www.socialexclusionunit.gov.uk

Social Inclusion

Social inclusion is achieved when individuals or areas do not suffer from the negative effects of unemployment, poor skills, low income, poor housing, crime, bad health, family problems, limited access to services and rurality, (e.g. remoteness, sparsity, isolation and high costs).

Centre for Economic and Social Inclusion
www.cesi.org.uk

objectives to address these linked problems:

1 Prevent social exclusion happening in the first place – by reducing risk factors and acting with those who are already at risk

2 Reintegrate those who become excluded back into society

3 Deliver basic minimum standards to everyone – in health, education, in-work income, employment and tackling crime

But there are other ways of looking at social exclusion. It has an affective component, which can cause people who suffer exclusion:

'... to feel depressed, cheated, bitter, desperate, vulnerable, frightened, angry, worried about debts or job and housing insecurity; to feel devalued, useless, helpless, uncared for, hopeless, isolated, anxious, and a failure:

Exercise

Social inclusion can also be defined in terms of admittance to a full sense of citizenship, with social connectedness and support.

• Do you feel that there is a tension between this sense of inclusive citizenship (going back to the foundational activity to establish the welfare state), and the individualist ideologies of consumerism that could be seen as running through some aspects of current health and social policy?

• Where do you stand with respect to this?

these feelings can dominate people's whole experience of life ... the material environment is merely the indelible mark ... of one's social exclusion and devaluation as a human being.'

Social Exclusion Unit, 2001

In addition, it could be argued that use of a rhetoric of social exclusion might work to stigmatize the poor as a problematic group who refuse to join in. This could become a form of 'blaming the victim', further excluding people and justifying enforced participation (e.g. by converting Incapacity Benefit into Job Seekers Allowance). A common strand in some SEU documents seems to be about 'getting people into jobs' while perhaps leaving structural inequalities unaddressed: for example, the unequal distribution of resources, or the fact that socially excluded groups face significantly poorer access to services such as GPs (Wilkinson, 1996).

Social inclusion can be defined more dynamically, as a process more than a state:

'... social inclusion comprises the processes by which efforts are made to ensure that everyone, regardless of their experiences and circumstances, can achieve their potential in life. To achieve inclusion, income and employment are necessary but not sufficient. An inclusive society is also characterised by a striving for reduced inequality, a balance between individuals' rights and duties and increased social cohesion.'

Centre for Economic and Social Inclusion

You might wish to explore the website of the Centre for Economic and Social Inclusion at www.cesi.org.uk to further explore these issues.

Mental health and social exclusion

'Poor health is a key cause of social exclusion. It is also a consequence of exclusion – with the most under-resourced services often located in the poorest areas.'

Department of Health, 2000a

Despite people with mental health problems being demonstrably a socially excluded group, the report produced by the SEU in 2001 had little to say specifically about their social inclusion needs. It was not until 2003 that the document 'Mental Health and Social Exclusion' was published.

This has since been followed by a highly practical guide entitled *Action on Mental Health* (Social Exclusion Unit, 2004), which contains twelve booklets that can be read in parallel with this resource, outlining policy direction and a range of grass roots action.

Both documents are included in PDF format on CD-ROM 2, and are available online at www.socialexclusionunit.gov.uk/trackdoc. asp?id=134&pId=257 ('Mental Health and Social Exclusion') and at www. socialexclusionunit.gov.uk/trackdoc.asp?id=300 &pId=257 (*Action on Mental Health*).

Even when concentrating wholly on the workplace, evidence suggests that discriminatory practices with regard to mental health persist. Mental health service users also report feeling stigmatized by the attitudes of the local service providers charged with working towards their social inclusion (Social Exclusion Unit, 2003).

As well as these institutional barriers, people with mental health issues are socially excluded and stigmatized by negative images and discrimination. 'Counting the Cost' (a survey conducted for MIND in 2000) highlighted the extent to which stigmatizing images adversely affect people with mental illness – for most respondents to the survey, the social stigma was harder to deal with than the symptoms of their particular condition. Some key results, according to MIND (2000), are:

- 73% of those surveyed felt that the media had been unfair, unbalanced or very negative over the past three years
- 50% claimed that poor media coverage had a negative impact on their mental health
- 24% experienced some hostility from neighbours and their local communities as a result of media reports

Although people with mental health problems are far more likely to be victims of violent crime than the general population (Walsh et al, 2003), a research project centred on the media found the overwhelming majority of both fictional and non-fictional representations of people with mental illness characterized them as harming others (Glasgow Media Group, 2001).

The GMG project also showed that even personal experience of knowing somebody with mental health problems did not assuage fears of violence regarding other people with mental health problems, and that 40% of the general population believed that serious mental illness was associated with violence and cited media representations as the source of their belief. Do you think that this makes the curtailing of the liberty of 'high-risk patients' under a revised Mental Health Act more, or less, likely? On a policy level, it could be argued that many of the proposed Mental Health Act reforms are based on a preoccupation with 'risk'.

Exercise

- Are you aware of a mental health promotion forum in your locality?
- Can you think of ways that a local campaign might result in popular media coverage?

'Key issues that influence individuals' experience of the world – gender, race, religion, culture, class, sexuality, disability, age – must … be incorporated into service planning, delivery and evaluation.'

Department of Health, 2002b

To date, the Department of Health is developing strategies to address the needs of three such groups – people from ethnic minority communities; people who are deaf; and women.

Minority ethnic communities

People from minority ethnic communities may be disproportionately exposed to risk of social exclusion, according to the Social Exclusion Unit (2001), because:

- they are more likely to live in deprived areas and in overcrowded housing
- they are more likely to be poor and to be unemployed
- Pakistani, Bangladeshi and African-Caribbean people are more likely to report suffering ill-health than white people

The National Institute for Mental Health in England (NIMHE) and the Department of Health, in their joint publication *Inside Out*, have reported that:

> 'There does not appear to be a single area of mental healthcare in this country in which black and minority ethnic groups fare as well as, or better than, the majority white community. Both in terms of service experience and the outcome of service interventions, they fare much worse than people from the ethnic majority do.'
>
> *National Institute for Mental Health in England and Department of Health, 2003b*

The NIMHE publication *Inside Outside* (2003b) (included in PDF format on CD-ROM 2, and available online at www.dh.gov.uk/assetRoot/04/01/94/52/04019452.pdf) reports on mental healthcare, as experienced by a service user from an ethnic minority, in these terms:

- it has an over-emphasis on institutional and coercive models of care
- professional and organizational requirements are given priority over individual needs and rights
- institutional racism exists within mental healthcare

Patients from minority ethnic groups are more likely to be prescribed drugs and electro-convulsive therapy (ECT), rather than 'talking treatments' such as psychotherapy and counselling; they spend (on average) longer periods of time within hospitals and are less likely to have their social care and psychological needs addressed (Sainsbury Centre for Mental Health, 2002).

Changing this situation is a complex and difficult task – but, even without the obvious moral and ethical considerations, there is an explicit legal duty to do so, as enshrined in the Race Relations (Amendment) Act (2000).

Inside Outside advocates two key approaches in ensuring a culturally competent and capable workforce:

> 'First, it is recommended that all staff working within mental health services should receive mandatory training in Cultural Awareness. Secondly, there should be an emphasis on recruiting staff (professionals as well as in other capacities, for example, cultural mediators) from diverse cultural backgrounds so that the workforce in mental health reflects the population it serves as well as the population it treats.'
>
> *NIMHE and Department of Health, 2003b*

Physical disability: the example of deaf people

A qualitative study conducted by Naish and Clark in 1996 highlighted the generally poor communication between general practitioners and deaf patients – despite the Disability Discrimination Act (1995) having stated that 'reasonable steps' have to be taken to facilitate the use of services by disabled people. The Act explicitly uses the example of providing a sign language interpreter as a means of facilitation (Section 21, 4).

In an attempt to address the mental health needs of deaf people the Department of Health has published the consultation document *A Sign of the Times* (2002c), included in PDF format on CD-ROM 2, and available online at www.dh.gov.uk/assetRoot/04/07/67/64/ 04076764.pdf.

It specifically recommended the development of primary care services – particularly with respect to making available appropriate communication support, providing training in Deaf Awareness, promoting the recognition of mental health problems, and establishing links with social and NHS mental health services.

Women

'Mental ill health in women, as in men, is common. It differs however in both presentation and character. Currently, much mental healthcare is not organised to be responsive to gender differences and women's needs consequently may be poorly met.'

Department of Health, 2002b

The document from which the above is taken ('Women's Mental Health') seeks to take forward the commitment of *The NHS Plan* to reducing inequalities and developing a comprehensive health service designed around the needs and preferences of patients. It argues that:
- gender issues should be acknowledged and addressed as a fundamental part of organizational culture and the inter-relationship between the organization, the practitioner and the service user
- an aware and informed workforce is essential
- leadership in organizations should make a clear commitment to address gender issues
- clinical governance arrangements should include gender and other inequalities

The Department of Health publication 'Women's Mental Health' is included in PDF format on CD-ROM 2, and is available online at www.dh.gov.uk/assetRoot/04/07/54/87/04075487.pdf.

With a view to this, the following are recommended to be available across all health service settings:
- access to women staff and women-only interventions and therapy groups, with acknowledgement of women's caring responsibilities (e.g. through the provision of childcare facilities, transport and flexible appointment times)

- access to a female doctor for physical healthcare
- physical examinations to be undertaken by a female member of staff or with a female chaperone present
- a female member of staff to be present if restraint is used

Department of Health, 2002b

Exercise

Consider the following:
- Is this kind of service available in the primary care settings which you have experienced?
- *The NHS Plan* stated that 'by 2004, services will be redesigned to ensure that there are women-only day-centres in every health authority' (Department of Health, 2000a). Are you aware of where such a centre may be, local to you?

As primary care services will continue to see the majority of mental ill health in women, primary care practitioners need to have appropriate training and support to ensure that depression, anxiety, eating disorders, self-harm, substance misuse, and experience of violence and abuse are detected and appropriately dealt with. It is important to remember that some of these factors may interact (e.g. domestic violence leading to depression), and to be aware of the possibility that some women may be dealt with as if the problem was personal (perhaps depression), when the underlying issue (domestic violence or abuse) is neglected or simply not inquired into. Primary care mental health workers are envisaged as being at the forefront of this care provision, by providing brief psychological interventions of proven efficacy.

The three instances given here – ethnic minorities, deaf people, and women – are only examples of populations affected by social exclusion; there are other populations whose mental health needs may be similarly obscured or unmet. Other examples include older people, people with learning disabilities, gay people,

Exercise

Can you think of any other distinctive groups, and how they might be socially excluded? Your answers might include the following:

- Older people
- People with learning disabilities
- Gay people
- People with HIV and AIDS

What practical measures could be put in place in primary care to move towards their social inclusion? Is it possible that organic initiatives within each stigmatized group (such as the activities of 'Survivors Speak Out' and 'Mad Pride' with respect to the user movement) could point a way forward?

and people with HIV and AIDS. Each population – in common, generally, with people who suffer from mental health problems – is in some degree stigmatised; they seem to possess 'an undesired differentness from what we had anticipated' (Goffman, 1963, p15).

Section summary

- Social inclusion and exclusion can be defined within a number of contexts
- Mental health service users tend to suffer stigmatization (often reinforced by media coverage) and consequent social exclusion
- The Department of Health is developing strategies specifically to address the needs of three groups within society:
  - ∞ people from minority ethnic communities
  - people who are deaf
  - women

References

Department of Health (1999c). *The National Service Framework for Mental Health*. London: HMSO.

Department of Health (2000a). *The NHS Plan: a Plan for Investment, a Plan for Reform*. London: HMSO.

Department of Health (2002b). *Women's Mental Health: Into the Mainstream – Strategic Development of Mental Health Care for Women*. London: HMSO.

Department of Health (2002c). *A Sign of the Times: Modernising Mental Health Services for People who are Deaf*. London: HMSO.

Disability Discrimination Act (1995). Available online at www.direct.gov.uk (search for 'DDA')

Glasgow Media Group (2001). 'Media and Mental Illness' in Davey, B., Gray, A., and Seale, C. (eds), *Health and Disease; A Reader*. Buckingham: Open University Press.

Goffman, E. (1963). *Stigma: Notes on the Management of Spoiled Identity*. New Jersey: Prentice Hall.

Implementation of the Race Relations (Amendment) Act (2000). www.homeoffice. gov.uk/documents/race-relations-amendact-150501?version=1.

MIND (2000). *Counting the Cost*. London: MIND.

Naish, S. and Clark, S. (1996). 'Profoundly Deaf Patients and General Practitioners: A Qualitative Study Looking at Communication and its Difficulties'. Unpublished document, University of Birmingham: quoted in Department of Health (2002c).

National Institute for Mental Health in England and Department of Health (2003b). *Inside Outside – Improving Mental Health Services for Black and Minority Ethnic Communities in England*. London: HMSO.

Sainsbury Centre for Mental Health (2002). *Breaking the Circles of Fear: A Review of the Relationship between Mental Health Services and the African and Caribbean Communities*. London: SCMH.

Social Exclusion Unit (2001). *Preventing Social Exclusion: Report by the Social Exclusion Unit*. London: SEU.

Social Exclusion Unit (2003). *Mental Health and Social Exclusion: Consultation Document*. London: SEU.

Social Exclusion Unit (2004). *Action on Mental Health*. London: SEU.

Walsh, K., Nicholson, J., Keough, C., Pridham, R., Kramer, M. and Jeffrey, J. (2003). Development of a group model of clinical supervision to meet the needs of a community mental health nursing team. *International Journal of Nursing Practice*, 9, 33–39.

Wilkinson, R. (1996). *Unhealthy Societies: the Afflictions of Inequality*. London: Routledge.

Recommended reading

Department of Health (1998b). *A First Class Service: Quality in the New NHS*. London: HMSO.

Department of Health (2000d). *NHS Implementation Programme*. London: HMSO.

Department of Health (2001d). *Safety First: Five-year report of the National Confidential Inquiry into Suicide and Homicide by People with Mental Illness*. London: HMSO.

Test yourself

 To check your progress, locate this section on CD-ROM 2 and work through the interactive questions at the end.

Chapter 2.2
The Expert Patient, advocacy and health promotion

Aim

To provide a critical and practical understanding of the Expert Patient Programme and of Chronic Disease Self-Management; and a comprehensive understanding of the principles behind advocacy, how those principles may be put into practice, and what challenges may arise; and to provide in-depth knowledge and a critical understanding of mental health promotion and principles of self-help.

Learning outcomes

By the end of this Chapter, the reader will be able to:

- Give an account of the development of the Expert Patient Programme (EPP) and the thinking behind it
- Discuss the model of the Chronic Disease Self Management Programme (CDSMP) as developed by Professor Kate Lorig at Stanford University, and consider its impact in the primary care arena
- Give an account of the background to advocacy and critically discuss its fundamental principles
- Critically discuss models and styles of advocacy
- Give a reasoned account of the possible challenges faced in advocacy work
- Discuss the possible functions of a user involvement worker
- Identify and critically discuss ways in which user and carer involvement can be incorporated into mental health promotion
- Critically consider the idea of self-help and empowerment in relation to mental health promotion

Introduction

The three areas of activity covered in this Chapter are conceived of as illustrative of the general theme of involvement in healthcare practice settings.

The Expert Patient Programme is an example of policy into action, promoting user involvement, remaining largely instigated by healthcare professionals and retaining some degree of being professionally led.

Advocacy is an example of hearing users' voices, and is largely instigated independently and led externally from healthcare services.

Health promotion is an example of health intervention amenable to effective alliances and partnership working, which need not require input of healthcare staff.

Chapter 2.2 content is as follows:

1 The Expert Patient Programme
2 Advocacy and the user involvement worker
3 Health promotion and the principles of self-help

Section 1: The Expert Patient Programme

This section is divided into four parts:
1 Background: the task force and the report
2 Models of chronic disease self-management
3 Current issues: 'mainstreaming', setting up courses
4 Conceptual and practical problems

'The expertise of patients themselves is a largely untapped resource in the effective

management of chronic disease.'
Department of Health, 2001b, p33

'The concept of patients forming partnerships with healthcare professionals does not exist universally no matter how easily the rhetoric embraces it.'
Wilson, 1999, p772

Background: the Task Force and the report

The current disease pattern in England, as in most other developed countries, is predominantly one of chronic or long-term illness (Department of Health, 2001b). The amount of health-related information available has increased (especially through electronic media), contributing to an informed population of service users who constitute an untapped resource with respect to their own health issues. However, it must be remembered that older generations and financially disadvantaged people (often those most highly represented among service users) are less well-informed, and less well placed to articulate choice. There is, however, an increasing body of evidence that self-management programmes are clinically effective on a variety of health outcomes and in a range of chronic illnesses (Lorig et al, 2001).

A plan for the establishment of an Expert Patients Programme was announced in the 1999 Health Strategy White Paper, *Saving Lives – Our Healthier Nation*, and later reaffirmed in the *NHS Plan* (Department of Health, 2000a). An Expert Patients Task Force was set up in late 1999, under the chairmanship of the Chief Medical Officer, to explore models, review evidence, consider barriers and recommend a programme that would bring together the work done by patient and clinical organizations in developing self-management initiatives in chronic disease.

The Task Force included representatives from the medical profession, non-governmental organizations, and experts in the fields of self-management training and research. Its report – *The Expert Patient: A New Approach to Chronic Disease Management for the 21st Century* – was

published in September 2001.

It recommended action over a six-year period to introduce lay-led self-management training programmes for patients with chronic diseases within the NHS in England – starting with a pilot phase between 2001 and 2004. *The* *Expert Patient* is included in PDF format on CD-ROM 2, and is available online at www.dh.gov.uk/assetRoot/04/01/85/78/04018578.pdf.

By January 2003, 144 PCTs had joined the Expert Patient Programme. The concept of the 'expert patient' now seems firmly embedded in UK healthcare policy, along with the admission that 'taken in the round, the NHS is not nearly as strong as it could be in meeting the needs of people with chronic disease' (Department of Health, 2001b, p19). However, most of the examples used in *The Expert Patient* are based on the care of physical conditions (e.g. asthma, arthritis, multiple sclerosis, back pain, diabetes, epilepsy), although some mention is given to the work done by the Manic Depression Fellowship and the Depression Alliance.

Models of chronic disease self-management

The Expert Patient recognizes two main types of self-management programme:

'Those which concentrate upon improving people's ability to adhere to their treatment regime. They are usually condition-specific, and led by health professionals ... [And those which] are user-led and move beyond the medical view ... They look at how the illness impacts upon daily life and the ways in which people can take greater control over their condition on a day-to-day basis.'
Department of Health, 2001b, p19

User-led self-management programmes have a development history stretching back at least twenty years. The Chronic Disease Self-Management Program (CDSMP), developed at Stanford University by a team headed by Kate Lorig, recognizes that people with chronic illnesses deal with broadly similar issues. These issues include:

Exercise

Consider the following:

- Do you think that a service user with a mental health issue can be an 'expert patient'?
- Are there additional issues involved?
- Is their 'expertise' likely to command as much respect?
- Is there any connection between issues of discrimination and the extent to which mental health service users are stigmatized and constructed as 'different', as discussed in Chapter 2.1, Section 2, 'Mental Health and Social Exclusion'?
- Are you aware of any Expert Patient Programmes in your local area?
- How would you find out where the nearest/most relevant programmes are for a specific patient?

- symptom management
- relaxation
- problem solving and action planning
- exercise and nutrition
- managing fatigue
- communication
- engaging with healthcare professionals

To manage these issues, the CDSMP treats certain skills as core. These include:

- problem-solving
- decision-making
- resource utilization
- forming patient–professional partnership
- taking action

Lorig et al, 2000

The course, as run within the NHS, typically comprises six weekly sessions, each of 2½ hours: a key element to the programme is the use of trained lay people with chronic illnesses as tutors. It is an assumption of the CDSMP that the process of a training programme is as important as the subject that is taught.

The aim of a chronic disease self-management programme is not simply about educating

Revisiting Nigel

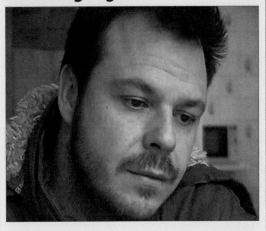

Nigel was introduced in Part 1. He is a 45-year-old man, recently separated from his wife. He presents with low mood and reduced energy. His GP has recommended that he commence antidepressant medication, but Nigel is reluctant to do so as he believes that 'taking tablets means that I am weak and a failure'.

Nigel usually enjoys his job as a clerical officer at the local county council, but has been struggling more recently. He has been on sick leave for the past three weeks and is anxious about his return to work.

 CD-ROM 2 includes three video clips, showing Nigel as he introduces himself, as he visits Dr Rushforth, his GP, and as he reflects on the meeting. Transcripts of the clips follow.

patients about their condition or giving them relevant information. The CDSMP is intended to develop the confidence and motivation of health service users in the use of their own skills, and in accessing information and professional services as appropriate, in order to take effective control of their lives (gain 'self-efficacy'). The training seeks to identify and tackle those factors which impact negatively upon individual's self-efficacy and confidence; as such, it resonates with many action-oriented and emancipatory models of learning and praxis.

An important concept within the programmes is that of 'concordance': this is defined in *The Expert Patient* as 'an agreement reached after negotiation between a patient and a healthcare professional, that respects the wishes and beliefs of the patient. Concordance assures the patient a proactive role in treatment decisions' (Department of Health, 2001b, p22). The concept of 'concordance' should not be mistaken for 'compliance', which means that the patient does what the clinician wants or thinks is best, especially in terms of medication. Such contradiction is often evident in the psychiatric literature regarding medication – where the terms adherence, compliance and concordance are often used interchangeably, as if shared meaning is implied. Concordance is also addressed in Chapter 1.3, Section 5.

Medication is one of the key issues for service users where disempowerment and lack of involvement are grounded in their unequal relationship with professionals: some of these ideas are picked up in the video clips included on CD-ROM 2. Transcripts of the videos are included in the following pages, and these transcripts may also be printed from CD-ROM 2.

Video: Introducing Nigel (Depression)

Nigel: I haven't been feeling very good since Jenny, my wife, left me for another man. I think I caused all that, I never took her out or anything. I never told her how nice she looked, and she did look nice. No wonder someone else fancied her, and she went off at the first opportunity. They were together for years and I didn't even notice. Now I can't stop thinking about it, I can't get it out of my head. I know it's all my fault, what I deserved, but now I can't eat or sleep properly. I haven't been able to concentrate at work, so I've been on the sick now for the past three weeks. That's bothering me too, because I'm never off, and I'm worried about what my colleagues think of me, but to be honest I just can't face it right now. I'm waking up about 4 o'clock every morning and I find it impossible to get back to sleep. I'm so exhausted during the day that I can't

be bothered to do anything, never mind drag myself into work. When I was there, I didn't seem to be able to do very much anyway. I sometimes wonder whether I'd be better off dead to be honest, but I wouldn't do anything, I couldn't do it to the kids. I should be able to handle this. I can't even tell Jenny I've been diagnosed with depression. What would she think of me? She'd see me as pathetic and weak for sure. I'm going to see Dr Rushforth today. She's really nice but I just can't imagine why she wants to bother with me.

Video: Issues about concordance – part 1

Dr Rushforth: Nigel, I know you are not keen on taking pills, but I'd really like you to give the antidepressants a shot. What do you think?

Nigel: No, I don't think so. I don't think tablets can really help with depression. I didn't think I would ever really need to take tablets. It feels pathetic to me.

Dr Rushforth: I know, but in my experience they can really help. There's no shame in it. It's a bit like taking pills for a physical illness, and you would do that wouldn't you?

Nigel: Yes.

Dr Rushforth: I've written you a prescription. I think these could really help you. What I want you to do is think it over. You're seeing the mental health worker in a couple of days. Why don't you talk it over with him, and have a think about it? What do you say?

Nigel: I don't think so, I don't really want to take tablets.

Dr Rushforth: Okay, well think it over in the next couple of days, but good luck.

Video: Issues about concordance – part 2

Nigel: You see, the thing is, I'm not normally like this, I usually would see the doctor if I was ill, and then take the medicine or whatever they said ... go to the hospital appointment. This is different. I can't get this prescription made up at the chemist, I just can't. The chemist would know what the medicine was and she'd think I was pathetic too, like a drug addict or something. Someone who can't cope without tablets, and Jenny might find out about them, then she would know. What would she think of me? I'd hate it if the kids found out.

There's all this stuff now, in the news and in the doctor's surgery, about working in partnership with the staff at the practice, letting them know how you feel about your treatment. It all sounds really good, but you feel as if you should do what they say, that they must know best. They probably do know best, well better than me. That wouldn't be difficult.

I wonder what she put on that sick note? Bloody hell! Moderate Depression! Moderate Depression? What's moderate about it? If I hand this in at work, then everyone will know. I'm never off sick, so they'll all be looking at the note in the office to see what's wrong with me. Why couldn't she have covered it up and put something else, like a virus or something? Everyone else seems to get a virus. It isn't a virus though, is it? It's not coping, being pathetic, and not remembering anything, like a right sicko. I won't take these tablets though. I don't care what the practice think of me. I'm not taking them.

Exercise

Consider the following:
- Did Nigel feel that he had a choice?
- How difficult was it for him to go against the professional advice he was given?
- And how does this leave him feeling?

Current issues: 'mainstreaming', setting up courses

In the United Kingdom, research into the benefits of user-led self-management programmes

has been carried out by the Long-Term Medical Conditions Alliance (LMCA: www.lmca.org.uk). With the assistance of the Living with Long-term Illness Project (Lill), it has set up and managed its own programmes using the CDSMP model. The experiences gained have fed into the work of both the Expert Patient Task Force and the Living Well Project. The Living Well Project aims to sustain and further develop high-quality, lay-led self-management programmes for people living with long-term conditions by providing information, advice, consultancy, central coordination and tutor support. Furthermore, the Lill Project has set up a national Self-Management Network for organizations who use a range of self-management interventions (not only the Chronic Disease Self-Management Programme).

The LMCA has produced a resource pack to facilitate the setting-up of courses, entitled 'Supporting Expert Patients'. The pack is 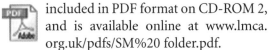 included in PDF format on CD-ROM 2, and is available online at www.lmca. org.uk/pdfs/SM%20 folder.pdf.

In addition, a National Resource for Expert Patients (NREP) is being developed to provide support and up-to-date information to the expert patients, volunteer tutors and EPP trainers who have been trained in the self-management of chronic disease.

Conceptual and practical problems

In common with much current thinking that seeks to validate the input of users of healthcare services, the Expert Patient Programme is based on a shift in the traditional power relations between provider and recipient of care. The Expert Patient Programme aims to bring expert patients centre stage, where they will 'interact more vigorously with all the personal and community sources of care and support, so that they can manage life with a chronic condition successfully and healthily' (Jafri et al, 2003, p19).

However, this positive view has to be balanced against the backdrop of a survey conducted around the same time that the Expert Patient Task Force was launched, which found that:
- only 21% of the doctors surveyed were in

favour of the Expert Patient proposals
- 56% thought the proposals would increase their workload
- only 24% thought the proposals would yield better health outcomes, while
- 37% thought the proposals would lead to a deterioration in doctor–patient relationships

Association of the British Pharmaceutical Industry (ABPI), 1999

Some commentators have questioned whether a professional understanding of 'expert' and a patient's demonstration of 'expertise' are, in any meaningful sense, reconcilable – arguing that a policy which focuses on the rights and responsibilities of patients needs to be linked to a strategy that is designed to challenge the long-standing assumptions of professionals (Wilson, 2001). The question 'how large is the gulf between the professions and patients – and are they even speaking the same language?' (Eaton, 2002a, p16) becomes especially relevant in the case of chronic diseases such as Chronic Fatigue Syndrome or Myalgic Encephalomyelitis. This conceptual gulf is mirrored elsewhere in the tensions between the self-help strategies championed by user-led groups (such as The Hearing Voices Network) and the bio-medical model in psychiatry. Psychosocial approaches, located within a philosophy of therapeutic alliance, may enable appropriate engagement with service user perspectives; but, in practice, many services are still organized in such a way that a much narrower (medical) view is privileged.

An Expert Patients Stakeholder Conference held in July 2000 also pinpointed the risk of excluding certain groups and that self-management programmes need 'to reach the right people', such as:
- people living in a rural location
- people whose ethnicity or culture might present language barriers
- people with specific communication needs or 'low literacy'
- people on the lowest incomes

Thought will also need to be given to working jointly with social care providers, and to providing courses with the flexibility to offer and evaluate

Meet Tim

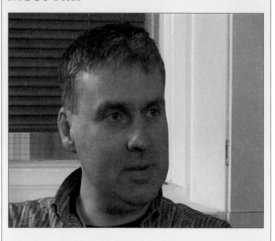

Tim is a 46-year-old man who lives with his partner John. Tim works for an IT company as a website designer. The company he works for has been undergoing financial difficulties which have resulted in a number of redundancies. Although Tim's job is not under immediate threat, he has seen a marked increase in his workload with the departure of a number of his close colleagues. He finds that he is having to come in to work earlier and regularly works late in an attempt to meet tight deadlines on projects. He feels that his job is under-resourced and that the expectations placed on him are unrealistic. He feels unable to discuss these issues with his boss as he has a substantial mortgage and would be in real financial difficulty if he lost his job. He finds that he has little time for anything other than work, which is even interfering with his weekends. He hasn't had a holiday for over a year. He bites his nails, has trouble concentrating, suffers frequently from indigestion and has difficulty getting to sleep at night. He smokes heavily, has a high caffeine intake, and lives on junk food as he gets home so late that he lacks the energy to cook a meal and rarely takes the time to go food shopping.

 CD-ROM 2 includes a video clip in which Tim introduces himself, and an audio clip of a meeting between Dr Mehra, Tim's GP, Katie, the primary care mental health worker, and Steve, an Expert Patient. Transcripts of the clips follow.

variations in specific needs (Department of Health, 2001b).

There are additional hurdles to be aware of in the planning of Expert Patient Programmes:

- Patients may not wish to participate: they may find the implicit change in their role threatening
- The approach is relatively time-consuming
- Is recruitment of self-management tutors from all sections of the community viable?
- Are accessible venues available?
- Is there a training issue for staff around the role of expert patients, and appropriate professional boundaries?
- Does previous negative experience of service provision make people more likely or less likely to participate? Will they be motivated to make a difference, or demoralized and lacking in trust that their contribution will be valued?
- There are important funding issues. Are people appropriately (financially) valued for their contribution? Will this negatively affect statutory benefits for those on low incomes?

Video: Introducing Tim (Stress)

Tim: My main problem is stress at work. I'm a web designer. Used to think I was quite good at it, thrived on the stress, but now I feel so anxious all the time. I seem to keep working to try and get it all right, but it just doesn't help. To be honest, even though I'm putting in all the hours that I can, I think I'm under-performing. I find it hard to concentrate and I keep forgetting what I need to do, where I need to be, where I put things.

My job has always been stressful, but now things are different because the company has been going through some financial difficulties, and some people have ended up losing their jobs. I've been lucky so far, although sometimes I wonder if I am that lucky, what with all this stress.

I find it so hard to switch off when I do eventually get home, and I'm not sleeping that well, especially getting off to sleep, and sometimes I wake up in the middle of the night and I can't get back off to sleep. I'm smoking like a chimney too which isn't helping.

My eating has all gone to pot. I tend to skip lunch and then just survive on coffee all day, and get a takeaway on the way home or see what John's left for me; but whichever, it still means I end up eating late, and then I end up with indigestion and that doesn't help my sleep. It's a vicious circle, and I've also got this permanent headache that I just can't shift.

I've had to cancel arrangements to see friends at the weekend because I had to work part of the time, then I was just so exhausted I couldn't face going for a game of squash then drinks.

And John is getting fed up with not seeing me, and when we do have any time together, well, I have no desire at all to have sex. He seems to think I don't love him anymore but that just isn't true, I'm just so stressed out that it's the last thing on my mind.

Dr Mehra took my blood pressure and told me it was a bit high, which is a bit of a worry, and he thinks the stress I'm under is making me susceptible to these colds and stuff I've been getting lately. He thinks I should consider a holiday. I nearly laughed when he said that. How am I going to find time to take a holiday when I can't even find time to get down the gym for an hour?

Anyway, it's all come to a head, and I'm feeling so low, I'm even tearful at times, and I just don't think I can cope anymore, so I've come to the practice for some help and I have been seeing the mental health worker and my GP.

I've haven't been prescribed any tablets from the GP though. Anyway, I was on the internet the other day, looking for some information about stress, and how to cope, and I found out about these Expert Patients. It's a new programme I think, where people who have a problem like diabetes or stress can give advice to people who aren't coping, on exactly how they've coped, which I suppose is the position I need to be in. Then I found out that the practice I go to is part of a Primary Care Trust that has signed up for this Expert Patient idea. So I asked the mental health worker, Katie, about it. I think she was pretty impressed actually, and then I noticed that there were leaflets and posters all round the practice telling everybody about it, and I just hadn't seen them. Anyway, she arranged for me to see someone called Steve, and actually he was great. He told me that he'd been trained and everything, and he really seemed to understand. I suppose he's been through it all himself, and he's a bit like me in a way in that he looks at all angles of things, and he gave me some really good advice about diet and supplements that you can have when you're feeling low and stressed, Omega-3 and Selenium. You can get extra Selenium from Brazil nuts, so I've been trying to eat a couple of them every day, and I get Omega-3 from oily fish apparently, or, in my case, from tablets from the health food shop, because my diet just doesn't include oily fish at the moment. So I'm going for the tablets and … I'm still smoking really heavily, but at least Steve's advice has helped me feel as if I'm doing something positive for myself about my problem.

Anyway, I went back to see Dr Mehra last week, and he asked me how I was getting on with the stress, and seeing Katie, and I told him about Steve, the Expert Patient, and the advice he had given me about the Omega-3 and Selenium, and Dr Mehra seemed a bit concerned about it; not about me going to see Steve per se, but about him not being informed about the advice I was given. He said some of these diet supplements can be dangerous and lots of people

are allergic to nuts, which I suppose is true, but the stuff that Steve recommended is completely natural so I can't really see what all the fuss is about.

Tim has been referred to the Expert Patient, Steve, by Katie, the mental health worker attached to the practice. The central issue in the transcript below is the potential for conflict between the Expert Patient role and the role of healthcare professionals. Note Dr Mehra's reaction to the advice the expert patient has given.

Audio: The potential for conflict between the roles of Expert Patients and healthcare professionals

Mental health worker (Katie): Thanks for your message, Dr Mehra. I understand that you wanted to talk to Steve and I about the advice given to Mr Monday.

GP (Dr Mehra): Yes, thank you for coming to see me. Basically I'm really pleased Tim went to see you, Steve. He obviously found it very beneficial, but I do have some concerns about patients in the practice being advised to take alternative medicines and dietary supplements, especially when I'm responsible for their physical and emotional well-being.

Expert Patient (Steve): The advice I gave to Tim was evidence-based. There is evidence that Selenium and Omega-3 can help people who are stressed and a bit low, and, as you know, Tim hasn't been eating properly of late.

Dr Mehra: Yes, but we don't know if those things work. What if Tim were allergic to Brazil nuts and he didn't know? Would you be able to explain an anaphylactic reaction to him? And also, he's not prescribed any medication at the moment, but the situation may well change, and if I don't know what other members of the team in the practice have advised him, and what sort of advice they have given, I wouldn't know how best to proceed, would I? I do hope you can understand my position, Steve. As it happens, I don't think there were any adverse effects reported, but the principle remains the same. The advice was given from this practice, where I am also working, and seeing Tim regularly. I wasn't informed that Tim was taking these supplements, or that you had recommended them to him.

Steve: I gave the advice in good faith. It was something that had helped me in the past, and I know has helped other people. Tim told me that he wasn't eating very well, and I felt he needed to know that there is evidence to suggest that these supplements can help.

Katie: Dr Mehra, is it fair to say that you are happy about Steve supporting Tim?

Dr Mehra: Oh yes, I am very positive about Steve's involvement. However, I think any advice on dietary supplements should be checked with me first.

Steve: So the real problem is that we didn't discuss the situation?

Dr Mehra: It would have been helpful to do so.

Katie: It does sound to me like communication is the real issue here. So, perhaps in future I could let you know, Dr Mehra, if I've arranged for a patient to see Steve, and then Steve can feed back to all the other practice staff involved in a patient's care. How would that be?

Steve: Well, that's fine with me, I can see the importance of it; but it does need to work both ways. It's been quite hard setting up the new role here at the surgery. I've felt that some of the staff see the Expert Patient Programme as making more work for them, and getting in the way of their relationship with the patients. That's not what its all about at all. I want to support the patients, and could even decrease your workloads, by helping people to manage their conditions themselves, without having to call on practice staff for help and support all of the time. Sometimes I find it difficult to approach the clinical staff, because I feel they resent me being here. I'm not saying that I am an expert, as you both might see

an expert, like a psychiatrist, but that I have expertise, through my own experience of mental health problems.

Dr Mehra: I appreciate your frankness, Steve; most of us working within the Trust were not trained in this way. I know that some of my colleagues were very sceptical at first, but the bottom line is that the Primary Care Trust is fully committed to the Expert Patient Programme and we here at the practice are committed to supporting it.

Katie: I feel like I've learnt a lot today about the difficulties that can arise for both clinicians and expert patients, and I think it might be really helpful to raise this at the practice meeting. I'm quite keen to do that actually. So, would either of you be willing to talk about it a bit?

Steve: I'd like the opportunity to speak to other members of staff about some of the things that have been raised today.

Dr Mehra: That seems like a positive way forward.

Exercise

In the context of the discussion between Steve, Katie and Dr Mehra, consider the following:

- How would these problems be worked through in your clinical practice?
- Discuss the problem with your peers.
- Do you think that the expert patient should be someone a patient may expect to be speaking to in confidence, as they would probably have a different relationship with a 'lay' person who shares their experiences, than with their doctor?
- What difficulties might arise here, and how could they be addressed?

The Expert Patient Programme is not the only government healthcare policy initiative that seeks to promote service user involvement. An example from the field of health and social care research is INVOLVE (previously known as Consumers in NHS Research: www.invo.org.uk).

Section summary

- The Expert Patient Programme is policy in action. It promotes user involvement, and is professionally led, the main driver being healthcare services. There are some potential difficulties associated with this emerging role
- User-led self-management programmes have a twenty-year history and are one example of promoting user involvement
- Concordance with medication or treatment plans is a recurring issue for people who have mental health problems

References

Association of the British Pharmaceutical Industry (1999). *The Expert Patient – Survey October 1999.* London: ABPI. www.abpi.org.uk.

Department of Health (1999d). *Saving Lives: Our Healthier Nation.* London: HMSO.

Department of Health (2000a). *The NHS Plan: A Plan for Investment. A Plan for Reform.* London: HMSO.

Department of Health (2001b). *The Expert Patient: A New Approach to Chronic Disease Management for the 21st Century.* London: HMSO.

Eaton, L. (2002a). The road to consensus. *Health Service Journal,* 12 (5789) 24 January, 16–17.

Jafri, T., Jones, R., Taylor, D. and Wakeling, M. (2003). *Future Partnerships: Primary Care in 2020?* University of London: The School of Pharmacy.

Lorig, K.R., Holman, H.R., Sobel, D.S., Laurent, D.D., González, V.M. and Minor, M.A. (2000). *Living a Healthy Life With Chronic Conditions (2nd edition).* Boulder: Bull.

Lorig, K.R., Ritter, P., Stewart, A.L., Sobel, D.S., Brown, B.W., Bandura, A., González, V.M., Laurent, D.D. and Holman, H.R. (2001). Chronic Disease Self-Management Program: 2-Year health status and health care utilisation outcomes. *Medical Care,* 39 (11), 1217–1223.

The Long-term Medical Conditions Alliance (2001). *Supporting Expert Patients: how to develop lay led self-management programmes for people with long-term medical conditions.* London: LMCA.

Wilson, J. (1999). Acknowledging the expertise of patients and their organisations. *British Medical Journal,* 319, 18 Sept, 771–774.

Wilson, P.M. (2001). A policy analysis of the Expert Patient in the United Kingdom: self care as an expression of pastoral power? *Health and Social Care in the Community,* 9 (3), May, 134–142.

Test yourself

 To check your progress, locate this section on CD-ROM 2 and work through the questions at the end.

Section 2: Advocacy and the user involvement worker

This section is divided into four parts:
1 Definitions of advocacy
2 Models of advocacy and the Advocacy Charter
3 Challenges of advocacy
4 Advocacy and the user involvement worker

'Even if benign and well-intentioned, mental health and learning disability services often involve a reduction in autonomy for the patient, for example through loss of liberty and a lack of choice.'

Royal College of Psychiatrists, 1999, p7

Definitions of advocacy

The word 'advocate' originates from the Latin 'advocatus', meaning legal advocate or counsellor – in Scotland, an advocate is still a term for a legal barrister. In a mental health context, an advocate is someone who undertakes to support a service user in the expression of their views, needs, wishes and worries – especially if the service user does not feel that they can do this directly.

Mental health advocacy has a long history: the pamphlet of 1620 entitled *The Petition of the Poor Distracted People in the House of Bedlam* is often cited as an early example (Campbell, 2001, p10). Until the early 1980s, however, there was no great focus on independent advocacy for health and social care; this situation changed with the rise of service user action groups.

Currently, advocacy may be summed up as an active process that helps people to:
- express their needs and concerns

Advocacy is partisan: 'by siding with the weaker party in the client/healthcare professional relationship, the advocate tries to create a situation in which there can be a discussion between more equal parties' (Curran and Grimshaw, 2000, p28).

Take some time to reflect on this statement, then consider closely the following questions:

- Shouldn't 'professional' input be enough to ensure that a service user is getting what they want or need?
- Why do we need independent advocates?
- Can a health professional act as an advocate?
- What are the positives and negatives of independent advocacy?

- safeguard and promote their rights and responsibilities
- obtain the information and services they need
- explore the choices available to them and express their wishes

An advocate informs, empowers and enables service users to obtain a more responsive, accessible and appropriate service. They are someone who listens, takes their partner's truth as valid and is wholly 'on their side' ('partner' being the preferred terminology for a service user in many advocacy settings); someone who helps them to get information, to say what they want to say, and to make informed choices.

The advocate works to ensure that the service user's unadulterated view is presented and their chosen objectives pursued. The advocate does not superimpose their views on the issues at stake. Importantly, the advocate does not subject the individual's view or expressed wishes to an appraisal of 'best interest', whereas care staff with a responsibility to assess risk may act on the grounds of personal or public safety. It may be that a person's wishes are judged irrational – but still, the advocate will present them as the

person's view, and support the individual to express themselves. This is one of the issues that can cause tension between advocacy and healthcare staff, if the latter fail to appreciate that it is the advocate's role to support the expression of people's views as they are, and not alter them in any way.

Models of advocacy and the Advocacy Charter

Advocacy services can be conceptualized as a continuum occupied by the principle of protection at one end and by that of empowerment at the other. An advocacy situation, where an individual is unable to communicate their needs adequately (as a result of, for example, dementia), may be termed 'non-instructed'/ 'non-directed' (or, sometimes, 'best-interest' advocacy); 'instructed advocacy' comprises a situation where an individual has the potential to express their needs, but there is a block to them doing so effectively. This second type of advocacy encompasses much of the work undertaken by mental health advocates, and several common styles of advocacy are situated at this end of the continuum. Leader and Crosby (1998) list six types of advocacy (see **page 100**).

Henderson and Pochin (2001) list and describe the various forms of advocacy, along with their historical development in the UK. An alliance of over 75 advocacy schemes based in London has compiled an Advocacy Charter. The alliance, which claims to define a set of core principles for advocacy schemes (see the Action for Advocacy website, www. actionforadvocacy. org.uk), has been adopted by schemes outside the capital (e.g. in Leicestershire and Rutland), and by schemes serving specific populations (e.g. PACE for lesbian, gay, bisexual and transgendered people, and RNIB for blind people). The Charter states: 'Advocacy is taking action to help people say what they want, secure their rights, represent their interests and obtain services they need. Advocates and advocacy schemes work in partnership with the people they support and take their side. Advocacy promotes social inclusion, equality and social justice.'

The Advocacy Charter details the principles

Six types of advocacy

Self-Advocacy An individual speaking for himself or herself and regaining control over their life. This type of advocacy is often the explicit goal of much mental health advocacy.

Peer Advocacy Advocacy offered by people with a similar background or experience to that of the individual concerned. These types of advocates may, for example, be trained volunteers or members of a user-run group.

Group Advocacy A group of people working together to speak up for what they want (e.g. a group of older people lobbying local service providers).

Citizen Advocacy This kind of advocacy finds commonest expression in the field of learning disability, referring to the activities of trained volunteers working with service users over the longer term to exercise or defend their rights as citizens.

Formal/Professional Advocacy This usually refers to services offered by voluntary groups that are not user-led, or to schemes where an advocate is paid to work with whoever needs their service. Formal advocacy addresses a specific situation or crisis.

Bilingual Advocacy This includes the practice of interpreting – but this type of advocate also undertakes to relay their client's cultural, religious and social context and challenge discrimination.

Leader and Cosby, 1998

of advocacy schemes under ten headings (see Box opposite).

A Code of Practice relating to advocacy has been developed by the United Kingdom Advocacy Network in conjunction with the Mental Health Task Force User Group (UKAN, 1997).

Under the proposed Mental Health Act reforms, there will be a right to advocacy for those people subject to compulsion. Barnes et al (2002) have written core standards for good practice guidelines for the Specialist Mental Health Advocacy Role. These are included in PDF format on CD-ROM 2, and are available online at www.dur.ac.uk/resources/sass/research/SASsummary 02_06_21.pdf.

The authors conducted a systematic consultation with a diverse group of relevant stakeholders, aimed at identifying consensus about advocacy, its purpose, principles for practice, and how it should be organized; the document is intended as a starting point for further consultation and discussions about the future shape of such services.

Challenges of advocacy

Challenges that may arise in 'instructed' advocacy often do so from the way in which the relationship between the advocate and the service user is conceived – either by the advocate and service user themselves, or by health and social care workers. In all cases, clarity of role and goal are key: boundaries and expectations should be clear to all parties. It should be explicit, for example, that the long-term goal of an advocacy relationship is self-advocacy (so that the service user does not become dependent on the advocate, and so, disempowered). The service user should be clear that the advocate is not a trained counsellor or social worker. In the practice of instructed advocacy, it is important that an advocate does not:

- give advice – an advocate helps a service user to explore the options open to them
- make decisions or choices for their client – the patient is the best judge of their best interest
- dominate their client – the service user is always the 'senior partner' in the relationship (inverting the most common power relation within healthcare provision)
- participate in an advocacy relationship where a conflict of interest could be perceived

The principles of advocacy schemes (taken from the Advocacy Charter)

Clarity of Purpose	The advocacy scheme will have clearly stated aims and objectives and be able to demonstrate how it meets the principles contained in this Charter. Advocacy schemes will ensure that people they advocate for, service providers and funding agencies have information on the scope and limitations of the scheme's role.
Independence	The advocacy scheme will be structurally independent from statutory organizations and preferably from all service provider agencies. The advocacy scheme will be as free from conflict of interest as possible, in both design and operation, and actively seek to reduce conflicting interests.
Putting People First	The advocacy scheme will ensure that the wishes and interests of the people they advocate for, direct advocates' work. Advocates should be non-judgmental and respectful of peoples' needs, views and experiences. Advocates will ensure that information concerning the people they advocate for is shared with these individuals.
Empowerment	The advocacy scheme will support self-advocacy and empowerment through its work. People who use the scheme should have a say in the level of involvement and style of advocacy support they want. Schemes will ensure that people, who want to, can influence and be involved in the running and management of the scheme.
Equal Opportunity	The advocacy scheme will have a written equal opportunities policy that recognizes the need to be pro-active in tackling all forms of inequality, discrimination and social exclusion. The scheme will have in place systems for the fair and equitable allocation of advocates' time.
Accountability	The advocacy scheme will have in place systems for the effective monitoring and evaluation of its work. All those who use the scheme will have a named advocate and a means of contacting them.
Accessibility	Advocacy will be provided free of charge to eligible people. The advocacy scheme will aim to ensure that its premises, policies, procedures and publicity materials promote access for the whole community.
Supporting Advocates	The advocacy scheme will ensure advocates are prepared, trained and supported in their role and provided with opportunities to develop their skills and experience.
Confidentiality	The advocacy scheme will have a written policy on confidentiality, stating that information known about a person using the scheme is confidential to the scheme and specifying any circumstances under which confidentiality might be breached.
Complaints	The advocacy scheme will have a written policy describing how to make complaints or give feedback about the scheme or about individual advocates. Where necessary, the scheme will enable people who use its services to access external independent support to make or pursue a complaint.

Conflicts with health and social care workers may arise around the concept of 'best interest'. In instructed advocacy, the advocate is there to help the patient find their own voice, and is always aware of the danger of pressure being brought to bear by professionals to accede to 'what is best' for an individual service user. The advocate is always independent of service providers, and works explicitly to the instructions of the service user. This can make things difficult for other workers – by the advocate insisting on longer or more frequent meetings, for example; but these difficulties can (hopefully) be resolved assertively and without confrontation.

Exercise

Consider the following scenario:

A patient in primary care has been prescribed medication for severe depression, which he says, is causing unpleasant side-effects. He wants to stop taking the tablets and not to consider admission to hospital. The mental health worker in his practice would like him to see a psychiatrist, but he is unwilling to do so. He has called in a local advocacy service to put forward his point of view. What would you expect an advocate to do?

[The following should be considered:
• Hear the patient's story in full, being committed to his viewpoint
• Avoid getting drawn into any debate about the 'real' nature of the side-effects.
• Ensure that the patient knows his legal position and talk through with him the consequences of ceasing the medication and refusing a psychiatric assessment.
• Establish what points he wants to put to the primary care team and help him to articulate his needs and views.]

The user involvement worker

The role of the user involvement worker is constituted differently in various health arenas. It is important to remember this, as they may be linked to (or employed by) statutory services. They do not fulfil the same role as an independent advocate. Some service user involvement workers may work directly with individual service users to help them address local issues. Some may focus on developing a liaison role between healthcare providers and user groups, aiming to facilitate an inclusive communication framework, so that service users and carers are involved and supported. Funding can come from various local or national organizations. Key components of the role are:

• User involvement workers are generally concerned with moving user (and carer) involvement from a peripheral role to being central to the mental health agenda
• It involves assessing local need, identifying obstacles and finding solutions to specific barriers to user and carer involvement
• One component of the role is often the shifting of user involvement from an ad hoc approach to being more coordinated and integral to service delivery
• User and carer involvement includes explicitly addressing difficult issues such as 'representativeness' and tokenism
• A component of the role is often mental health promotion. In some circumstances, this can be more implicit than explicit: health promotion is not a direct goal of the activity, but participants or members of a user forum (for example) can grow in self-esteem and confidence and become more resilient to threats to their well-being, because of the involvement in an empowering group with associated values and goals
• The role may be designed to support the development of advocacy services and to challenge discrimination

However, it is important to remember the value of organizing and funding user involvement work independently of service providers, and of supporting the organic growth of such activity in local communities (this will be stressed again in Chapter 2.3, Section 1, 'Dilemmas in practice').

Section summary

- Advocacy is usually independently instigated and is a way of hearing the voice of users who are not in a position to effectively speak for themselves
- It is useful to view advocacy services as a continuum with protection at one end and empowerment on the other
- Under proposed Mental Health Act reforms there will be a statutory right to advocacy

References

Barnes, D., Brandon, T. and Webb, T. (2002). *Independent Specialist Advocacy in England and Wales: Recommendations for Good Practice.* Durham: University of Durham. Also available at the Department of Health website, www.dh.gov.uk/Home/fs/en.

Campbell, P. (2001). From petitions to professionals. *Openmind*, 107 Jan/Feb, 10.

Curran, C. and Grimshaw, C. (2000). Advocacy. *Openmind*, 101, Jan/Feb, 28.

Henderson, R. and Pochin, M. (2001). *Right Result? Advocacy, Justice, and Empowerment.* Bristol: Policy Press.

Leader, A. and Crosby, K. (1998). *Power Tools – Resource Pack for Mental Health Advocacy.* Brighton: Pavilion.

Royal College of Psychiatrists (1999). *Patient Advocacy: Council Report CR74.* London: RCP.

United Kingdom Advocacy Network (UKAN) (1997). *Advocacy – A Code of Practice.* London: NHS Executive Mental Health Task Force User Group.

Test yourself

 To check your progress, locate this section on CD-ROM 2 and work through the interactive questions at the end.

Section 3: Health promotion and principles of self-help

This section is divided into six parts:
1 Defining mental health promotion, and the philosophical and practical approaches to mental health promotion
2 How does mental health promotion work, how can users and carers be incorporated?
3 Distinguishing between prevention and promotion in mental health, including individual and population programmes
4 Delivering standard one of the National Service Framework – user and carer involvement
5 Empowerment in relation to health promotion and self-help
6 Self-help

Defining mental health promotion: practical and philosophical approaches

In common with the World Health Organisation definition of health (World Health Organisation (WHO), 1946), in this section 'mental health' is referred to as a state that is determined not only by an absence of mental illness, but also by a sense of well-being.

It is important to consider mental health and physical health holistically – interventions which seemingly primarily target physical health (such as exercise and recreational activity) can positively influence mental health; and the chronically mentally unwell can experience disproportionate levels of physical ill-health.

In order to develop critical thought about promoting mental health and well-being, it is useful to establish a shared understanding of what it is to be mentally healthy and to experience well-being. To date, much of this debate has focused on mental illness rather than on mental health – being concerned with conditions such as anxiety, depression and schizophrenia. Less consideration has been given to issues which threaten a sense of well-being – such as isolation and loneliness, low self-esteem and fear – which are often debilitating and have direct effects on people's mental and physical health. Mental health is directly affected by the conditions in which individuals and communities live and interact, as well as by predisposition (Department of Health, 2001e). 'Well-being', especially in terms of mental health, can be a nebulous concept – easy to define in terms of its absence, hard to define in positive terms.

The WHO has been most influential in defining health promotion, its Ottawa Charter (WHO, 1986) being the most important document in health promotion. This represents a philosophical and practical guide to health promotion identifying five key strategies:

1 reorienting health services
2 developing personal skills
3 building a healthy public policy
4 strengthening community action
5 creating supportive environments for health

According to the WHO, all policy and practice (whatever its focus) should give full attention to:

- equity – the equal right to healthcare
- community participation – the involvement of people in the planning and implementation of decisions involving their healthcare (especially users and carers)
- intersectorial collaboration – a recognition of the complexity of factors that affect health and the need for different agencies to work together

The charity Mentality is the first and only charity dedicated solely to the promotion of mental health. It works with the public and private sectors, user and survivor groups and voluntary agencies, to promote the health of individuals, families, organizations and communities. It considers (Mentality, 2002: Mentality's publications are available on www.mentality.org.uk) that mental health promotion is primarily concerned with:

- how individuals, families, organizations and communities think and feel
- the factors which influence how we think and feel collectively
- the impact that this has on overall health and well-being

How does mental health promotion work; how can users and carers be involved?

According to Mentality, health promotion works at three levels (each level is relevant to whole populations, to individuals, vulnerable groups and people with mental health problems).

At each level, interventions may focus on strengthening factors known to protect mental health (e.g. social support, job control) or to reduce factors known to increase risk (e.g. unemployment, violence).

Mentality asserts that mental health promotion contributes to overall health gain. Interventions – to reduce stress in the workplace, to tackle bullying in schools, to increase access to green, open spaces and to reduce fear of crime – all contribute to health gain through improving mental well-being. Results of a survey of 6000 adults show that stress appears to be a major health problem (Rainford et al, 2000). Stress is highest in the age group 25–54, peaking at 35–44. Stress is also covered in Chapter 3.1, Section 3.

Mental health promotion aims to prevent certain mental health problems, notably depression, anxiety, substance abuse and behavioural disorders. However, mental health promotion also promotes recovery and quality of life for people with mental health problems.

Examples of evidenced-based mental health promotion activities

Reducing problematic alcohol consumption

Setting: Primary care
Level of action: Individual
Brief interventions in primary care (including taking an alcohol history and providing information and advice) are effective in reducing alcohol consumption in people drinking above the recommended levels. Routine or oppor-

tunistic screening for alcohol problems in Accident and Emergency departments should be followed by a brief intervention (Ashenden et al, 1997).

More than 6% of men and 25% of women consume more than what is regarded as a 'safe' level of alcohol – 2–3 units of alcohol a day for men, and 1–2 units of alcohol a day for women, with at least 2 alcohol free days a week.

Physical exercise
Setting: Primary care/Neighbourhood
Level of action: Individual
Evaluation of the Balance for Life scheme in Essex found that a 10-week programme of exercise significantly reduced depression and anxiety, and increased overall quality of life and self-efficacy. Of clinically depressed patients, 68% had depression scores that became non-clinical within three months (Darbisher and Glenister, 1998).

Distinguishing between mental illness prevention and mental health promotion

The prevention of mental illness is generally conceived of as a public health issue, in that it is concerned with populations rather than individuals. Public health practitioners usually divide preventive activities into three levels:
1 *Primary prevention* – the processes involved in reducing the risk that people in any given community will develop mental illness
2 *Secondary prevention* – the activities involved in reducing the duration of episodes of mental illness
3 *Tertiary prevention* – preventing complications where illness already exists, promoting rehabilitation and preventing relapse, so that the best possible level of mental health might be achieved

Prevention in practice

Primary prevention The workplace environment could be considered as a cause of mental illness exacerbated by stress. One approach to workplace stress is to focus on the individual. Another would be to consider the role of the organization. Cooper (1994) asserts that the way forward is to identify sources of workplace stress and then to intervene with a view to moving from treatment to preventative action.

Secondary prevention The argument for mental health screening (especially for identified vulnerable groups) includes the positive effect mental health has on quality of life and the potential for prevention of further deterioration.

Tertiary prevention There are social, economic and emotional costs to individuals and families, in the context of severe and enduring mental health problems (Brooker, 1990). With an estimated total of 100,000 people diagnosed with schizophrenia in Britain, there is a clear need to identify strategies for the promotion of health and the prevention of further deterioration. Evidence is being accrued to support psychosocial interventions based on the stress/ vulnerability model of psychosis.

Delivering standard one of the National Service Framework

The aim of standard one is to ensure that health and social services promote mental health and reduce the discrimination and social exclusion associated with mental health problems.

Health and social services should promote mental health for all, working with both individuals and communities (Department of Health, 1999c). They should combat discrimination against individuals and groups with mental health problems and promote their social inclusion. Meeting standard one requires action across whole populations, as well as programmes for individuals at risk.

Service users were consulted between 1997 and 1999 in relation to the creation of the National Service Framework for Mental Health. As a result of their experience in this consultation, a set of ten draft principles for user involvement was developed (Sainsbury Centre

for Mental Health, 2003). These principles are:

1 Make user involvement the norm
2 There must be a base of support and accountability
3 Power imbalances must be examined and dealt with
4 Outreach – professionals need to go where the service users are
5 Service users make their own decisions about involvement
6 Value the experience of service users and help them gain new skills and confidence
7 Be sensitive about paying users
8 Professionals need training in user involvement
9 Service users and carers are not interchangeable
10 Mental health organizations need to set up user involvement policies and programmes

Exercise

Consider a Health Promotion strategy with which you are familiar, and identify which of the above principles might be applied.

The concept of empowerment

The term 'empowerment' has entered the discourse of public policy, but is used to mean very different things (and at times appears to lack any real content). Nevertheless, many health promoters argue that empowerment is central to the process of health promotion. A working definition might be 'enabling others to take charge of their lives and destinies, and to feel in control of their circumstances'.

This approach can be based on a 'bottom-up' strategy: instead of the expert role, the health promoter acts as a catalyst who gets things going and then withdraws from the situation.

The Tones model of health promotion (Figure 5) claims to be an empowerment model, which as its cardinal principle has the goal of enabling people to take control of their own health. Education is seen as the key to

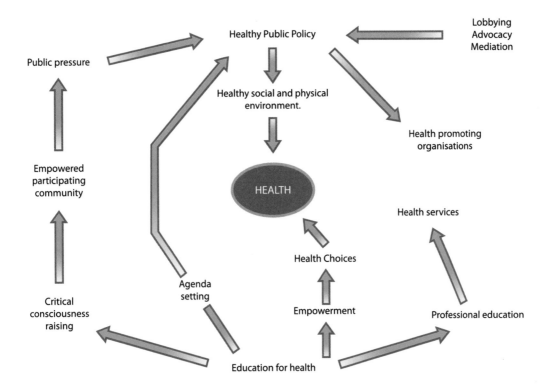

Figure 5: The Tones model of health promotion (Tones and Tilford, 1995)

empowering both lay and professional people, by raising consciousness of health issues. People are then more able to make choices and create pressure for healthy public policies (Tones and Tilford, 1995).

When considering empowerment, it is necessary to distinguish between *self*-empowerment and *community*-empowerment. Self-empowerment is used (in some cases) to describe those approaches which are based on counselling and which use non-directive, patient-centred approaches aimed at increasing people's control over their own lives. For people to be empowered they need to:

- recognize and understand their powerlessness
- feel strongly enough about their situation to want to change it
- feel capable of changing the situation through having information, support and life skills

Empowerment is also used to describe a way of working which increases people's power to change their 'social reality'. We will be looking at this in more depth in Chapter 2.3, Section 1.

The extent to which professionally-led initiatives can be truly empowering can be questioned, as allegiances to services and practices that are essentially part of the problem are so deeply ingrained.

Nevertheless, there are clear cases where professional staff do act wholeheartedly in support of service users' empowerment (often at personal cost), such as in instances of whistleblowing. Two service user activists have written booklets in conjunction with MIND and COHSE (later, renamed Unison), which have explored empowerment both in mental health practice and in advocacy (Read and Wallcraft, 1992, 1994). They raise the alternative possibility of service users' and staff's collective interests not being necessarily mutually exclusive, and argue for an empowered and motivated workforce as being best placed to support user empowerment and deliver high-quality services.

Self-help: individual and group

The concept and practice of self-help has a long history. The political connotations of the concept mean that many contemporary user groups would not describe themselves in this way (although they may find themselves described as such by others). Groups may acknowledge that self-help is a result, if not the prime purpose, of their actions (Barnes and Shardlow, 1997).

Barnes and Bowl (2001) argue that a distinction needs to be made between:

- separate action on the part of mental health service users, and
- action from within service systems which enables users to take part in the decision-making process

---

Exercise

What do you think are the strengths and weaknesses of these two positions? Do you, for example, agree with those who see user involvement within mental health services as compromised by the 'the paradox of empowerment?

Self-help is addressed in detail in Chapter 1.3, Section 4 and Chapetr 3.4, Section 4.

Barnes and Bowl go on to identify concerns:

- over the way in which service users are 'allowed' to exercise power, which is often determined by professionals
- about the continuing gradient of power between service users and professionals
- about the background of coercion that may underpin the work of such agencies

In contrast, self-help organizations are seen as seeking to empower in four ways, by:

1 providing models that emphasize the achievements and potential of service users (and hence counter stigma)
2 giving individuals access to resources and skills needed to reach personal goals
3 giving service users control over and responsibility for organizational policy
4 collectively seeking change in the wider society

Section summary

- Health promotion relies on partnership working and alliances built outside the healthcare arena
- Mental health promotion has a role in prevention of certain mental health disorders, such as anxiety and substance use problems, but also in recovery and quality of life for people with mental health problems
- Mental health promotion is enshrined in standard one of the National Service Framework: health and social services should promote mental health for all, working with individuals and communities
- Empowerment is central to the process of mental health promotion

References

Ashenden, R., Silagy, C. and Weller, D. (1997). A systematic review of effectiveness of promoting lifestyle change in general practice. *Family Practice*, 14, 160–175.

Barnes, M. and Bowl, R. (2001). *Taking Over the Asylum: Empowerment and Mental Health*. Basingstoke: Palgrave.

Barnes, M. and Shardlow, P. (1997). From passive recipient to active citizen: participation in mental health user groups. *Journal of Mental Health*, 6 (3), 289–300.

Brooker, C. (1990). The health education needs of families caring for a schizophrenic relative and the potential role for community psychiatric nurses. *Journal of Advanced Nursing*, 15 (9), 1092–1098.

Cooper, C. (1994). Finding the solution – primary prevention: identifying the causes and preventing mental ill health in the workplace, in *Mental Health in the Workplace*. London: HMSO.

Crowther, R., Bond, G., Huxley, P. and Marshall, M. (2000). Vocational training for people with severe mental disorders (Protocol for a Cochrane Review). *The Cochrane Library*, Issue 3, Oxford.

Darbisher, L. and Glenister, G. (1998). *The Balance for Life Scheme: mental health benefits of GP recommended exercise in relation to depression and anxiety*. Colchester: The University of Essex: Health and Social Services Unit.

Department of Health (1999c). *The National Service Framework for Mental Health.* London: HMSO.

Department of Health (2001e). *Making it Happen: A Guide to Delivering Mental Health Promotion.* London: HMSO.

Rainford, L., Mason, V. and Hickman, M. (2000). *Health in England 1998: Investigating the Links between Social Inequalities and Health.* London: HMSO.

Sainsbury Centre for Mental Health (2003). *On Our Own Terms: Users and Survivors of Mental Health Services Working Together for Support and Change.* London: SCMH.

Segal, S.P., Silverman, C. and Temkin, T. (1993). Empowerment and self-help agency practice for people with mental disabilities. *Social Work, 38* (6), 708.

Tones, K. and Tilford, S. (1995). *Health Education: Effectiveness, Efficiency and Equity* (Second Edition). London: Chapman and Hall.

World Health Organisation (WHO) (1946). *World Health Organisation Constitution.* Geneva: WHO.

World Health Organisation (WHO) (1986). *Ottawa Charter for Health Promotion.* Geneva: WHO.

Recommended reading

Advocacy Across London (2002). *The Advocacy Charter*, available online at www.advocacyacrosslondon. org.uk.

Department of Health (2004b). *Patient and Public Involvement in Health: The Evidence for Policy Implementation – A summary of the results of the Health in Partnership research programme.* London: HMSO.

Helman, C. (2000). *Culture, Health and Illness* (Fourth Edition). Oxford: Butterworth Heinemann.

National Institute for Mental Health in England (2004a). *Working With Carers: a handbook for professionals working with those who provide help and support to people with mental health problems.* London: HMSO.

Test yourself

 To check your progress, locate this section on CD-ROM 2 and work through the interactive questions at the end.

Chapter 2.3
The community and the voluntary sector

Aims

To provide an in-depth knowledge and critical understanding of the theory and practice of community development and to provide the information to apply this to mental health, and user and carer involvement; and provide an insight into the voluntary sector and its place in mental health provision.

Learning outcomes

By the end of this Chapter, the reader will be able to:
* Understand the origins of community development, and critically consider definitions
* Analyse issues of power and empowerment in relation to community development and mental health
* Discuss and critically evaluate issues of autonomy, advocacy and empowerment with respect to community development
* Critically discuss dilemmas in community development practice, especially in relation to mental health and user and carer involvement
* Have a critical understanding of the role of voluntary sector organizations and their place in mental health service mapping
* Have a critical understanding of the provision and position of secondary mental health services and their relationship to primary care, voluntary sector providers, and local authority provision
* Appreciate the role of the voluntary sector in addressing diverse/local needs, not necessarily best met by large organizational bureaucracies

Introduction

The focus of this Chapter is community development; it is important to remember this when thinking about issues such as advocacy and empowerment, which we touched on previously in Chapter 2.2, Section 2. There, the focus was primarily on healthcare practice settings. In this Chapter, we are concerned more with the organization and funding of user involvement work, independently of service providers, and with how the organic growth of such activity in local communities can be encouraged and supported.

Chapter 2.3 content is as follows:

1 Community development models
2 Voluntary sector resources and mapping

Section 1: Community development models

This section is divided into five parts:
1 Defining community
2 Community development
3 The relationships between community development, power and empowerment
4 Advocacy, autonomy, empowerment and mental health in relation to community development
5 Dilemmas in practice

'The increased involvement of communities and greater patient participation and person-centred approaches support the promotion of mental health through engagement and inclusion.'

Mentality, 2004

Defining community

The New Public Health, the self-help movement and the women's movement were all strongly associated from the 1970s with a shift in power from the experts to people themselves. By the late 1980s, the terms 'community development', 'community participation' and 'community empowerment' were all central to the health promotion (and wider emancipatory) discourse.

The idea that communities could identify their health needs and take action to control them signalled a definite shift in approach; community care is particularly important in relation to mental health, because it has long been seen as the favoured way of delivering mental health services.

Before looking in depth at what community development means, we must consider what is meant by the term 'community'. The concept of community is often used in debates about health and social care, and is generally considered to be a 'good thing' when contrasted to state or bureaucratic organization. It is assumed that services provided by, and in, the community will be more appropriate and sensitive. There are other ways of considering 'community' than as the distinction between state and non-state provision, of course. Among these are: opposition between a solidaristic sense of community and the idea of disconnected, isolated individuals; and the contrast between collective goals and self-interest. This raises the question of the relationship between a sense of community and contradictory trends and social forces (such as consumerism–individualism).

However, with respect to the different ways of defining community, the most commonly cited factors are:

- **Geography** A community may be defined on a geographical or neighbourhood basis; for instance, many studies have been done on the East End of London. This way of defining community is based on the assumption that people living in the same area have the same concerns, due to their geographical proximity.

- **Culture** Here, shared cultural traditions outweigh geographical or other barriers, and unite otherwise scattered groups of people. Examples are 'the Jewish community' or 'the Chinese community'. Members of a cultural community may be more likely to share resources and, generally, to support one another.

- **Social stratification** A community may be based on shared socio-economic position (although there are many other forms of social stratification). We might think in terms of 'working-class' or 'middle-class' groupings. This way of defining community is particularly important in relation to mental health primary care, because, as discussed in the section on Social Inclusion and Mental Health, our socio-economic position can impact dramatically on the way we experience health and illness and the way in which we access services.

Exercise

Think about what, if any, communities you feel you belong to, and identify any problems in conceptualizing community in the ways described above.

Thus, the meaning of the term varies greatly, but how we define 'community' is important because it impacts on how community representatives or users and carers may be identified.

Community development

An early definition of community development is one suggested by Ross in 1995:

'Community development is a process by which a community identifies its needs or objectives, orders (or ranks) these needs or objectives, develops the confidence or will to work at these needs or objectives, finds the resources (internal and or external) to deal with these needs and/or objectives, takes action in respect to them, and in so doing extends and develops co-operative and collaborative attitudes and practices in the community.'

Ross, 1995

We can see how this very early definition of community development can be taken and extended to include user and carer involvement. There are, however, some more contemporary concepts in community development that have relevance to mental health; these include concepts of social capital and social enterprise, and the development of social firms. Arguably, many community and voluntary-sector organizations would recognize explicitly 'social enterprise' descriptors as applying to themselves, or may even describe themselves in these terms.

A growing number of grant funders are sponsoring the growth of social firms/social enterprise; some now exist exclusively to promote this sort of activity. In some areas (such as the North West), Primary Care Trusts are supporting the development of health-related social enterprise; associated with this, regional development agencies are increasingly relating capital and employment initiatives to key health objectives.

There are various sociological accounts of the processes at stake in enacting social change, especially with regard to the best ways of achieving this through membership of groups. Traditional groups associated with aspirations for social change (political parties, trade unions, etc.) tend to be referred to as 'old' social movements – and these are sometimes criticised for a progressive dilution of radicalism and an inertia born of expanding bureaucracy. In contrast, so-called 'new' social movements are seen as more dynamic and in touch with grassroots expressions of radicalism and democracy. Such dichotomous analyses are often associated with anti-globalization and environmental politics, but they also include some feminist and anti-racist movements. Rogers and Pilgrim (1991) argue that the mental health service user movement can be perceived as an emergent 'new' social movement. These social movements are invariably associated with transformational political aspirations. Transformational leadership styles will be discussed in Chapter 2.4, Section 2, 'Styles of leadership and user involvement'.

Naidoo and Wills (2000) state that community development is both a philosophy and a method. As a philosophy its key features are:

- a commitment to equality and the breaking down of hierarchies and power relations
- an emphasis on participation and enabling all communities to be heard
- an emphasis on lay knowledge and the valuing of people's own experience
- collectivizing of experience and seeing problems as shared
- the empowerment of individuals and communities through education, skills development, sharing and joint action

The community development approach has been heavily influenced by the work of Paulo Friere in the 1970s. Friere was a Brazilian cleric and educator who believed that education (in this case basic literacy) was the means by which subordinate groups of peasants in Peru and Brazil could challenge the system behind their oppression, and so improve their position in life. He aimed to engage these people in critical consciousness-raising (what he called 'conscientization'), helping people to understand their circumstances and why they are oppressed.

This process begins with problem-posing groups that seek to break down barriers and establish dialogue between individuals, and between individuals and a facilitator. Eventually a state of praxis is reached in which there is common understanding and development of practice and action, whereby people can collectively transform their circumstances.

This process is summarized as:
- reflections on aspects of reality
- search and collective identification of the root causes of that reality
- an examination of their implications
- development of a plan of action to change reality

As Carey (2002) points out, we might well ask what relevance do techniques used in Brazil in the 1950s and 1960s have for us in the UK now? The connection is of not 'having a voice' and the accompanying reality of powerlessness. This is as common for many groups in the UK today (including users of mental health services) as it was for the Brazilian peasants in the 1960s.

Examples of community development

1 The User Involvement Project in the London Boroughs of Redbridge and Waltham Forest

Setting: Community and workplace
Level of action: Individual and community
Target: People with mental health problems, employers and service providers
Aims: To increase individual and collective empowerment through capacity building and training. To ensure the voice of the user is heard. To promote the involvement of users in planning and training provision.

The work includes:

- a service users' forum
- training users as co-trainers within health
- training users to monitor services
- ensuring that services have an explicit way of consulting with service users and formal ways for users to be involved
- users taking part in recruitment/ interviews

Department of Health, 2001e

2 The Bourneville Community Development Project

Between 1991 and 1993 a project called 'Look after your heart' was run on a deprived housing estate in Weston-super-Mare. Outcomes from the project were recorded in relation to participation, knowledge levels and access to health-promoting facilities. The project responded to issues local people saw as being most important. The major outcomes of the project were better access to health promoting facilities – such as a mother's group, a needle exchange scheme at the estate pharmacy, a local health centre, environmental improvements such as playgrounds, and a secure road crossing area. People living on the estate raised these issues, and, by having a strategy that addressed these concerns, the project led to a stronger sense of 'community' and a place where people wanted to live (Simnett, 1995).

Exercise

Consider the two examples above – one which directly addresses mental health, and the other which will contribute to improved mental health through the well-being approach, as discussed in Part 2.2, Section 3, 'Defining mental health promotion: practical and philosophical approaches'.

Identify and research two projects in your practice area, one of which takes a direct approach and the other that takes a well-being approach. Note the contrasting and comparable aspects in their ways of working.

The relationships between community development, power and empowerment

The community is the focus for a wide variety of health promotion and public health initiatives. Many individually focused behaviour change programmes have community settings, which are often strongly associated with general practice or community nursing. At the other end of the spectrum, the community is linked to sustainable development, as seen in Local Agenda 21 (United Nations, 1993) and in its mantra, 'think globally, act locally'.

It is now the responsibility of local authorities to develop strategies that aim to improve economic, social and environmental well-being (www. neighbourhood.gov.uk).

Simply placing a programme in a community setting does not necessarily lead to empowerment. In 1986, the Ottawa Charter placed empowerment at the heart of health promotion through community action:

'Health promotion works through concrete and effective community action, setting priorities, making decisions, planning strategies, and implementing them to achieve better health. At the heart of this is the process of empowerment of communities, their ownership and control of their destinies.'

World Health Organisation (WHO), 1986

One of the tenets of community action is for members of the community to be involved in the process from the outset.

One of the main problems with community development is that it is often top-down rather than bottom-up; that is, approaches are imposed on communities rather than coming from them. Top-down approaches can:

- provide easier access to 'expertise'
- provide easier access to resources
- be part of a broad, planned, health-promotion policy
- be evaluated more simply
- express power of the professionals over their patients
- draw attention away from macro or structural issues

In addition, well-meaning project leaders may not think sufficiently about how to involve individuals and communities, or do not go back to basics and concern themselves with the facilitation of bottom-up or organic community initiatives; organically-situated community groups often have really good ideas, but are frequently starved of resources to put them into action.

The move from top-down programming to a bottom-up process is particularly important for health visitors and other professionals working in primary care who wish to move beyond education and awareness into more empowering forms of community practice.

Advocacy, autonomy, empowerment and mental health in relation to community development

It is clearly desirable to support the idea of empowering individuals and communities to take control of their own health; but this presents particular issues in relation to a minority of people with mental health problems (although it could be argued that these very issues are the result of the views taken by professionals working within the medical model of care).

People who are assessed as having mental health problems may find themselves in situations where they receive medical treatment compulsorily. Resorting to the law in order to treat an individual against his or her will is justified by the risk that the person is thought to pose to themselves or to others.

Their competence to guide their own treatment effectively is therefore called into question, and, at this point, even a degree of empowerment on core treatment issues becomes more difficult to achieve. However, too interventionist an approach may undermine the principle of autonomy and lead to over-paternalistic interventions. It could be argued that a paternalistic approach is widespread in mental healthcare – indeed, in healthcare in general. It may need to be consciously and consistently challenged in all professional–patient encounters, so that it becomes possible to progress towards alternative ways of structuring healthcare interactions in order to attain respectful, egalitarian, and therapeutic alliances which maximize negotiation at the expense of autocratic authority.

Dilemmas in practice

The question of whether community development is involved in radical practice or in supporting the status quo is at the root of the ambiguity surrounding practice issues. Some voluntary-sector organizations have complained that the very expression 'community development' suggests that power differentials will be prolonged – that communities are to be 'developed' along particular preconceived lines, and that the expertise that already exists within communities will not be respected.

Common dilemmas surrounding practice relate to the following:

Funding

Most community development projects are funded by statutory agencies, such as health and education; sometimes they are jointly funded, or funded from sources such as national lottery monies. Other projects might be located in the voluntary sector and be funded from a range of sources, including government grants and independent fundraising. Most community development work tends to be short-term funded only. This lack of security can lead to problems in planning and evaluating work and to difficulty in establishing an evidence base for a project. Insecure funding can also mean that the project worker spends more time and energy fundraising than working on the project.

Accountability

All community development workers, be they involved as users or professionally appointed, have a dual accountability: to their communities, and to their employers. Funders expect projects to be accountable, and conflicts can arise where the interests of the community and that of the funding agency do not coincide. The focus of the community and the community worker may also differ. For instance, safety in a neighbourhood may be identified as a priority. The worker might suggest better lighting and a common responsibility to shared areas as part of the solution, whereas the community might want increased vigilance or even the exclusion of particular groups, families or individuals – and this conflict might be exacerbated when dealing with 'unpopular' groups, including stigmatized mental health service users.

This raises the question of whether a sense of community has been undermined by contradictory trends and social forces, such as consumerism/individualism. Also, there is the issue of who or what organization has led the development of the project. Is this a project born of a professional 'blueprint' and applied to a community, or has the idea grown up 'organically' from within the community – and what differences does this make with respect to accountability?

Acceptability

Community development might be seen as taking large amounts of time and resources for unclear results, which may be diffuse and not amenable to providing demonstrable benefit on which to base future resource allocation. Community development workers may be seen as allying themselves with dissent and thus 'betraying the interests' of the organization that is funding them. (This is not, of course, a prob-

lem for an organic, independently-funded initiative – and, in general, community development workers explicitly seek links and partnerships, not conflict and opposition.)

The role of the professional

The role of the community development worker is that of catalyst and facilitator, and practice should be based on egalitarianism and shared knowledge – as distinct from any notion of the professional as 'expert'.

Evaluation

Many projects report positive feedback from communities who have been involved in work around health issues, but, because of the local scale of such work, it is not widely disseminated. A report of the Hartcliffe Health and Environment Action Group, a group based in a deprived outer city housing estate in Bristol, states:

> 'From a health education point of view, this project can be seen to be instrumental in promoting people's health. A significant number of those involved would, in all probability, never otherwise have had access to information about health, health services and the support and opportunity for personal growth which has been presented through their participation in this group.'
>
> *Roberts, 1992*

A member of the Hartcliffe group said, 'I don't feel like an outsider now'. However, these kinds of outcomes, though worthwhile, are difficult to express concisely or to quantify.

Section summary

- There has been a gradual shift in power from 'experts' to people since the 1970s
- Community and community development are complex areas to understand and are only meaningful when there is real empowerment of people in the community
- Community development workers have to break the mould, and therefore their role is based on shared knowledge and egalitarianism, a move away from the notion of 'experts'

References

Carey, P. (2002). 'Community Health and Empowerment' in Kerr, J. (ed.) *Community Health Promotion.* London: Bailliere Tindall.

Department of Health (2001e). *Making It Happen: A Guide to Developing Mental Health Promotion.* London: HMSO.

Mentality (2004). *Participation promotes mental health.* London: Sainsbury Centre for Mental Health. www.scmh.org.uk (use Search to find report title).

Naidoo, J. and Wills, J. (2000). *Health Promotion: Foundations for Practice* (second edition). London: Bailliere Tindall.

Roberts, S.E. (1992). *Healthy Participation: an Evaluative Study of the Hartcliffe Health and Environment Action Group, a Community Development Project in Bristol.* Bristol: University of the West of England (unpublished MSc dissertation).

Rogers, A. and Pilgrim, D. (1991). Pulling down churches: accounting for the British mental health users movement. *Sociology of Health and Illness,* 13 (2), 129–148.

Ross, M. (1995). *Community Organisations: Theories and Principles.* New York: Harper.

Simnett, I. (1995). *Managing Health Promotion: Developing Healthy Organisations and Communities.* Chichester: Wiley.

United Nations (1993). *Earth Summit Agenda 21: the United Nations programme of action from Rio.* New York: The United Nations Department of Public Information.

World Health Organisation (WHO) (1986). *Ottawa Charter for Health Promotion.* Geneva: WHO.

Test yourself

 To check your progress, locate this section on CD-ROM 2 and work through the interactive questions at the end.

Section 2: Voluntary-sector resources and mapping

This section is divided into five parts:

1. Current policy
2. Mapping
3. Local services
4. Information sources and resources
5. Issues in practice

Current policy

In September 2004, the Department of Health published a strategic agreement between themselves, the NHS and the voluntary and community sector (Department of Health, 2004c). This document, *Making Partnership Work For Patients, Carers and Service Users*, acknowledges the contribution and history of voluntary-sector organizations in providing services directly to the community (and to specific groups within the community), and was based on a consultation exercise carried out in 2003. It is included in PDF format on CD-ROM 2, and is available online at www.dh.gov.uk/ assetRoot/ 04/08/95/16/ 04089516.pdf.

The strategic agreement reflects the shift towards service commissioning and funding by Primary Care Trusts (PCTs) and Care Trusts. As we have already seen, part of the Modernization Agenda is to ensure that services meet the needs of patients, and, in mental health, the strategy for achieving this includes joint commissioning with local authorities. The government has acknowledged that the large number of voluntary-sector providers reflects the diversity of need.

Mapping

There is a huge number of local authority, NHS and voluntary-sector organizations offering services to people with mental health problems – and their number is ever growing. This can be extremely confusing, especially when you are trying to work out who is responsible for what, and where they are based. A useful resource is the Mental Health Service Mapping for Working Age Adults 2004 (www.dur.ac.uk/service.mapping/ amh). Notice that the mapping project is monitoring the numbers of graduate primary care mental health workers, STaR workers and carers' support workers employed. You can also access local directories from this website, and a national service directory is planned. Some areas have their own local mapping of mental health services.

Exercise

Consider the following:
*   Does your Primary Care Trust (PCT) work in partnership with local voluntary-sector organizations?
*   What is the evidence in practice?
*   Do voluntary-sector providers in your area provide services for communities previously neglected by the NHS?
*   Why have voluntary-sector organizations taken on this health need when the statutory sector has not?

The overall aim of mapping exercises is to collect data and information using different methods, and to develop an overview of patterns in a particular area. A range of stakeholders will be consulted and information gathered from them, and this will include voluntary-sector groups, users and carers.

Local services

Mental health workers in primary care can use the Primary Care Profile workbook provided in PDF format on CD-ROM 1 to note local service providers, contact numbers, and individuals who either link to their practice, or provide a service that can be accessed by the users of their practice. Using the workbook as a foundation, it may be practicable to develop a primary care practice register or resource directory, to be shared with wider primary care teams and secondary services personnel. This type of resource will need an investment of time to keep it 'live' and up-to-date. Useful organizations for accessing this type of information include the National Council for Voluntary Organisations (NCVO: www.ncvo-vol.org.uk) and the National Association of Councils for Voluntary Service (NACVS: www.nacvs.org.uk).

It may be useful to contact some of the organizations to introduce yourself, let them know about your role, and find out more about what they provide.

Types of secondary services provided to people with mental health problems

Services for people experiencing mental health problems vary across the country. The Mental Health Trusts provide services in a number of areas.
*   Community Mental Health Teams (CMHTs) are available everywhere; some teams are very small and others more developed
*   Assertive Outreach Teams (AOTs) are available almost everywhere.
*   Crisis Resolution Teams (Home Treatment Teams) are available in about half of the country
*   Inpatient care: numbers of inpatient beds have been falling steadily, though mainly in long-stay facilities
*   Outpatient and Day Hospital care
*   Separate services for children and adolescents (CAMHS), and for older people

Social care

In 2000/1, 25.1 adults per 10,000 aged 18–64 were assessed by their local authority Social Services department for their social care needs, arising from a mental health problem. In 2000/1, 37.4 per 10,000 were receiving some kind of service, mainly in the community. The overwhelming providers of these services are independent, although funding comes from local authorities.

Funding for support and accommodation services comes from the borough in which a patient lives, or in some cases the borough with which the person has a significant connection.

Historically, there is more accountability in local authorities – in that service users elect local councillors to represent their views, and people working for the local boroughs are in turn accountable to the elected representatives, and to the public. This is not the case in the NHS.

Information sources and resources

Access to high-quality information about mental health problems is a way of empowering users to manage their own condition and to increase their sense of self-esteem and confidence, and their readiness to ask questions during consultations. There is evidence (Eaton, 2002b) that one third of Europeans and half of Americans use the internet to access health information.

Some patients are reluctant to use official-looking mainstream websites, and could be vulnerable to exploitation through unofficial sites – those offering medication for sale, for example. You may therefore wish to provide patients with a list of recommended websites, or offer printed information in your practice. The American Medical Association produces guidelines for assessing a website's usefulness for patients. This is a summary of its content:

- Check the site's ownership, quality of editorial content, date of posting and updating and sources of editorial content
- Advertising should not be on the same page as information about the same topic; sponsorship should be displayed
- Is the information given factually correct?

Other issues to take into consideration are:

- Do users and carers have any input to the site?
- Are voluntary sector organisations/ communities of interest contributing to the site?
- Is the site accessible and user-friendly?
- Does the site use patronizing language, or confusing medical terminology, which would exclude users and carers?
- Does the site provide links to sources of support?

DISCERN provides an online tool for assessing the quality of health information, including printed materials and web resources, on its website, www.discern.org.uk.

The internet is also a good source of information for mental health workers, and the Primary Care Trust you are working in will subscribe to some useful databases. Some of the websites recommended in this book are run by voluntary organizations.

Issues in practice

A number of situations could arise with regard to patient information. For example, the patient knows more about their condition than the practitioner – in which case, responses might be to:

- acknowledge the patient's expertise
- suggest that there are always different ways of looking at a problem
- use the patients' expertise as a resource to find solutions to their difficulties

On occasion the patient may not want to receive information or to be involved in decision-making – in which case responses might be to:

- consider why this might be; for example, confidence, self-esteem
- explain your motivation for including the patient
- assist the patient to be part of the process, being specific about options and avoiding vague responses to questions
- ask colleagues what they think

It is also important to consider when to give information, and how much to give. Information may reassure some people and provoke anxiety in others.

Section summary

- Joint commissioning between the voluntary sector, health and social services is an essential part of the strategy to meet patients' needs
- Understanding and using mapping techniques is a useful tool to understanding service provision and resources
- Primary Care and Social Services are major providers of mental healthcare
- The internet is an increasingly important resource for empowering patients and carers

References

Department of Health (2004c). *Making Partnership Work for Patients, Carers and Service Users*. London: HMSO.

Eaton, L. (2002b). A third of Europeans and almost half of Americans use internet for health information. *British Medical Journal*, 325, 989.

North East Public Health Observatory (2004). *Occasional Paper 2: Scoping Study of Mental Health Data: Key Messages.* www.nepho.org.uk.

Useful websites

Centre for Health Information Quality: www.chic.org.uk.

Commission for Patient and Public Involvement in Health: www.cppih.org.

Communities for Health: www.communitiesforhealth.net.

Department of Health: www.dh.gov.uk.

Developing Patient Partnerships: www.dpp.org.uk.

DIPEx: Database of Individual Patient Experiences: www.dipex.org.uk.

Expert Patient Programme: www.expertpatients.nhs.uk.

Health Voice Network: www.healthvoice-uk.net.

INVOLVE: www.invo.org.uk.

MIND: www.mind.org.uk.

National Association for Patient Participation: www.napp.org.uk.

National Electronic Library for Mental Health (NeLMH): www.library.nhs.uk/mentalhealth.

Patient UK: A database of patient information materials and contact information for patient organisations and support groups: www.patient.co.uk.

Rethink: www.rethink.org.

Sainsbury Centre for Mental Health: www.scmh.org.uk.

Recommended reading

Department of Health (2004b). *Patient and Public Involvement in Health: The Evidence for Policy Implementation.* London: HMSO.

Leeder, S. and Dominello, A. (1999). Social Capital and its relevance to health and family policy. *Australian and New Zealand Journal of Public Health*, 23 (4), 424–429.

Mentality (2002). *Mental Health Improvement: What Works? A Briefing for the Scottish Executive.* Edinburgh: Scottish Development Centre for Mental Health.

Test yourself

 To check your progress, locate this section on CD-ROM 2 and work through the interactive questions at the end.

Chapter 2.4
Quality issues, leadership and change

Aim

To provide: a critical awareness of the impact of user and carer involvement on matters relating to quality in healthcare; in-depth knowledge concerning important issues related to leadership; and a critical and practical understanding of organizational change and patient involvement.

Learning outcomes

By the end of this Chapter, the reader will be able to:

- Critically discuss the possible impact of user and carer involvement on quality, with respect to education, research and service delivery
- Analyse the impact of collaborative learning models on user and carer involvement
- Critically consider the nature and purpose of leadership
- Analyse partnership working in health and social care
- Identify the role of user involvement in relation to management and leadership
- Describe styles of leadership
- Consider ways in which service users can work with leaders and managers in mental health services (a case study)
- Critically consider the importance of the background to organizational change and the factors which influence it
- Critically evaluate the thinking behind and contribution of *Change Here!*
- Analyse the impact of change on individuals and the reasons why change may be resisted by both patients and professionals

Introduction

This part of the programme is essentially about the improvement of services. The first section is concerned with quality improvement (including collaborative learning models); the second section is concerned with leadership; and Section 3 is concerned with organizational change.

Chapter 2.4 content is as follows:

1 Quality Improvement Models, including collaborative learning models
2 Leadership
3 Organizational change

Section 1: Quality improvement models, including collaborative learning models

This section is divided into three parts:
1 The impact of user and carer involvement on quality in education and research
2 The impact of user and carer involvement on quality in service delivery
3 Communities of practice

The impact of user and carer involvement on quality in education and research

The education of potential practitioners and the production of relevant research are two areas that can have profound effects on quality of care. In each of these fields, the involvement of users and carers may have important and far-reaching benefits, some of which are summarized below.

Education

- User and carer involvement in education enables students to go beyond theory and learn from those with direct service experience. This can lead to a deeper understanding for the clinician, with new insights and changed attitudes.

- User and carer involvement brings to the fore the power relations always present in care delivery. It can bring into focus the implicit roles taken on by users, carers and professionals, and allow them to be creatively challenged.
- User and carer involvement can improve communication skills, helping to lessen barriers to effective communication such as professional jargon, and can facilitate reflective practice.
- For current developments, check resources such as the Mental Health in Higher Education (MHHE) website (www.mhhe. heacademy.ac.uk/), which includes case examples of best practice in different HE institutions.

Research

- Users and carers identify and prioritize issues differently from professionals, and may question the relevance and focus of the research design. Users and carers have different perspectives, ask different questions, and look at different outcomes.
- Users and carers can help with recruitment of their peers; response rates to questionnaires may be higher; interviewees may feel more comfortable talking to a fellow service user or carer. Users and carers can help access people who may be marginalized, such as people from minority ethnic communities.
- Users and carers can help interpret and disseminate the results of research (often providing an alternative perspective to findings), and can ensure that changes that result from research projects are actually implemented.
- Users and carers can help analyse research data and interpret research findings, providing an alternative perspective and potentially adding to the richness and validity of these processes.

- Users and carers can assist in disseminating the results of research.
- Service users can inform decision-making at all stages of the research process, which can involve very grounded and practical insights into the consequences for service users of particular decision-making.
- For current developments, check resources such as the INVOLVE website (www.invo. org.uk).

The impact of user and carer involvement on quality in service delivery

Many professional groups are currently examining the ways in which users and carers may be actively involved in their care. The *British Medical Journal* (*BMJ*) devoted an issue to this – 'The Patient Issue', 14 June 2003 (vol. 326, no. 7402). Contributors to that issue include Ian Kennedy (chairman of the public inquiry into paediatric cardiac surgery carried out at the Bristol Royal Infirmary and chair of the Healthcare Commission), Liam Donaldson (Chief Medical Officer) and Angela Coulter (who has written a book about ending paternalism in medicine, *The Autonomous Patient* (2002) – reviewed in the same article of the *BMJ*).

Exercise

Review the issue, perhaps starting with the 'Comment' section and 'Good patient' sections. Does it provoke any reflections on your own practice?

The care delivered by any healthcare organization can be only as good as the people who staff it. Users and carers can be included in the selection process of staff by:

- helping to shortlist
- contributing questions or rating criteria at interview
- helping create the job specification
- being on the interview panel

In April 2004, the Department of Health published a meta-analysis of research about patient and public involvement, in which 300,000 patients were asked about their experiences in 568 English NHS Trusts. The document, *Patient and Public Involvement in Health* (Department of Health, 2004b), is included in PDF format on CD-ROM 2, and is available online at www.dh.gov.uk/assetRoot/04/08/23/34/04082334.pdf.

Although the vast majority of patients were satisfied with the care they received, people with mental health problems, especially, said they would like more information about their care. Nearly a third of people visiting GPs said they were not as involved as they would like to be in decision-making about their care and treatment (Department of Health, 2004a).

Although this report is broadly positive about patients' experiences, it contrasts with a previous Commission for Health Improvement (CHI) report, *Unpacking the Patients' Experience: Variations in the NHS patient experience in England* (CHI, 2004), which demonstrated that involvement alone did not change things – and that information, communication and engagement skills have to be employed to promote positive change.

One interesting aspect of investigating the extent of patient involvement and its impact is the attitudes of professionals to user and carer involvement. There is much variance between disciplines, and people have different reasons for resisting involvement.

The report has some useful suggestions for improving patient involvement, including a checklist of questions and comments that facilitate involvement. In addition, a consistent finding from research into the views of mental health service users (e.g. Rogers et al, 1993) is that people want quality relationships, someone to talk to, and time to talk.

Communities of practice

This describes an approach to learning where an individual becomes a part of a 'community of practice'. It involves understanding the structure of communities and how learning occurs

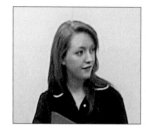

The nurse: *'I'm supportive of patient involvement, but I sometimes worry that the patient can't cope with the information I'm giving or might make the wrong decision for them.'*

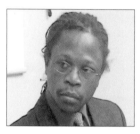

The doctor: *'I can't compromise on what I know to be the best technical decision. That seems unethical to me.'*

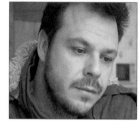

The patient: *'I need to know they are listening to me. If they're just tapping into the computer and I'm trying to say something really important to me, I just give up speaking in the end. What's the point?'*

in them; the idea was introduced by the Institute for Research on Learning, and developed by the Xerox Corporation in the United States.

'Communities of practice' are based on the following assumptions:
- Learning is a social activity, and people organize their learning around the communities they belong to.
- Knowledge is part of the life of communities that share values, languages and a belief system. Real knowledge is integrated in the doing, in social relations and in the expertise of these communities.
- The process of learning and membership of a community of practice are inseparable.
- You cannot separate knowledge from practice – you cannot learn without doing.

- Empowerment – the ability to contribute to a community – gives us potential for learning; hence, circumstances in which a person acts to try to improve or contribute to their community create the most powerful learning experience.

This approach strongly suggests that teachers are part of the community they are teaching in, and it is the 'collective intelligence' of that community that shapes services and progress. Communities of practice are also utilized in business, and there are many (mainly American) websites dedicated to different communities of practice, with the premise that knowing your market and your workforce will enhance product innovation and productivity.

Exercise

Consider the idea of communities of practice.
- How does this idea translate in primary care?

Section summary

- Users and carers can have an important influence on quality in education and research, allowing students and researchers to go beyond theory and learn from those with direct experience of services
- In research, users and carers have different perspectives and are interested in different outcomes
- Users and carers can be involved in the recruitment of staff, with the aim of recruiting user-focused staff
- Communities of practice are a useful means by which individual practitioners can reflect on and share good practice

References

British Medical Journal (2003). 'The Patient Issue', Volume 326 (14 June).

Commission for Health Improvement (CHI). (2004). *Unpacking the Patients' Experience: Variations in the NHS patient experience in England.* London: CHI.

Coulter, A. *The Autonomous Patient: Ending Paternalism in Medical Care.* London: Nuffield Trust, 2002.

Department of Health (2004a). *Patient and Public Involvement in Health: The Evidence for Policy Implementation.* London: HMSO.

Rogers, A., Pilgrim, D. and Lacey, R. (1993). *Experiencing Psychiatry: Users' Views of Services.* Basingstoke: Macmillan.

Test yourself

 To check your progress, locate this section on CD-ROM 2 and work through the interactive questions at the end.

Section 2: Leadership

This section is divided into five parts:
1 The nature and purpose of leadership
2 Partnership working as a response to demographic, cultural and organizational change
3 Service users, leadership and the new approach
4 Styles of leadership
5 Users and carers and leadership

The nature and purpose of leadership

Sofarelli and Brown (1998) argued that, in the past, no distinction was made between the terms 'manager' and 'leader'. Managers were viewed as leaders in the NHS, and this reflected the strong hierarchical nature of the organization where power and authority were determined by the position a person held in that organization. It is further argued that this lack of clarity about leadership is no longer tenable: changes taking place in the NHS have created a new environment requiring management and leadership to be separated as concepts. It has been observed that the NHS was over-managed but under-led. Furthermore, leadership would be assumed by senior clinicians without any relevant managerial training.

Sofarelli and Brown (1998) state that the difference between leaders and managers is that managers are concerned with power and control, while leaders are concerned with empowerment. The role of managers is to run organizations, while the role of leaders is to make changes.

The role of managers and leaders

Role of the manager
Create stability
Take control
Accomplish tasks
Possess authority
Hold power from their position
Plan, organize and control human and
    material resources
Enforce policy and procedures
Maintain hierarchical rule
Put the organization before people

Role of the leader
Be proactive
Have an ethical approach and sound integrity
Thrive on change
Challenge the status quo
Inspire followers
Have vision
Be willing to take risks
Value people
Develop relationships
Communicate effectively
Not hold power through position or authority
Empower others

Sofarelli and Brown

However, the arguments put forward above (although useful) fail to acknowledge the power held by particular professional groupings, especially the medical profession.

In the UK since the 1970s, an industrial model of management has been introduced to healthcare as well as to other public services (Gabe et al, 2004). Usually called New Public Management (NPM), the emphasis is on man-

agers taking control, setting performance targets and imposing budgetary and workload ceilings. In practice, this has set managers on a collision course with doctors – particularly because of doctors' claim to professional autonomy. The traditional dominance of medicine in the NHS has certainly constrained the march of NPM, but its impact on professionalism has still been significant, and the longer-term impact of such a transformation is yet to be seen.

Partnership working as a response to demographic, cultural and organizational change

Health and social care is facing a number of challenges in the 21st century that make effective leadership essential. The most important of these challenges are demographic, cultural and organizational.

Demographic change

The demographic map of the UK shows a marked trend to an older population, while at the same time there are fewer adults of working age to provide care services, either formally or informally. The real challenge is not only to provide services for a 'sicker' older population, but to ensure that the older population is a healthier population. Services will need to be organized and delivered in new and creative ways, which will require leaders who have the vision to achieve this. In mental health services, this will mean working closely with users and carers in the planning and delivery of services.

Cultural change

The general public have increasingly become discerning consumers of health and social care. The availability of advanced communication systems means that people have a much greater understanding of their physical and mental health, and their expectations of care are consequently greater than ever before. Professionals need to work in partnership with users and carers and to accept that users of services may often be better informed about their own care needs than the professionals. Leadership in this new consumer-oriented environment will be a crucial factor in helping to reorient health and social care priorities away from the service provider to the service user's needs.

Organizational change

As we have already observed, leadership in the NHS was traditionally based upon professional hierarchies and the positions held within the organization. In the 1990s, general management was used as a method to bring in a market culture, making professionals more accountable to consumers. The market-oriented health service of the 1990s led to a competitive culture far removed from the original ethos of the NHS. However, a review of the NHS following the election of the Labour Government in 1997 (Department of Health, 2000a) claimed that a return to the old order was not appropriate and a 'third way' should be envisaged. This vision was of a strong primary care base, supported by a modern secondary care service – not brought about through competition, but through collaboration and cooperation. The key to the future is seen as the development of social networks crossing agency boundaries, and of working partnerships between professionals and service users, and between health and social care.

Another major challenge is the effective management of resources. This includes the effective and efficient management of funding allocation, spending and achieving best value and high quality. It also involves ensuring sustainability (future staffing numbers) and boosting morale/motivation amongst the workforce.

Bowles and Bowles (1999) claim that effective leadership in this new context seeks collaboration and cooperation across different agencies and different professions, with the user at the centre.

Service users, leadership and the new approach

The concept of user involvement has now been promoted by the government for over two decades.

Newman and Clark (1994) argue that the consumerist developments of the 1980s and 1990s cannot necessarily be equated with a commitment to the empowerment of users and carers, and that leaders are no more likely to be committed to the objectives of the users/survivors movement than nurses and doctors.

> 'Management/Leadership has been identified as a transformational force counterpoised to each of the old modes of power. By contrast with the professional, the manager is driven by the search for efficiency rather than abstract professional standards … Unlike the politician, the manager inhabits the 'real world' of 'good business practices', not the realms of doctrinaire ideology. In each of these areas, the manager is also more 'customer-centred' than concerned with the maintenance and development of organisational empires.'
>
> *Newman and Clark, 1994, p23*

Although managerialism in the health service may indeed have had limited benefit for user involvement, it is important to remember that the explicit rebuttal of ideology often raises suspicions concerning the ideological allegiances of the author. Nothing is culture- or value-free. Criticism of an opponent's rhetoric and ideology often reveals the implicit ideology of the critic. You might wish to consider what the various ideological tensions may be in the competing discourses that engage with user involvement.

Current research suggests a gap between rhetoric and the reality of user involvement in many instances (Ham and Alberti, 2002; Pilgrim and Waldron, 1998; Milewa, 1999). Research by Rutter et al (2004) examined user involvement in the planning of adult mental health services. They carried out qualitative case studies of user involvement in two mental health provider Trusts in London. Semi-structured interviews were conducted with a variety of stakeholders (including Trust staff at all levels and user group members) to compare the expectations of diverse stakeholders and the extent to which these were being achieved. The researchers found that user involvement remained in the gift of provider managers/leaders, who retained control over decision-making and expected users to adopt Trust policy and conform to Trust management practices. Users wanted to achieve concrete changes to policies and services, but had broader aspirations to improve the status and condition of people with mental health problems – whereas leaders were unlikely to have such aspirations.

Milewa (1999) demonstrated the frustrations felt by service users when the consultation forums they belonged to were unable to get a response from managers with regard to many proposals concerning funding priorities. Milewa argues that this illustrates how difficult it is for service users to gain a voice within the health sector – because, despite the rhetoric of change, there is continuing managerial and clinical control.

Barnes and Bowl (2001) argue that such contradictions are consistent with a number of other analyses of the way in which the mentally ill are 'managed' in society, and the way in which social policies and professional and management practices (including leadership/management practices) reflect different understandings of what mental illnesses are. Clearly we need to understand how psychological distress can affect individuals, but this cannot be disentangled from the responses they receive from both lay and professional people. It could be argued that this reflects the dominant discourse within which mental illness is defined and negotiated, and in which mental health services operate.

Styles of leadership and user involvement

Four types of leadership and their relationship to user involvement will now be considered.

Transactional leadership

This is the style traditionally adopted in the NHS and is one that reflects the hierarchical nature of the organization. In this model, leadership is seen as synonymous with management; transactional leadership involves maintaining the status quo of the organization. This was well suited to the early days of the NHS, where stability was important. Through planning, organizing and controlling both human and material resources, leaders were able to achieve their primary task of accomplishing the goals of the organization. Leaders were expected to lead through possession of power and authority derived from their position. Followers responded to the leader in this scenario in terms of exchange, such as services for salary.

Transformational leadership

'Transformational leadership is a style which is ideally suited to the present climate of change, because it actively embraces and encourages innovation and change' (Sofarelli and Brown, 1998, p203). The NHS Executive (1999) also states that the argument for transformational leadership in the current climate of change is strong. This style stresses the interpersonal nature of leadership and encompasses four competencies:

1 Management of attention: This involves having a vision for the future. The leader is able to make connections, so that people can see the 'big picture' while dealing with the micro level. The leader ensures that followers have all the information required to help them work towards the shared vision, and helps them develop skills to make decisions.

2 Management of meaning: As Sofarelli and Brown (1998, p204) state: 'To be effective, a leader must fulfil many functions, but one of the most important is the management of meaning and the effective articulation of their dreams to their followers in order to inspire them to accept and be committed to the vision.'

3 Management of trust: A relationship of trust must be developed between leader and followers. To achieve this, a leader must possess integrity, be honest, be reliable and be highly visible.

4 Management of self: Leaders need to have high self-esteem and be self-aware. This will give them the confidence and ability to

encourage others, help them take risks and be willing to learn. Leaders value learning both for themselves and others, viewing mistakes as opportunities to learn.

The main strengths of transformational leadership lie in the focus on change and the empowerment of people. The leader in this model leads informally by consensus, rather than gaining power and authority by position in the organization.

Renaissance leadership

This term is used by Cook (1999) to describe a renewed interest in nursing leadership in Australia. He claims that nursing leadership has been weak in Australia, but that the present climate is one of turbulence and, from this climate, leaders are emerging. The focus of this leadership is on influencing healthcare policy. Previously, little attention has been given to the issue of power and influence beyond the boundaries of the leader/follower relationship.

Connective leadership

Cook (1999) also identifies connective leadership within the American context. This is a collaborative and persuasive way of working, with the main focus on building networks. The focus of the literature on transformational leadership tends to ignore the importance of networks in building alliances between different professional groups and service users. Studies tend to discuss leadership in relation to specific occupational groups rather than in an interdisciplinary way, and the issue of service users is ignored – or at best neglected. Leaders need to work across boundaries if they are to influence policy-making.

It is suggested that renaissance and connective styles of leadership provide a useful direction for theory to develop, but that they do not necessarily replace the need for transformational leadership. Transformational leaders will need to adopt such an outward-looking and collaborative approach to be successful in the future.

Exercise

Carefully consider the styles of leadership described above and:
- identify the types, or combination of types, of leadership that you have experienced in your professional life
- reflect on your own responses to different styles of leadership which you have experienced and critically consider why you have responded in the way you have
- consider which would be most conducive to user and carer involvement, and the reasons for your choices

Users, carers and leadership

Rutter et al (2004) developed a series of case studies to illuminate user involvement in the planning and delivery of mental health services. They provide insights into three areas:

1 models and impact of user involvement used in the study
2 perspectives on user involvement of all significant parties in the study
3 positive and negative factors influencing user involvement

Models and impact of user involvement

In both of the Trusts that Rutter and colleagues researched, it was clear that leaders/managers retained the option to consult with users or not. A senior manager stated, 'We are paid to take decisions'. Another stated, 'There may be an inability to understand why something is being offered, or to accept why something else is not. Patient power could pervert what was on offer … The art of psychiatry is to get the users to want what they need.' The research also found considerable disparity in the spread of user involvement capacity. Most areas had one or more user groups and, where there was little user activity, statutory agencies had come together to fund a user development consultant or had commissioned the voluntary sector to generate user forums.

Positive and negative factors influencing user involvement:

Positive outcomes of user involvement include:

- Campaigning against Trust plans: for example, the opposition to plans for inpatient unit re-provision (with inadequate single-sex and Intensive Treatment Unit (ITU) provision) alerted regional and local politicians. The outcome was delay to re-provision, and the building was improved with users consulted throughout.
- Refurbishing of inpatient units: users had significant impact when consulted about environment and activities.
- Contract specification and monitoring of 'hotel' services: users involved in decisions about catering, cleaning and security services.
- Policy, practice and information about women's safety: users joined with staff to design policy and advice leaflets to develop women's support services and women-only wards.
- Integration of health and social services: users involved in planning and implementing joint services.

Rutter et al (2004) concluded that Trust staff and users did cooperate to improve services, but the focus was different. Where users focused on extension of their influence over day-to-day services and wanted more control over the agenda for change, leaders and managers focused on the process of involvement and sometimes did not appear to recognize that user groups might exist for their own purposes, rather than as tools of management. In the two Trusts studied, the researchers noted that consultation rather than partnership was an apt description of 'involvement':

> 'The balance of power remains firmly with provider Trusts, and the new arrangements of forms and surveys for giving patients 'a voice' may serve to institutionalise and legitimise arrangements which do not give mental health service users the power they want.'
>
> *Rutter et al, 2004*

Stakeholders' perspectives on the objectives, limits and goals of user involvement

Common to all staff

Objectives: improved quality
Limits: user involvement should be limited

Nursing staff

Objectives: misplaced political correctness
Additional issues: added 'burden' on nurses; users' views given more credibility than nurses'; Government ignores nurses' views; objections to local users on employment panels

Leaders/managers

Objectives: support managerial function; help resist bureaucratic and financial constraints; help justify decisions
Limits: 'users are involved in everything'; lack of expertise; managers are paid to be the ones to take responsibility
Goals: inviting users to meetings seen as good practice

Users and voluntary sector

Objectives: empowerment of oppressed groups; improved self-esteem; respect for patients; promotion of citizenship and civil rights; countering stigma, social exclusion and coercive controls; desire to change services; preference given to user-identified issues rather than Trust agenda
Limits: believe they 'add value' to Trust decision-making; recognize they are more likely to be consulted about discrete, time-limited and material developments rather than policies or long-term planning
Goals: the concrete outcomes of involvement are emphasized and considered rare
Additional issues: frustrated by resistance; critical of consumer analogy, because they have no choice but to consume services

Rutter et al, 2004

Section summary

- In the modernized NHS, the nature and purpose of leadership needs to be transparent and responsive to demographic, cultural and organizational change
- Leaders need to recognize the positive outcomes that user and carer involvement can bring
- General management conflicts with doctors' claim to professional autonomy
- There is a gap between the rhetoric and the reality of user and carer involvement
- Research studies have demonstrated that some leaders or managers believe that user and carer involvement is optional

References

Barnes, M. and Bowl, R. (2001). *Taking over the Asylum: Empowerment and Mental Health.* Basingstoke: Palgrave.

Bowles, N. and Bowles, A. (1999). Transformational leadership. *Nursing Times* (Learning Curve Supplement) 3 (8), 2–5.

Cook, M. (1999). Improving care requires leadership in nursing. *Nurse Education Today*, 19 306–312.

Department of Health (2000a). *The NHS Plan: a Plan for Investment, a Plan for Reform.* London: HMSO.

Gabe, J., Bury, M. and Elston, M.A. (2004). *Key Concepts in Medical Sociology.* London: Sage.

Ham, C. and Alberti, K. (2002). The Medical Profession, the Public and the Government. *British Medical Journal*, 324, 838–842.

Milewa, T. (1999). Community participation and citizenship in British health care planning: narratives of power and involvement in the British welfare state. *Sociology of Health and Illness*, 21 (4), 445–465.

Newman, J. and Clarke, J. (1994). 'Going about our Business? The Managerialisation of Public Services', in Clarke, J., Cochrane, A. and McLaughlin, E. (eds). *Managing Social Policy.* London: Sage.

NHS Executive (1999). *Leadership for Health: the Health Authority Role.* Leeds: NHS Executive.

Pilgrim, D. and Waldron, L. (1998). User involvement in mental health service development: how far can it go? *Journal of Mental Health*, (1) 95–104.

Rutter, D., Manley, C., Weaver, T., Crawford, M. and Fulop, N. (2004). Patients or partners? Case studies of user involvement in the planning and delivery of adult mental health services in London. *Social Science and Medicine*, 58, 1973–1984.

Sofarelli, D. and Brown, D. (1998). The need for nursing leadership in uncertain times. *Journal of Nursing Leadership*, 6, 201–207.

Recommended reading

Mental Health in Higher Education (2004). Learning from experience: involving service users and carers in mental health education. Available online in PDF format at www.mhhe.heacademy.ac.uk/ docs/lfeguide/Learningfromexperience.pdf (in its entirety) or http://www.mhhe.heacademy.ac.uk/docs/lfeguide/Executivesummary.pdf (as an executive summary).

Test yourself

 To check your progress, locate this section on CD-ROM 2 and work through the interactive questions at the end.

Section 3: Organizational change

This section is divided into four parts:

1 The background to organizational change
2 The range of change factors which influence organizations
3 Organizational change and the Audit Commission report *Change Here!*
4 The impact of change and resistance to it

The background to organizational change

> 'Organisations simply must poise themselves to innovate, to change, or they risk decline and death.'
>
> *Peters, 1990, p9*

Any discussion of change in health and social care is set against a background of a service in which service users, patients and a variety of providers in both the state and independent sectors have an increasing role as stakeholders. Important factors to consider include:

- The need for negotiation in health and social care services is born out of the fact that, in a democratic society, wherever change is being implemented there will be a number of competing interests at play. The NHS offers an example of how contrasting perspectives on an important social development gave rise to competing interests. When policy is applied in an atmosphere of competition, there will always be winners and losers. As Ham (2004, p5) states: 'It is questionable whether or not such a competitive model of change management is conducive to social policy development.'

- Politics: The UK's political system, through its legislative machine and prevailing political ideologies, plays a major part in the decision-making process in our health and social services. Handy (1995, p13) states: 'Over the last ten years, this process of change has accelerated violently. Under Thatcher and Reagan greed was good ... but there is a curvilinear logic in the universe. Prosperity cannot last forever. Empires and organisations flounder. The world must be reinvented. We can now be certain only of uncertainty. And to plan for the future we must learn to think differently.'

Reference to Thatcher and Reagan shows the influence that political ideologies, electoral systems, and even personalities can exert on organizations, and the effect of politics on organizational change.

If people involved in, and in receipt of, health and social services are to feel they are partners in change rather than victims of it, then it is essential that they are able to identify and understand the factors that are driving change.

Factors that influence organizations

One mechanism traditionally used for the analysis of change factors in organizations is the political, economic, social and technological (PEST) inventory. Developed from this is the Bowman and Asch (1989) model which identifies four major environmental factors that influence organizational change.

1 Governmental influences

The Modernization Agenda in health and social care has seen a massive restructuring of services with a strong emphasis on partnership working (Department of Health, 1997). Partnership is perceived in the new, modern NHS as the means by which professional barriers are broken down and a more inclusive form of management, which includes all stakeholders.

2 Economic and demographic influences

Since the industrial revolution, shifts in population and the effect of poverty in society have had an impact on the development of society and the health of its citizens.

The relationship between poverty and population shift exerts an influence on modern policy-makers, because of the inequalities in wealth and health that have developed at regional, national and global levels (Bartley, 2004). On the basis of this argument, establishing equitable healthcare is as important as setting up services in themselves.

In the area covered by the East London and City NHS Trust, mental illness is one of the two top causes of illness, disability and preventable death. The Trust has therefore decided to invest in action to improve mental health as part of its Health Action Zone (HAZ) programme. HAZ has identified priorities for action, which include:

- improving health and reducing inequalities by focusing on mental health
- improving advocacy and interpretation services
- opening up opportunities for local people to take part in decisions about health

The work streams include community involvement, access to information and advocacy, and access to care, all of which reflect the importance placed on patient involvement in such local initiatives.

3 Organizational cultures and relationships

In an increasingly multicultural society, the mix of values, beliefs and attitudes which confront providers of health and social care is complex. Sensitivity to the cultural needs and aspirations of patients is only part of the work that needs to be undertaken to produce a system of health and social care that has the potential for creating and accommodating change. However, it is essential that health and social care organizations are able to analyse and understand the component parts of their own culture, if they are to respond to change in a way that is inclusive. Research has shown that, among some patients, consultation and participation is marginalized. They are expected to fit into the existing organizational culture of traditional mental health agencies (Lord et al, 1998). Church (1996, p39) argues that adherence to established norms within consultation exercises serves to maintain existing power differences – 'dominant professional groups maintain their position by teaching user groups codes of behaviour … which sublimate anger, for example, into non-political forms of action.'

The South West London and St George's Mental Health Trust embarked on a User Employment Project, through which barriers to the employment of service users within the service were removed by reframing experience of mental health problems as an asset to the employer (Perkins et al, 1997). Employing service users in a range of clinical posts makes it less likely that user involvement can be bypassed.

4 Technological influences

Technology has radically changed the operating environment of health and social care organizations, and has altered the expectations of consumers of health and social care. In terms of knowledge management, there are more opportunities for the sharing of acquired knowledge. The Department of Health (1997) identified changes that could be achieved through information technology:

- making patient records available when they are needed
- using the NHSnet and the internet to bring patients quicker test results, to enable on-line booking of appointments and to provide up-to-date specialist advice
- enabling accurate information about finance and performance to be available promptly
- providing knowledge about health, illness and best practice to the public through the internet and emerging public access media
- developing telemedicine to ensure specialist skills are available to all parts of the country

However, it should be noted that technology, especially medical technology, can get in the way of better service user–clinician relationships; and that many individuals do not have access to more advanced information technologies.

Organizational change

The Audit Commission aims to promote the best use of public money by helping those responsible for public services to achieve economy, efficiency and effectiveness. *Change Here!* (2001) examines organizational change in public services. The essence of the report's findings are summarized thus: 'Without knowing anything about the people who use your services, how can you begin to understand their needs? Without hearing what they want from you, how can you focus on what really matters to them? Without an accurate picture of their experience, how can you be sure that you fully understand what works and what needs fixing, especially when your contribution is part of an extended process involving other agencies as well as your own?' (Audit Commission, 2001, p64).

The Audit Commission points out that a change programme to improve public services, that does not begin and end with customers, is unlikely to deliver its full potential. User focus does not mean that all customer demands can be satisfied.

As discussed earlier, it is the role of the political

process (at both local and national level) to reconcile user expectations with the resources available to deliver them. The commission goes on:

> 'It is only by focusing on users' experience that public services can deliver improvements that are relevant and add public value. This means that successful change programmes must begin and end with an understanding of what matters to users.'
> *Audit Commission, 2001, p64*

Such aspirations may be very hard to turn into reality – but examples do exist.

Joining up services for users: a case study

Background

In 1997 the Housing Department of the London Borough of Hammersmith and Fulham found evidence of a rising demand for support for tenants with mental health problems, and of dissatisfaction with existing service provision. At the same time, housing officers were concerned about high rates of tenancy breakdown, with persistent problems of rent arrears and neighbour complaints. There was also concern from health and social services over the standard of housing being offered to mental health patients leaving hospital.

Approach

A new Mental Health and HIV Housing Team, which consulted with patient representatives, was set up, bringing together staff from a range of areas to respond more flexibly to diverse patient needs. A survey of mental health accommodation projects helped to establish a profile of patients and their needs. A hospital liaison officer was appointed to work closely with Charing Cross Hospital to meet the housing needs of inpatients, and to prevent delays in discharge. Performance indicators are now used to track improvements and fine-tune the service.

Impact

Over a three-year period, the number of new patients helped more than doubled. The weekly total benefits being paid following team intervention rose and rent arrears were reduced. Over the same period, hospital discharge referrals provided with accommodation rose from 26% to 46%. The proportion helped to return to their own homes increased from 13% to 27%. Patient surveys showed a high level of satisfaction, and feedback from housing officers indicated that they were much happier with the support they received for tenants with mental health problems.

The critical factors which led to the success of the initiative described above, were:
- keeping in touch with the changing needs of patients
- building partnerships with other agencies

Conclusion

Without actively listening to patients and feeding back information to staff and managers, services can become static and out of touch. Public services have at their disposal a number of methods for collecting feedback, including focus groups, panels and surveys. Thoroughly understanding patient experience provides the basis for setting targets and measuring the things that patients think are important. In implementing a change programme, it is necessary to keep checking that the vision makes sense to patients and resonates with what patients consider to be important.

The impact of change and resistance to it

Iles and Sutherland (2001) suggest that the NHS is characterized by three defining features:
1 range and diversity of stakeholders (including patients)
2 complex ownership and resourcing arrangements
3 professional autonomy of many staff

The NHS is a large organization employing and serving people with a wide range of talents, perspectives and passions. Its complexity is further complicated by diverse cultures and norms arising from:

Exercise

- Identify a change situation in your practice that you have witnessed, or which you might witness, and analyse the extent to which the above preconditions have been or might be met, and the strategies adopted.
- Describe a scenario involving change and consider how you, as a mental health worker, might work to facilitate patient involvement at either an individual or group level

- different socialization processes of the professions
- needs and expectations of different patient groups
- the different histories of different institutions
- local priorities, resource allocation, and performance management

Eccles (1994) suggests that, to create change successfully, eight preconditions must be met:
1 pressure for change
2 a clear and shared vision of the goal
3 effective liaison and trust between those concerned
4 the will and power to act
5 capable people with sufficient resources
6 suitable rewards and accountabilities
7 actionable first steps
8 a capacity to learn and to adapt

Assuming that the need for change is established, Taylor (1994) identified eight successful strategies:
1 goals – must be specific and measurable
2 vision – must be clear to all participants
3 organization – managers must have structures and be accountable
4 culture – must be clear communication of values
5 quality – to succeed, this must be measured against the best
6 performance management – every partici-

pant to be involved in delivering a high-quality product
7 innovation – harness creativity, do new things, do things differently
8 partnership and networks – trust and cooperation with external agencies

One major factor to be considered when examining organizational change is the history and culture of that organization (Ward, 1994). In 1992, Ashworth Hospital Authority was the subject of a major enquiry (Health Advisory Service, 1995). One of the main findings was the presence of a negative and damaging culture. A vivid picture emerged of life in a brutalizing, stagnant, closed institution. There was an oppressive subculture that persistently undermined therapeutic approaches. It was concluded that the changes that the hospital aspired to could not be achieved in the climate existing at the hospital at that time; although, interestingly, the rehabilitation centre of the hospital was remarked upon as having a distinctly different culture – and was referred to in the original Inquiry Report as 'an oasis of therapy'.

Once an organization has been able to identify such factors, the challenge is to consider how the restraining forces can be weakened to inhibit their negative effects, and conversely how the driving forces can be strengthened to increase the likelihood of successful change.

It may be argued that the example of

Key forces at Ashworth Hospital
Driving forces
Commitment to change
Additional funds
Stated values of the organization
Desire for demonstrable improvements

Restraining forces
Negative staff and patient culture
Resistance to change
Poor leadership
Inadequate funding
Poor industrial relations
Poor record of previous successful change

Ashworth is not necessarily representative of change management in general, as change was brought about as a result of scandal and external scrutiny. Indeed, within six years, the hospital was rocked by another Public Inquiry into equally shocking but different malpractices, although the initial inquiry recommendations did usher in some progressive practices (such as independent advocacy and better support for relatives). Arguably, further progress has been made since, and many caring and skilled staff work there, but it is very difficult to change culture in such institutions: a text which addresses many of these issues is Mason & Mercer (1998).

Stages of emotional response to change

Stage	Response
Denial	Unwillingness to confront reality. Hope it will go away.
Anger	'Why are you doing this to me?' Turn on those 'responsible'.
Bargaining	Attempt to negotiate. 'What if I do it this way?'
Depression	'It's hopeless, there's nothing I can do now'.
Acceptance	Come to terms with the situation. 'How am I going to move forward?'

Individuals within a large and complex organization may find change traumatic and stressful. It has been argued that such individuals' emotional response can be likened to that identified by Kubler-Ross (1969) in relation to death and dying.

Section summary

- Organizational change is profoundly influenced by a broad range of factors which include: government, economic, demographic, technology relationships and cultures
- Resistance to change arises because of the stressful nature of change itself
- There are preconditions for change, and if the need for change is established, strategies have been identified that can help to achieve this change
- The Audit Commission has stated that a change programme to improve public services that does not include consumers is unlikely to succeed

References

Audit Commission (2001). *Change Here! Managing Change to Improve Local Services.* London: Audit Commission. www.audit-commission.gov.uk.

Barnes, M. and Bowl, R. (2001). *Taking over the Asylum: empowerment and mental health.* Basingstoke: Palgrave.

Bartley, M. (2004). *Health Inequality: Theories, Concepts and Methods.* Oxford: Polity.

Bowman, C. and Asch, D. (1999). *Strategic Management.* London: Macmillan.

Church, K. (1996). Beyond 'Bad Manners': the Power Relations of Consumer Participation in Ontario's Mental Health System. *Canadian Journal of Community Mental Health,* 15 (2), 27–44.

Department of Health (1997). *The New NHS: Modern, Dependable.* London: HMSO.

Eccles, T. (1994). *Succeeding with Change: Implementing Action-Driven Strategies.* London: McGraw Hill.

Ham, C. (2004). *Health Policy in Britain* (Fifth Edition). London: Macmillan.

Handy, C. (1995). *Beyond Certainty.* London: Hutchinson.

Health Advisory Service (1995). *With Care in Mind, Secure.* London: HMSO.

Iles, V. and Sutherland, K. (2001). *Managing Change in the NHS: Organisational Change.* London: National Coordinating Centre for NHS Service Delivery and Organisation Research and Development. www.sdo.lshtm.ac.uk.

Kubler-Ross, E. (1970). *On Death and Dying.* London: Tavistock.

Lord, J., Ochoka, J., Czarny, W. and MacGillivray, H.

(1998). Analysis of change within a mental health organisation: a participatory process. *Psychiatric Rehabilitation Journal*, 21 (4), 327–329.

Mason, T. and Mercer, D. (1998). *Critical Perspectives in Forensic Care: Inside Out*. London: Macmillan.

Perkins, R., Buckfield, R. and Choy, D. (1997). Access to employment: a supported employment project to enable service users to obtain jobs within mental health teams. *Journal of Mental Health*, 6 (3), 307–318.

Peters, T. (1990). Get innovative or get dead, *California Management Review*, Fall, 9–26.

Taylor, B. (ed.) (1994). *Successful Change Strategies: Chief Executives in Action*. Hemel Hempstead: Fitzwilliam.

Ward, M. (1994). *Why your Corporate Culture Change isn't working and what to do about it*. Aldershot: Gower.

Recommended reading

Consumers in NHS Research Support Unit (2000). *Involving Consumers in Research and Development in the NHS: Briefing Notes for Researchers*. Eastleigh, Hampshire: CNHSR Support Unit.

Wykurz, G. and Kelly, D. (2002). Learning in practice – developing the role of patients as teachers: literature review. *British Medical Journal*, 325 (12 Oct), 818–821.

Test yourself

 To check your progress, locate this section on CD-ROM 2 and work through the interactive questions at the end.

Part 3
Clinical skills for primary care mental health practice

Authors: Pamela Myles and David Richards

Chapter 3.1
Common mental health problems

Aim

To develop knowledge and understanding of common mental health problems in primary care.

Learning outcomes

By the end of this Chapter, the reader will be able to:
- Recognize common mental health problems seen in primary care
- Understand the diagnostic criteria for these common mental health problems
- Identify emotional, physical, cognitive and behavioural symptoms of these problems

Introduction

The term 'common mental health problems' refers to psychological difficulties that are experienced by a significant number of the population at some time in their lives. These problems are more frequently experienced than 'serious mental health problems' such as schizophrenia and bipolar affective disorder, etc., which are far more likely to be managed in the secondary care setting, as more in-depth and longer-term treatment is likely to be required.

Eighty per cent of people who go to see a professional about their psychological difficulties will suffer from a common mental health problem such as depression or anxiety, the symptoms of which most of us are very familiar with. These types of problems are mainly treated in the primary care setting through the use of guided self-help, medication and low-intensity, evidence-based therapeutic interventions. However, in some instances, symptoms can be more severe and referral to secondary services may be required.

In this Chapter, the following disorders will be covered in some depth: depression; anxiety, including Panic Disorder, phobias, and Generalized Anxiety Disorder; stress, sleep problems and anger problems. These problems have been chosen as they are some of the most common problems encountered by mental health workers in primary care, and how to help people overcome these problems is likely, therefore, to be clinically relevant to workers based in that setting. Each problem will be described and case examples given; this will be followed through in further sections to illustrate specific evidence-based treatment strategies. Further recommended reading appears at the end of each section and in the complete reading list.

Chapter 3.1 content is as follows:

1 Depression
2 Anxiety disorders
    2a Panic disorder
    2b Phobias, including:
        Specific phobias
        Agoraphobia
        Social phobia
    2c Generalized Anxiety Disorder
3 Other difficulties
    3a Stress
    3b Sleep problems
    3c Anger problems

Section 1: Depression

Introduction

Depression is extremely common and frequently encountered in the primary care setting. Depression is differentiated from normal changes in mood by its severity, the symptoms experienced and their duration. Depression can seriously disrupt a patient's functioning and is associated with negative emotional, physical, cognitive and behavioural symptoms, sometimes with devastating consequences. Unfortunately, suicide is not an uncommon outcome of depression. Depression and schizophrenia are associated with 60% of suicides.

When someone is depressed, they typically suffer from lowering of mood, loss of interest and pleasure in previously enjoyed activities, and reduced energy levels. These are the key symptoms of depression. The patient's low mood is generally un-reactive to positive changes in circumstances and is likely to remain low throughout the course of the day, although some people find that their mood is at its lowest on waking and experience gradual improvement throughout the day, only to find that their mood is low again on waking the next day. Some people do find that they can have a temporary lift in mood to positive changes in circumstances, but these elevations in mood are generally not sustained for any great length of time. Commonly, because of this reduced pleasure, interest and energy levels, patients tend to be less active.

Depressed patients also typically experience a number of behavioural and physical symptoms including social withdrawal, disturbed sleep (especially early morning wakening), change in appetite (usually a reduction, sometimes leading to significant weight loss), reduced sex drive, fatigue, and reduced activity levels. Cognitive symptoms include lowered self-esteem, loss of confidence, feelings of helplessness, poor concentration, and negative thoughts about oneself, one's world, one's past and the future. Even in the mildest of depressions, people may experience a sense of guilt and worthlessness. Apart from lowering of mood and tearfulness, emotional symptoms often include increased irritability and anxiety.

The causes of depression can include a major life event (e.g. bereavement, relationship breakdown, losing one's job, moving house, etc.), family history of depression, childbirth, menopause, diagnosis of diseases or disability, alcohol and substance misuse, and some side-effects of medications (e.g. oral contraceptives, corticosteroids, etc.). Often depression results from exposure to multiple, minor stressors rather than to a single life event.

Prevalence

Depression is the most common mental health problem in community settings, affecting about 121 million people worldwide. Globally, depression is projected to be the second biggest cause of disability after coronary heart disease by 2020.

At the present time, depression is already the second biggest cause of disability in 15–44-year-olds. It is estimated that 5.8% of men and 9.5% of women will experience a depressive episode in a given year. The lifetime risk of experiencing a major depressive episode is approximately 12% for men and 25% for women. It has been estimated that 75% of psychiatric hospital admissions can be accounted for by depression.

Prognosis

If untreated, many people will experience short-lived symptoms and make a spontaneous recovery. For others, however, the depression may persist for six months or longer. Depressed people may experience an increasing sense of hopelessness and despair and may also be subject to suicidal thoughts. For some patients, persistent depression can lead to chronic disability.

Depression is highly treatable and, with appropriate intervention, the majority of patients will make a complete recovery. Most patients can be treated successfully for depression in the primary care setting. However, some patients may require more intensive and lengthy treatment, which is more appropriate for secondary care. Antidepressant medication and brief, structured, low-intensity interventions are effective for 60–80% of those suffering from depression and can be delivered in primary care.

Diagnostic criteria

For the diagnosis of depression to be made, the patient must exhibit certain symptoms.

Most patients will explain their symptoms to you. However, it is important to ask about associated symptoms which they might not disclose.

Key symptoms

The key symptoms that must be met for a diagnosis of depression and determining its degree of severity are:
- Persistent sadness or low mood; and/or
- Loss of interests or pleasure
- Fatigue or low energy

At least one of these, most days, most of the time for at least two weeks.

If any of these key symptoms are present, ask about associated symptoms:
- Disturbed sleep (initial, middle or late insomnia; sometimes increased sleep)
- Poor or increased appetite
- Poor concentration or indecisiveness
- Agitation or slowing of movements
- Decreased libido
- Low self-confidence
- Suicidal thoughts or acts
- Guilt or self-blame

Number of symptoms
4 = Mild
5–6 = Moderate
≥7 = Severe

Then ask about past, family history, employment, associated disability and availability of social support. A patient may have a past history of depressive episodes or a strong family history of depression. Lack of a job outside the home, concurrent physical or psychological problems and lack of confiding and supportive relationships have also been found to be vulnerability factors for depression; therefore, it is important to ask patients about these.

For more detailed information on diagnosis, see ICD-10 (International Classification of Diseases) or DSM-IV-TR (Diagnostic and Statistical Manual of Mental Disorders).

Depression checklist

		Yes
A	Low mood/sadness	☐
B	Loss of interest and pleasure	☐
C	Decreased energy and/or increased fatigue	☐

If YES to any of the above, continue below

1	Sleep disturbance Difficulty falling asleep Early morning wakening	☐
2	Appetite disturbance Appetite loss Appetite increase	☐
3	Concentration difficulties	☐
4	Psychomotor disturbance or agitation	☐
5	Decreased libido	☐
6	Loss of self-confidence or self-esteem	☐
7	Thoughts of death or suicide	☐
8	Feelings of guilt	☐

Summing up
Positive to A, B or C and at least four positive from 1–8, all occurring most of the time for two weeks or more. Indication of depression

Reference
World Health Organisation (2000). *WHO Guide to Mental Health in Primary Care*. The Royal Society of Medicine Press Limited. Reproduced with permission.

Depression checklist

The Depression checklist (see Box; the Checklist is also included in PDF format on CD-ROM 3) can also be used as a handy tool for diagnosing and measuring depressive symptoms.

Degrees of severity

A depressive episode may be classified as mild, moderate or severe, depending on the number and severity of symptoms experienced. See

Diagnostic criteria (above) for further description.

- In mild depression, the patient will have some symptoms of depression and they will need to make an extra effort to do the things they need to do. Mild depression usually results in only slight impairment to occupational and social functioning (e.g. feelings of sadness, reduced motivation).

- In moderate depression, the patient will have some occupational and social impairment which is somewhere between that seen in either mild or severe depression. The patient will have many symptoms of depression that are likely to keep them from doing the things they need to do (e.g. reduced energy levels, early morning wakening).

- In severe depression, the patient will have marked impairment to occupational and social functioning. The patient will have nearly all the symptoms of depression and it will almost always keep the patient from doing regular daily activities (e.g. feeling unable to go to work, social withdrawal). Somatic symptoms are also commonly present in severe depression (e.g. extreme fatigue, muscle pains). Severe depression can be associated with a vegetative state, which will result in the person being unable to engage in therapeutic work.

The risk of suicide

Suicide is among the top ten causes of death in every country. The lifetime risk of suicide in people with mood disorders (mainly depression) is 6–15%. If a person sees themselves as worthless, as a burden to others, and believes that there is no hope of their circumstances ever changing, then suicide can be a major risk factor. Even mildly depressed individuals can commit suicide if they feel hopeless about the future. If you suspect a patient could be hopeless or suicidal then you must discuss this with their GP as a matter of urgency. How to assess suicidal risk and what action should be taken will be discussed later in Part 3.3.

Psychosocial assessment of depression

In addition to the diagnostic symptoms, patients with depression report a wide range of disturbance. As well as confirming diagnosis using the diagnostic checklist, it is helpful to group symptoms into four areas and identify the connections between these symptom areas. This information can then be used to help guide treatment. These four areas are emotional, physical, cognitive and behavioural symptoms, and are shown on page 142, with diagnostic criteria symptoms highlighted in bold.

A simple model can be used to demonstrate the connections between these four symptom areas. This model (Figure 6; see page 143) can be used in two ways: as a summary of the problems faced by the patient; and to analyse in detail a specific time when the patient's mood has been affected. This model can be shared with patients to help them understand their problems, the connection between symptoms, and to help guide appropriate treatment.

Note: The symptom grouping is taken from *Depression: management of depression in primary and secondary care*, published by the National Institute for Health and Clinical Excellence (NICE) and the *Enhanced Services Specification for depression under the new GP contract* published by the National Institute for Mental Health in England (NIMHE) North West Development Centre (2004). Both these documents are included in PDF format on CD-ROM 3, and are available online at www.nice. org.uk/download.aspx?o=236667 &template=download.aspx (the NICE guideline) and kc.nimhe.org.uk/upload/nGMS1.pdf (the Enhanced Services Specification).

NICE guidelines

The National Institute for Health and Clinical Excellence (NICE) suggests the following overall treatment plan:

Emotional, physical, cognitive and behavioural symptoms of Depression

Emotional symptoms	**Low mood** **sadness** Variation of mood over the day (it is often worse in the morning, and improves as the day goes on – but the pattern can be the other way around) Feelings of anxiety Tearfulness for no reason Irritability
Physical symptoms	**Disturbed sleep**, usually waking early in the morning and being unable to get back to sleep **Lack of energy** **Fatigue** **Loss of appetite or overeating** **Reduced desire for sex** **Agitation**
Cognitive symptoms	**Loss of interest** **Lack of pleasure** **Poor concentration** Negative thinking **Indecisiveness** Forgetfulness Negative thoughts about the future **Feelings of guilt and self-blame** Loss of identity **Low self-esteem** Feelings of hopelessness and despair Unrealistic sense of failure Feelings of loneliness, even when amongst people **Loss of confidence** Feelings of worthlessness Loss of motivation Brooding over the past **Suicidal thoughts**
Behavioural symptoms	**Slowing of movement** Reduced activity Social withdrawal Loss of routine Feeling slowed down Decreased productivity **Suicidal acts**

1   Factors that favour general advice and watchful waiting:
   • Four or fewer of the diagnostic symptoms
   • No past or family history
   • Social support available
   • Symptoms intermittent or less than two weeks duration
   • Not actively suicidal
   • Little associated disability

Revisiting Nigel

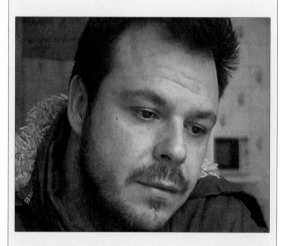

Nigel was introduced in Parts 1 and 2. He is a 45-year-old man, recently separated from his wife. He presents with low mood and reduced energy. His GP has recommended that he commence antidepressant medication, but Nigel is reluctant to do so as he believes that 'taking tablets means that I am weak and a failure'.

Nigel usually enjoys his job as a clerical officer at the local county council, but has been struggling more recently. He has been on sick leave for the past three weeks and is anxious about his return to work

 CD-ROM 3 includes three video clips, showing Nigel as he introduces himself, as he visits Dr Rushforth, his GP, and as he reflects on the meeting. Transcripts of the clips follow.

NICE guidelines continue on opposite page.

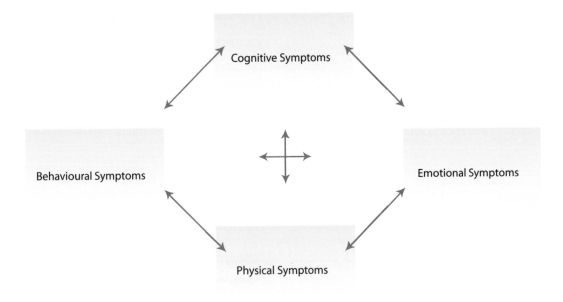

Figure 6: The connections between symptom areas

2 Factors that favour more active treatment in primary care:
- Five or more symptoms
- Past history or family history of depression
- Low social support
- Suicidal thoughts
- Associated social disability

3 Factors that favour referral to a mental health professional:
- Poor or incomplete response to two interventions
- Recurrent episode within one year
- Patient or relatives request referral
- Self neglect

4. Factors that favour urgent referral to a psychiatrist:
- Actively suicidal ideas or plans
- Psychotic symptoms
- Severe agitation accompanying severe (more than 10) symptoms
- Severe self neglect

The treatment of depression will be covered in depth in Part 3.4.

Video: Introducing Nigel (Depression)

Nigel: I haven't been feeling very good since Jenny, my wife, left me for another man. I think I caused all that, I never took her out or anything. I never told her how nice she looked, and she did look nice. No wonder someone else fancied her, and she went off at the first opportunity. They were together for years and I didn't even notice. Now I can't stop thinking about it, I can't get it out of my head. I know it's all my fault, what I deserved, but now I can't eat or sleep properly. I haven't been able to concentrate at work, so I've been on the sick now for the past three weeks. That's bothering me too, because I'm never off, and I'm worried about what my colleagues think of me, but to be honest I just can't face it right now. I'm waking up about 4 o'clock every morning and I find it impossible to get back to sleep. I'm so exhausted during the day that I can't be bothered to do anything, never mind drag myself into work. When I was there, I didn't seem to be able to do very much anyway. I sometimes wonder whether I'd be better off dead to be honest, but I wouldn't do anything, I couldn't do it to the kids. I should be able to handle this. I can't even tell Jenny I've been diagnosed with depression. What would she think of me? She'd see me as pathetic and weak for sure. I'm going to see Dr Rushforth today. She's really nice but I just can't imagine why she wants to bother with me.

Revisiting Sarah

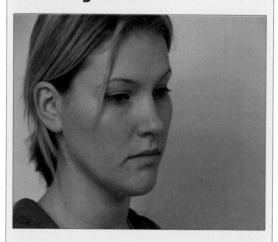

Sarah was introduced in Book 1. Age 24, she has been feeling increasingly depressed over the last three months since she lost her job as a secretary. Her mood is low and she is tearful a good deal of the time. She has done little to find another job and, despite her flatmate's encouragement, her social life is now non-existent.

She is very negative about the future, finding it difficult to see herself getting another job. She has recently started having thoughts of suicide but has dismissed these so far.

 A video clip in which Sarah introduces herself is included on CD-ROM 3, and a transcript of the clip follows.

Exercise

Watch the video clip about Nigel, or read the transcript.

- Using the Emotional, Physical, Cognitive and Behavioural Symptoms of Depression list, consider which of the symptoms in the list Nigel presents with.
- Then use the model on page 143 as a guide to help you demonstrate these links in a diagrammatic form.

Video: Introducing Sarah (Depression)

Sarah: I've been feeling more and more down over the past three months or so. It all started when I lost my job at Myles and Kelly Builders. I really liked my job, it was a good laugh and the work was easy. I know it probably sounds stupid, but I can't stop crying about it. Sometimes I just start crying and don't even know why. I haven't done anything about getting another job just yet, I haven't been able to face it.

Now I just sit around all day doing nothing apart from drinking tea and watching telly. I just don't feel up to doing anything. I feel really guilty about it. I'm just so tired though, I think that's why I can't be bothered. I'm not sleeping well either. I'm waking up really early, and I just can't get back to sleep.

Karen, my flatmate, she's been really great about it, but it's not fair that she's having to do everything. She tried to drag me out the other night, she's always doing that, but I can't face going out any more. God, I can't even face eating half the time, never mind going on a night out.

I can't see how things are going to get any better. Dr Mehra has put me on some tablets which he reckons might help. I'm going to give them a go. Let's hope they help. He's also asked me to see a mental health worker at the practice. I think he thinks I could do with someone to talk to. I think I might find that helpful.

Exercise

Watch the video clip about Sarah, or read the transcript.
- Using the Emotional, Physical, Cognitive and Behavioural Symptoms of Depression list, consider which of the symptoms in the list Sarah presents with.
- Then use the model on page 143 as a guide to help you demonstrate these links in a diagrammatic form.

Section summary

- Depression is extremely common
- When someone is depressed, they experience a range of varying emotional, physical, cognitive and behavioural symptoms
- Suicidal intent should be dealt with immediately
- Depression tends to be related to loss, whether perceived or real
- ICD-10 and DSM-IV-TR illustrate the diagnostic criteria to be met to warrant a diagnosis of depression

References

American Psychiatric Association (2000). *Diagnostic and Statistical Manual of Mental Disorders: DSM-IV-TR: Fourth Edition Text Revision*. Washington DC: American Psychiatric Association. www.psych.org.

National Institute for Health and Clinical Excellence (2004a). *Depression: Management of depression in primary and secondary care*. London: National Institute for Health and Clinical Excellence. www.nice.org.uk.

National Institute for Mental Health in England North West Development Centre (2004). *Enhanced Services Specification for depression under the new GP contract*. Hyde, Cheshire:

NIMHE North West Development Centre.

World Health Organisation (1994). *ICD-10 International Statistical Classification of Diseases and Related Health Problems*. Geneva: World Health Organisation. www.who.int.

World Health Organisation (2000). *WHO Guide to Mental Health in Primary Care*. London: The Royal Society of Medicine Press Ltd.

Recommended reading

Burns, D.D. (2005). *Feeling Good. The New Mood Therapy (Third Edition)*. New York: Penguin.

Gilbert, P. (2000). *Overcoming Depression. A self-help guide using Cognitive Behavioural Techniques*. London: Robinson.

Greenberger, D. and Padesky, C.A. (1995). *Mind Over Mood, A Cognitive Therapy Treatment Manual for Clients*. London: Guilford Press.

Simon, G.E. and Von Korff, M. (1995). Recognition and management of depression in primary care. *Archives of Family Medicine*, 4, 99–105.

Williams, C.J. (2001). *Overcoming Depression: A Five Areas Approach*. London: Arnold.

Test yourself

 To check your progress, locate this section on CD-ROM 3 and work through the interactive questions at the end.

Section 2: Anxiety

Introduction

Everyone knows what it feels like to be anxious, whether it be the way our hearts pound when we perceive that we are facing a potentially dangerous situation or it's the butterflies experienced on a first date. It is a normal emotion to experience in certain instances and a necessary part of day-to-day life, acting as a basic survival mechanism. The anxiety response is commonly known as 'fight or flight', which refers to the physical and emotional response to real or perceived danger. The body is preparing itself either to tackle the focus of the danger or to run away from it. There are many situations that

Anxiety checklist

Yes

A **Feeling tense or anxious?** ☐
B **Worrying a lot about things?** ☐

If **YES** to any of the above, continue below
1 **Symptoms of arousal and anxiety?** ☐
2 **Experiences intense or sudden fear unexpectedly or for no apparent reason:**

Fear of dying	☐	Feeling dizzy, lightheaded or faint	☐
Fear of losing control	☐	Numbness or tingling sensations	☐
Pounding heart	☐	Feelings of unreality	☐
Sweating	☐	Chest pains or difficulty breathing	☐
Nausea	☐	Trembling or shaking	☐

3 **Experiences fear/anxiety in specific situations:**

Leaving familiar places ☐
Travelling alone, e.g. train, car, plane ☐
Crowds, confined places/public places ☐

4 **Experiences fear/anxiety in social situations:**

Speaking in front of others ☐
Social events ☐
Eating in front of others ☐
Worrying a lot about what others think, ☐
or being self-consciousness

Summing up

Positive to A, B and 1, recurring regularly, and negative to 2, 3 and 4: **Indication of Generalized Anxiety Disorder**
Positive to 1 and 2: **Indication of Panic Disorder**
Positive to 1 and 3: **Indication of Agoraphobia**
Positive to 1 and 4: **Indication of Social Phobia**

Reference

World Health Organisation (2000). *WHO Guide to Mental Health in Primary Care*. The Royal Society of Medicine Press. Reproduced with permission.

come up on a day-to-day basis in which it is both appropriate and reasonable to experience some degree of anxiety. If someone is anticipating an experience that has some level of risk or potential danger, then it is realistic to feel anxious about the potential harm that could come about. However, for some people anxiety may occur to such a degree as to cause distress to the person. Usually, this is when it happens too frequently (e.g. when someone gets anxious when not faced with real danger), it is too intense (e.g. leading to panic attacks), or it lasts too long (e.g. going on longer than the stressful situation triggering the anxiety). Therefore anxiety, whilst normal and necessary for our survival, is unhelpful and debilitating when it is too frequent, too intense or of excessive duration. Such circumstances would be considered to be indicative of an anxiety disorder.

Fight or flight

The 'fight or flight' response is a fundamental physiological reaction which is the body's primitive, automatic, inborn response that prepares the body to 'confront' or 'run away' from perceived attack, harm or threat, to make survival possible. This reaction is related to an area of the brain called the hypothalamus which, when stimulated, triggers a sequence of nerve cells and chemical releases that prepare the body for fighting or fleeing. It is these nerve cells and chemical releases which cause the body to undergo a series of dramatic changes. Respiratory rate increases and blood is directed away from the digestive tract and rerouted into the major muscle groups and limbs because extra energy and fuel are needed for fighting or running away. Pupils dilate and sight sharpens as the person scans the environment for the 'enemy', awareness intensifies, reactions quicken, and perception of pain reduces. In effect, the person is getting prepared, both physically and psychologically, for fight or flight.

When in a state of fight or flight, everything in the environment is perceived as a possible threat to survival. While in this state of alertness, a person will perceive almost everything in their world as a potential threat and be on the look-out for every possible danger, while narrowing focus on things that are potentially harmful.

Anxiety disorders

A number of anxiety disorders are covered in this section, each with their own distinct features, namely: Panic Disorder; phobias, including Specific Phobias, Agoraphobia with and without Panic, and Social Phobia; and Generalized Anxiety Disorder.

In Panic Disorder, the predominant problem is recurrent panic attacks which can occur in almost any situation. In Specific Phobias, the predominant problem is anxiety confined to a single feared object or situation (e.g. spiders, heights, flying, etc.). In Agoraphobia, the predominant problem is anxiety related to being far from perceived safety and can be related to a number of situations, namely crowded areas, supermarkets, public transport, etc. In Social Phobia, the predominant problem is fear of negative evaluation, criticism and rejection by others, and is particularly focused on social situations (e.g. speaking, eating, drinking and writing in public). In Generalized Anxiety Disorder, the predominant problem is excessive and unrealistic anxiety and worry about various life circumstances and not related to anticipation of panic attacks.

NICE guidelines

The National Institute for Health and Clinical Excellence has published guidelines for the management of anxiety. *Management of anxiety (panic disorder, with or without agoraphobia, and generalized anxiety disorder)* (NICE, 2004b) is included in PDF format on CD-ROM 3, and is available online at www.nice.org. uk/guidance/CG22#documents.

The boxes offer a handy reference for the predominant problems for each anxiety disorder, and a checklist for diagnosing and measuring anxiety symptoms. The checklist is also included in PDF format on CD-ROM 3.

Anxiety disorders and their predominant problems	
Panic Disorder	Recurrent panic attacks which can occur in almost any situation with few symptoms of anxiety between attacks
Specific Phobia	Anxiety confined to a single feared object or situation (e.g. spiders, heights, flying, etc.)
Agoraphobia	Anxiety associated with being far from perceived safety and can be related to a number of situations, namely crowded areas, supermarkets, public transport, etc.
Social Phobia	Fear of negative evaluation, criticism and rejection by others and is particularly focused on social situations (e.g. speaking, eating, drinking and writing in public)
Generalized Anxiety Disorder	Excessive and unrealistic anxiety and worry about various life circumstances and not related to the expectation of panic attacks

References

National Institute for Health and Clinical Excellence (2004b). *Anxiety: Management of anxiety (panic disorder, with or without agoraphobia, and generalized anxiety disorder) in adults in primary, secondary and community care.* London: National Institute for Health and Clinical Excellence. www.nice.org.uk.

World Health Organisation (2000). *WHO Guide to Mental Health in Primary Care.* London: The Royal Society of Medicine Press Ltd.

Recommended reading

American Psychiatric Association (2000). *Diagnostic and Statistical Manual of Mental Disorders: DSM-IV-TR: Fourth Edition Text Revision.* Washington DC: American Psychiatric Association. www.psych.org.

Wells, A. (1997). *Cognitive Therapy of Anxiety Disorders. A Practice Manual and Conceptual Guide.* Chichester: John Wiley & Sons.

World Health Organisation (1994). *ICD-10 International Statistical Classification of Diseases and Related Health Problems.* Geneva: World Health Organisation. www.who.int.

Section 2a: Panic Disorder

Introduction

The main feature of Panic Disorder is recurrent and severe attacks of panic, which do not occur in response to exposure to specific objects or situations as in phobias, and which, therefore, seem unpredictable. Panic attacks start suddenly, are extremely distressing, and last for several minutes, sometimes longer. However, if a patient states that they 'panicked all day' they are usually describing feeling very anxious all day rather than describing a panic attack.

In panic attacks, bodily symptoms are misinterpreted in a catastrophic way. For example, the feeling of lightheadedness could be interpreted as a sign of imminent collapse, increased heart rate as the start of a heart attack, breathlessness as suffocation, racing thoughts as going mad and so on. The initial trigger of the panic can be an internal cue (e.g. a thought, image or bodily sensation), or an external cue (e.g. a crowded shop), which is perceived as threatening.

An internal or external cue which is considered to be threatening will result in anxiety with associated physical symptoms. If these symptoms are then misinterpreted as being catastrophic then the anxiety increases, and this continues in a vicious circle with the symptoms continuing to escalate, until the person has a panic attack.

Panic attacks are not restricted to specific or predictable situations, but can occur at any time and are commonly followed by persistent concern about future panic attacks.

Prevalence

About 20% of adults will experience at least one panic attack in their lifetime. In any one year, about 2% of the population will experience panic attacks of a frequent enough nature to meet diagnostic criteria for Panic Disorder. Panic Disorder is more frequent in women.

Prognosis

If left untreated, panic attacks can occur several times a week, or even daily. Panic Disorder can continue for years and may ultimately lead to Agoraphobia. If this is the case, there may be periods of partial or complete remission. Panic Disorder is highly treatable and has been found to respond particularly well to psycho-education and Cognitive Behavioural Therapy (CBT) approaches.

Diagnostic criteria

For the diagnosis of Panic Disorder to be made, the patient must exhibit certain symptoms. The patient will have experienced several panic attacks within a one-month period. These attacks:

- Occurred in circumstances where there is no real danger
- Were not just confined to known or predictable situations (otherwise, see Specific Phobias or Social Phobia)
- There were few symptoms of anxiety between panic attacks (although anxiety in anticipation of further panic attacks is common)
- Did not occur as a result of physical exertion, a general medical condition (e.g. hyperthyroidism) or substance use (e.g. drugs of abuse, medication)

For more detailed information on diagnosis see ICD-10 (International Classification of Diseases) or DSM-IV-TR (Diagnostic and Statistical Manual of Mental Disorders).

Emotional, physical, cognitive and behavioural symptoms of Panic Disorder

Emotional symptoms	Anxiety Panic
Physical symptoms	Palpitations Hyperventilation Tingling Trembling or shaking Sweating Shortness of breath Dizziness Lightheadedness Choking or smothering feeling Feeling faint Hot or cold flushes Dry mouth Nausea Muscle tension Blurred vision Chest pain
Cognitive symptoms	Fear of some catastrophe occurring (e.g. heart attack, collapsing, fainting, going mad, dying, losing control) Perception of oneself or of the environment as unreal Urge to escape Difficulty gathering thoughts Preoccupation with thoughts about future panic attacks
Behavioural symptoms	Escape from situations when experiencing panic symptoms Safety behaviours Avoidance of places where panic attacks have occurred

Maintenance factors

Once the panic cycle is established, three key factors act to maintain the problem: selective attention, avoidance and safety behaviours.

Exercise

For the next two or three minutes focus your attention on your left hand. Do not move it, just concentrate on what sensations you experience during the exercise. You can close your eyes to help you concentrate, or you may want to look at your hand during the exercise. When the time has elapsed, answer the following questions:

- Did you experience any of the following symptoms: heaviness, warmth, tingling, shakiness, other, nothing?
- Were you aware of any of the sensations prior to the exercise?

If you experienced any sensations during this exercise that you had not noticed before, then this highlights how selective attention works. If you experienced no sensations, then try the exercise again but for a little longer this time. Try focusing on another part of your body as well (e.g. your feet, eyes, etc.) and see what happens.

1 Selective attention

Because the symptoms are so frightening, the person may start to look out for them. This hypervigilant behaviour is called 'selective attention', which means that bodily changes, which most other people would probably not even notice, are detected and accepted as further evidence that something is seriously wrong.

2 Avoidance

A person with panic attacks will often try to avoid the circumstances that tend to trigger anxiety symptoms. Therefore, specific situations may be avoided (e.g. supermarkets; rush-hour traffic) or even certain activities (e.g. strenuous exercise). These avoidance behaviours help to maintain the problem, as the person never has the chance to find out that anxiety in these situations does not lead to the catastrophe they dread. Panic attacks can sometimes lead to agoraphobic avoidance of situations where escape may be difficult or help may not immediately be at hand. Therefore, Panic Disorder can be classified as being with or without Agoraphobia.

3 Safety behaviours

Safety behaviours refer to what a person does to stop the feared catastrophe from happening. The problem with these behaviours is that they prevent the person from discovering what will happen naturally. More often than not the outcome would not be catastrophic. For example, a woman in a busy shopping centre experiences lightheadedness and thinks that she had better sit down or otherwise she will faint. Once she has sat down, she feels some relief and the symptoms start to pass, and – crucially – she does not faint. She may then erroneously believe, 'If I hadn't sat down at that moment I would have fainted'. Once this type of thinking is established, she is likely to repeat the behaviour of sitting down every time she feels lightheaded. She is therefore unlikely to face up to her symptoms, and so does not discover that anxiety does not result in fainting or indeed any other kind of physical disaster.

In some instances, safety behaviours can actually make symptoms worse. For example, someone who tries to control their breathing by taking deep breaths can actually end up hyperventilating as a result, which serves to intensify bodily symptoms of panic.

Therefore, safety behaviours help to maintain panic symptoms in two important ways: by stopping the person ever finding out that what they fear will not in fact happen; and some safety behaviours can actually make symptoms worse.

What if the catastrophe has actually happened?

Be prepared for patients occasionally telling you that the feared catastrophe has actually occurred (e.g. the patient has fainted). This kind of information should be assessed in

Meet Alison

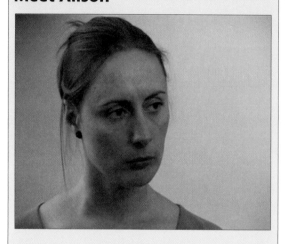

Alison is a 31-year-old single mother who works at a local travel agents. She developed panic attacks five months ago, which tend to occur when she is in crowded places or in shops where she believes there is no quick exit. Recently she has had a couple of panic attacks at work and is finding it increasingly difficult to go there. When she is having a panic attack, she believes that she is about to have a heart attack, which is extremely distressing for her. Her main physiological symptoms are racing heart, shortness of breath, tingling down her left arm and chest pain. She is becoming increasingly pre-occupied with concerns of future panic attacks. Alison's father died suddenly last year from a heart attack. She was very close to her father and initially had difficulty coming to terms with his death. Her mother lives nearby. They have a close relationship. Her daughter Chloe is six years old and doing well at school.

 A video clip in which Alison introduces herself and discusses her panic attacks is included on CD-ROM 3, and a transcript of the clipfollows.

depth. Some patients who have fainted on occasions may have fainted in a different context and may be confusing some of the symptoms of panic with the symptoms of fainting. It is highly unlikely that the patient will have fainted during a panic attack. For someone to faint, they must first experience a sharp drop in blood pressure. During a panic attack blood pressure rises. Therefore, the two states are incompatible. It can be useful to compare and contrast the symptoms of fainting and of panic attacks to acknowledge the similarities (e.g. feeling lightheaded), but also to highlight the differences (e.g. feeling sleepy when about to faint and feeling a sense of heightened alertness during a panic attack).

Note: There is one exception to the fainting rule. Although the normal physiological response to anxiety is for blood pressure to rise, people with blood/injury phobia also experience a rapid drop in blood pressure. Consequently, patients with blood/injury phobias will faint on the sight of blood.

Psychosocial assessment of Panic Disorder

In addition to the diagnostic symptoms, patients with Panic Disorder can report a wide range of disturbance. As well as confirming diagnosis using the diagnostic criteria from ICD-10 or DSM-IV-TR, it is helpful to group symptoms into four areas and identify the connections between these symptom areas. This information can then be used to help guide treatment. The model presented on page 143 can be used to help us understand the connections between symptoms presented by a client with Panic Disorder. These four areas are emotional, physical, cognitive and behavioural symptoms.

Video: Introducing Alison (Panic Disorder)

Alison: I've been having these panic attacks. It's really getting me down, it's a huge problem for me. They used to just happen in the shops. They're really bothering me, now they're happening at work as well, and my

daughter Chloe, if we're in the shops and it happens, I need to get out and she doesn't understand.

So I went to the doctors. I spoke to the doctor about it, she says it's panic attacks. I'm not so sure. My father, he had a heart attack, and the symptoms that I get are the same as the symptoms he had. I get shortness of breath, I get tingling in my arm, my heart's pounding, I've got pains in my chest. I think it could be a heart attack. When it happens, if I'm in Sainsbury's, I just have to grab Chloe and I have to get out and she doesn't understand that. She gets upset about it. I can't use Sainsbury's any more because it's too scary, as soon as I get near there, I feel like I'm going to have one of these attacks, one of these panic attacks. So I'm going to Tesco, it's further afield and it's a real pain.

Sometimes when it happens, if I dig my nails into my hands, then I can make it go away. It works occasionally but it doesn't work all the time.

The doctor, she says she's going to get my heart checked out, so she must think that it might be a problem with my heart, and what with what happened with my father and everything, I think it probably is. She's also said, though, that I should see a mental health worker, and I'm going to do that next week.

Exercise

Watch the video clip about Alison, or read the transcript.
- Using the Emotional, Physical, Cognitive and Behavioural Symptoms of Panic Disorder list, consider which of the symptoms in the list Alison presents with.
- Then use the model on page 143 as a guide to help you demonstrate these links in a diagrammatic form

Section summary

- The trigger for a panic attack can be internal or external
- Once the panic cycle is established, three key factors act to maintain the problem (selective attention, avoidance, and safety behaviours)
- If left untreated, Panic Disorder can continue for years and may ultimately lead to Agoraphobia

References

American Psychiatric Association (2000). *Diagnostic and Statistical Manual of Mental Disorders: DSM-IV-TR: Fourth Edition Text Revision.* Washington DC: American Psychiatric Association. www.psych.org.

World Health Organisation (1994). *ICD-10 International Statistical Classification of Diseases and Related Health Problems.* Geneva: World Health Organisation. www.who.int.

Recommended reading

Clark, D.M. (1986). A cognitive model of panic. *Behaviour Research and Therapy,* 24, 461–470.

National Institute for Health and Clinical Excellence (2004b). *Anxiety: Management of anxiety (panic disorder, with or without agoraphobia, and generalised anxiety disorder) in adults in primary, secondary and community care.* London: National Institute for Health and Clinical Excellence. www.nice.org.uk.

Silove, D. and Manicavasagar, V. (2000). *Overcoming Panic. A self-help guide using Cognitive Behavioural Techniques.* London: Robinson.

Wells, A. (1997). *Cognitive Therapy of Anxiety Disorders. A Practice Manual and Conceptual Guide.* John Wiley & Sons: Chichester.

Test yourself

 To check your progress, locate this section on CD-ROM 3 and work through the interactive questions at the end.

Section 2b: Phobias

Introduction

Phobias are extremely common; you might even have one yourself. To other people who don't have the same phobia, they can seem strange and difficult to understand, but to the sufferer they can cause extreme distress. Phobias are irrational fears of particular objects or situations (e.g. spiders, heights, flying, being far away from home). It is often not clear why someone has developed a fear; however, we do know what helps maintain the problem, which is mainly avoidance. Avoiding the feared object or situation gives immediate relief, but in the long term avoidance merely helps to keep the phobia going and ultimately increases the fear. To break the cycle of fear and avoidance it is crucial for the person to gradually learn to face their fears.

We all have an in-built mechanism to cope with fear, which is vital to our survival. It is something we are all familiar with. When we feel in danger or under threat, our hearts beat fast, our mouths go dry and we do our utmost to get out of that situation as quickly as we can. This feeling is anxiety and is completely normal. It is known as the fight or flight response. Basically, our bodies are preparing to fight, or to run away from whatever is frightening us. Without it, we would have no way of knowing whether we were in danger or not.

Patients with phobias will experience severe anxiety when faced with the focus of their fears, and will attempt to avoid the objects or situations which trigger the anxiety. Unfortunately, this avoidance only serves to make the phobia worse as the patient never learns that there is nothing to fear. It can result in the person's life being completely dominated by what they have to do to avoid coming into contact with triggers of their anxiety.

Patients with phobias are usually only too aware that they are in no real danger and may even feel embarrassed for having their fear, but they feel helpless to do anything about it.

There are three main categories of phobias: Specific Phobias; Agoraphobia; Social Phobia.

Specific Phobias

Specific Phobias are irrational fears of highly specific objects or situations, such as heights, certain animals, birds or insects, flying, enclosed spaces, certain types of food, thunder, hospitals, going to the dentist, the sight of blood or injury, etc. The patient with a Specific Phobia will present with an intense fear of a specific object or situation and marked avoidance of it. They will experience intense symptoms of anxiety and distress when faced with, or even the contemplation of being faced with, the focus of their phobia. Feelings of anxiety are absent when the patient is not in contact with the object of their fear or is not thinking about it. Phobias can interfere with the person's life and cause marked distress.

Blood/injury phobias are a special case, in that, contrary to other phobias, the person will generally faint when confronted with blood or injury. A patient presenting with this type of phobia should be referred for specialist treatment.

Prevalence

Specific phobias are very common, with 8% of the population having a diagnosable Specific Phobia, although only approximately 1% will present for treatment. Specific phobias are almost twice as common in women than men.

Prognosis

Many phobias begin in childhood but generally disappear without ever requiring treatment. Those specific phobias that develop later in life usually take a more chronic course. Specific phobias generally respond very well to psycho-education and graded exposure.

Diagnostic criteria

For the diagnosis of Specific Phobia to be made, the patient must exhibit certain symptoms, including:
- Persistent and irrational fear of a particular object or situation

---

Emotional, physical, cognitive and behavioural symptoms of Specific Phobias

Emotional symptoms	Fear Anxiety Panic
Physical symptoms	Palpitations Trembling or shaking Breathlessness Dry mouth Sweating Nausea Urge to go to the toilet
Cognitive symptoms	Distressing thoughts about thefeared stimuli, whether in anticipation of facing them or in real life
Behavioural symptoms	Avoidance of the feared object or situation Escape from situations when faced with phobic stimuli

- An immediate anxiety response when in contact with the stimulus
- Avoidance of the stimulus or extreme anxiety during exposure
- Fear, avoidance or distress interfere with the individual's normal life and social activities

Warning: Differential diagnosis

Whilst most specific phobias do not have a specific onset incident, some do. Where this is the case and the patient has more general levels of arousal and intrusive images about the onset of the event, then it may be that the patient is presenting with Post Traumatic Stress Disorder (PTSD). If this is the case, then they should be referred for specialist treatment.

- The fear is recognized as being irrational or excessive

Meet Lorraine

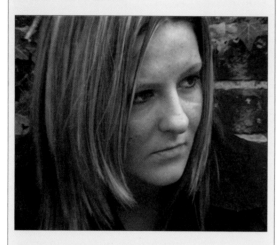

Lorraine is a 22-year-old single woman living with her parents. She has a six-month history of a phobia of driving, following a minor road traffic accident. There was no serious injury to any party involved. Post Traumatic Stress Disorder has been ruled out. This problem is causing great inconvenience to Lorraine as she either has to be driven to work by her mother or take the bus. She is keen to overcome her difficulties but terrified about even sitting in the driving seat of a stationary car. She even gets anxious when travelling as a passenger, but forces herself to do this. Symptoms include palpitations, shaking, breathlessness and intense thoughts about being involved in a crash. Her Mum tries to push her to drive, but has yet to be successful in persuading her to do this.

 A video clip in which Lorraine introduces herself and discusses her phobia is included on CD-ROM 3, and a transcript of the clip follows.

For more detailed information on diagnosis see ICD-10 (International Classification of Diseases) or DSM-IV-TR (Diagnostic and Statistical Manual of Mental Disorders).

Psychosocial assessment of Specific Phobias

In addition to the diagnostic symptoms, patients with specific phobias can report a wide range of disturbance. As well as confirming diagnosis using the diagnostic criteria from ICD-10 or DSM-IV-TR, it is helpful to group symptoms into four areas and identify the connections between these symptom areas. This information can then be used to help guide treatment. The model presented on page 143 can be used to help us understand the connections between symptoms presented by a client with Specific Phobia. These four areas are emotional, physical, cognitive and behavioural symptoms.

Video: Introducing Lorraine (Driving Phobia)

Lorraine: I'm having real problems with my driving. I have done for the past six months, since the car accident. It wasn't that serious or anything, nobody was even badly hurt. The car wasn't even that damaged. I was at a roundabout and I should have gone as there were no cars coming, but I stalled. Anyway, the bloke in the car behind me wasn't really paying any attention and bumped into the back of me. I got minor whiplash but that soon went, but I got a real fright.

I don't have nightmares or anything, although I did for the first couple of nights, but I certainly haven't had any for ages now. I used to love driving but it literally terrifies me now. I can't even sit in the driver's seat when it's stationary without getting really terrified.

When I get worked up like that, I get these palpitations, I start to shake and I find it hard to catch my breath. I also get all these thoughts coming into my head that I'm going to be in another crash.

I asked Dr Attenborough if she could give me something to help. I'd read about beta-blockers, but she said that she didn't think that tablets were the answer. She's getting me to see someone instead who she thinks might be able to help.

Exercise

Watch the video clip about Lorraine, or read the transcript.
- Using the Emotional, Physical, Cognitive and Behavioural Symptoms of Specific Phobias list, consider which of the symptoms in the list Lorraine presents with.
- Then use the model on page 143 as a guide to help you demonstrate these links in a diagrammatic form

---

Agoraphobia with or without Panic

Agoraphobia is more complex than a Specific Phobia as it is less well defined. Some patients with Agoraphobia also have an associated Panic Disorder, and it is not unusual for depressive features to be present. The main characteristic of Agoraphobia is anxiety about being somewhere from which escape is difficult, or in which immediate help is not available if a panic attack should occur. The patient with Agoraphobia may experience a number of related fears, including fear of: leaving home, going into shops, crowded places, using public transport, crossing bridges, using lifts, etc.

Patients with Agoraphobia are usually highly avoidant and use 'safety behaviours' to help them cope. A major factor in Agoraphobia is the anxiety experienced by being far away from 'safety' (often their home is where most patients feel safe). There is a common misunderstanding that Agoraphobia means a fear of open spaces, whereas it actually translates as 'fear of the marketplace'. Patients with Agoraphobia are far more likely to be anxious in crowded places such as department stores, public transport and supermarkets than in open spaces (though this is not unheard of).

Patients with Agoraphobia, when entering a feared situation, will commonly look for escape routes. Common fears include losing control and fainting or collapsing.

Patients with Agoraphobia sometimes find that, if they are accompanied by someone they trust, they are more able to cope; even being accompanied by a child can help. They may also use safety behaviours such as carrying an umbrella or tablets in a pocket, or pushing a pram, as these props can be seen by the person as helping them cope. When assessing a patient with Agoraphobia, be sure to ask about props like this.

Onset of Agoraphobia commonly occurs after the patient has experienced a panic attack. However, once Agoraphobia has developed, panic attacks may not necessarily continue. For example, if the patient avoids feared situations, anxiety will be lower and, therefore, panic symptoms are less likely to occur. However, the agoraphobic avoidance frequently continues despite the absence of panic attacks, as the fearful anticipation of experiencing a panic attack continues.

Prevalence

In any one year, Agoraphobia with or without Panic Disorder affects around 2% of the population. Agoraphobia is more common in women than men.

Prognosis

If untreated, Agoraphobia can take a chronic course and become seriously disabling for the person. Avoidance can cause significant interference in a person's work and social functioning. Most patients with Agoraphobia can be successfully treated using CBT approaches.

Diagnostic criteria

For the diagnosis of Agoraphobia to be made, the patient must exhibit certain symptoms. These include:
- the anxiety occurs mainly (or only) in at least two of the following situations: crowds; public places; travelling away from home; and travelling alone

- avoidance of the feared situation is prominent

Emotional, physical, cognitive and behavioural symptoms of Agoraphobia

Emotional symptoms	Fear Anxiety Panic
Physical symptoms	Palpitations Breathlessness Lightheadedness Dry mouth Dizziness Sweating Chest pain Nausea Numbness and tingling Urge to go to the toilet Shaking
Cognitive symptoms	Distressing thoughts about the feared stimuli, whether in anticipation of facing them or in real life Fear of losing control Fear of fainting Fear of collapsing Feelings of helplessness
Behavioural symptoms	Avoidance of feared situations (usually crowded places where escape is difficult) Escape from these situations Engaging in safety behaviours (e.g. holding onto a pram, carrying tablets, etc.) Dependence on others

---

For more detailed information on diagnosis see ICD-10 (International Classification of Diseases) or DSM-IV-TR (Diagnostic and Statistical Manual of Mental Disorders).

Revisiting Deborah

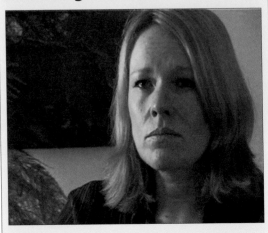

Deborah was introduced in Part 2. She is a 42-year-old married woman who lives with her husband and 19-year-old son. She has difficulty leaving home unaccompanied for fear that she will faint, despite having no history of fainting. The anticipation of going out unaccompanied makes her feel extremely anxious and leads to lightheadedness, palpitations and trembling. She is worried that her problem is deteriorating.

 A video clip in which Deborah introduces herself and discusses her Agoraphobia is included on CR-ROM 3, and a transcript of the clip follows.

Psychosocial assessment of Agoraphobia

In addition to the diagnostic symptoms, patients with Agoraphobia can report a wide range of disturbance. As well as confirming diagnosis using the diagnostic criteria from ICD-10 or DSM-IV-TR, it is helpful to group symptoms into four areas and identify the connections between these symptom areas. This information can then be used to help guide treatment. The model presented on page 143 can be used to help us understand the connections between symptoms presented by a client with Agoraphobia. These four areas are emotional, physical, cognitive and behavioural symptoms.

Video: Introducing Deborah (Agoraphobia)

Deborah: I suppose my problems started a few months ago when I was in hospital. I had this funny virus; anyway I was in hospital for a while and when I came home, when I came out of hospital, I couldn't go anywhere, I couldn't go out and then when I could go out, it seemed like I couldn't. Well, whenever I went out, I'd get this really, really dry mouth and felt that I couldn't swallow. My heart was beating so loud, it was almost like I thought people could hear it, and I just felt like I couldn't swallow, I had to hang onto things. I sometimes felt I was going to be sick or I'd faint. It was just awful and it was much, much worse when I went into crowded places. If I went on the bus, or if I went on the tube and it was crowded, it just made me feel like I would faint at any moment. It just was awful, and then I found that I couldn't even go into the supermarket which meant that Paul, my husband, had to do all the shopping and everything outside of the house because I just haven't been able to go out at all really. I just can't see it getting any better.

It's like, whenever I even think about going out, I start to feel really nervous and it's like a feeling of having lost all your confidence, having no confidence at all. If it hadn't been for Paul, I just don't know what I'd have done because he's been so fantastic. He's really done everything for me and everything that I have to do inside the house is fine but anything to do with going out, he's doing all of it and I just don't know how long he can carry on doing that, because it must be really difficult for him, and that worries me a lot.

I've been seeing my GP, and he referred me to a mental health worker at the practice and that's actually been quite helpful I think, but now the mental health worker wants to see Paul and I together today and that's what we're going to do. I do hope it goes okay.

Exercise

Watch the video clip about Deborah, or read the transcript.

- Using the Emotional, Physical, Cognitive and Behavioural Symptoms of Agoraphobia list, consider which of the symptoms in the list Deborah presents with.
- Then use the model on page 143 as a guide to help you demonstrate these links in a diagrammatic form.

Social Phobia

Like Agoraphobia, Social Phobia is much more complex and debilitating than Specific Phobias. The key characteristic of Social Phobia is the fear of being scrutinized or evaluated negatively by others. The person will worry that they may do something embarrassing or act in a way that may be humiliating in some way, including showing any obvious symptoms of anxiety. The fear may be restricted to certain situations or it may have generalized to most social situations. The fears of socially anxious patients are more subtle than those in Specific Phobias or Agoraphobia as they are unseen (e.g. negative judgements of others). Some patients are unable to write in public for fear that others will be watching and their hands will shake. Others have difficulty eating or drinking in front of others. Public speaking also commonly causes difficulty, as can using public toilets. Many of these situations may be avoided, or the patient may have developed safety behaviours to help them cope (e.g. tensing an arm when taking a drink of coffee, avoiding eye contact to decrease the chance of having to engage in conversation, etc.). A major aspect of Social Phobia is the upsetting negative thoughts related to fear of negative evaluation and rejection by others, although the person recognizes that their fears are irrational or excessive. Avoidance is far more difficult in Social Phobia, as most of us are faced with

Emotional, physical, cognitive and behavioural symptoms of Social Phobia

Emotional symptoms	Fear Anxiety Panic
Physical symptoms	Palpitations Breathlessness Dry mouth Dizziness Sweating Nausea Vomiting Urge to go to the toilet Shaking Blushing
Cognitive symptoms	Distressing thoughts about one's own performance Fear of criticism and negative evaluation by others Mind going blank
Behavioural symptoms	Avoidance of feared situations Escape from social situations Engaging in safety behaviours (e.g. avoidance of eye contact)

Revisiting Andrew

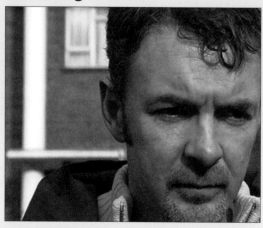

Andrew was introduced in Part 1. He is a 34-year-old single man who lives alone, and who is very nervous about meeting new people because of his worries that he will not know what to say and that people will think he is stupid because of this. In social situations he is prone to sweating, shaking and nausea; he has actually vomited occasionally.

 A video clip in which Andrew introduces himself and discusses his social phobia is included on CD-ROM 3, and a transcript of the clip follows.

numerous social interactions on a daily basis. For this reason, Social Phobias tend to be debilitating.

Prevalence

It is estimated that 2% of the general population suffers from Social Phobia. It is equally common in men and women. Social Phobia is generally a chronic disorder that may fluctuate over time.

Prognosis

If Social Phobia goes untreated, it commonly causes marked impairment in social or occupational functioning. Good outcomes have been found using CBT approaches.

Diagnostic criteria

For the diagnosis of Social Phobia to be made, the patient must exhibit certain symptoms, including:
- A marked and persistent fear of being scrutinized by others in one or more social or performance situations. The fear involves acting in a way that will be embarrassing or humiliating (including showing symptoms of anxiety)
- Exposure to the feared situation causes anxiety and may lead to a panic attack
- The fear is recognized to be irrational and excessive

- The fear leads to marked distress during exposure to the social situation or may lead to avoidance of that situation

For more detailed information on diagnosis see ICD-10 (International Classification of Diseases) or DSM-IV-TR (Diagnostic and Statistical Manual of Mental Disorders).

Psychosocial assessment of Social Phobia

In addition to the diagnostic symptoms, patients with Social Phobia can report a wide range of disturbance. As well as confirming diagnosis using the diagnostic criteria from ICD-10 or DSM-IV-TR, it is helpful to group symptoms into four areas and identify the connections between these symptom areas. This information can then be used to help guide treatment. The model presented on page 143 can be used to help us understand the connections between symptoms presented by a client with Social Phobia. These four areas are emotional, physical, cognitive and behavioural symptoms.

Video: Introducing Andrew (Social Phobia)

Andrew: I guess I'm kind of shy. The thing I find toughest though is meeting people for the first time. I never know what to say, I get all tongue-tied, my mind goes completely blank and I end up making a complete fool of myself. People just end up thinking I'm really stupid. You know, they can come across as the nicest person in the world and I'll still be like some kind of gibbering wreck. I try to avoid eye contact these days to reduce the chance that anyone will talk to me. I can just feel all the tension inside and start to shake really noticeably. I also start sweating like a pig. Sometimes I blush too, which I really hate. I can see how they must see me and just want to get away. There's no way they'll want to give me the time of day.

I've been sick a couple of times too, which is horrendous. Both were on family meals out when I just felt really self-conscious, being with all these aunties and uncles that I hadn't seen for ages, and I just couldn't eat while I was talking to them. It was a nightmare.

One of the times I remember, I'd ordered fish and chips because I thought that'd be easier to eat, but it came with peas. I plucked up the courage to eat some peas, but my hands shook that much that they went everywhere. I just ended up feeling sick and I had to go to the toilets where I actually vomited.

My mates drag me out every now and again, but I usually have to drink a couple of beers before I go out as I worry about my hand shaking in the pub. That does help, but I don't think it's good that I have to do that. I just try to avoid going if I can, or make some excuse and come away after an hour or so. I'm hoping that the person Dr Mehra has referred me to will be able to help.

Exercise

Watch the video clip about Andrew, or read the transcript.
- Using the Emotional, Physical, Cognitive and Behavioural Symptoms of Social Phobia list, consider which of the symptoms in the list Andrew presents with.
- Then use the model on page 143 as a guide to help you demonstrate these links in a diagrammatic form.

Section summary

- There are three main categories of phobias: Specific Phobias, Agoraphobia and Social Phobia
- Phobias are irrational fears of particular objects or situations
- Phobias are maintained by avoidance behaviours

References

American Psychiatric Association (2000). *Diagnostic and Statistical Manual of Mental Disorders: DSM-IV-TR: Fourth Edition Text Revision.* Washington DC: American Psychiatric Association. www.psych.org.

World Health Organisation (1994). *ICD-10 International Statistical Classification of Diseases and Related Health Problems.* Geneva: World Health Organisation. www.who.int.

Recommended reading

Butler, G. (1999). *Overcoming Social Anxiety and Shyness. A self-help guide using Cognitive Behavioural Techniques.* London: Robinson.

Marks, I.M. (2001). *Living With Fear (second edition).* London: McGraw-Hill.

Wells, A. (1997). *Cognitive Therapy of Anxiety Disorders. A Practice Manual and Conceptual Guide.* Chichester: John Wiley & Sons.

Test yourself

 To check your progress, locate this section on CD-ROM 3 and work through the interactive questions at the end.

Section 2c: Generalized Anxiety Disorder (GAD)

Introduction

The key characteristic of Generalized Anxiety Disorder (GAD) is excessive worry. The person with GAD tends to experience excessive or unrealistic anxiety and worry over many aspects of life which are commonly accompanied by some of these symptoms: muscle tension, disturbed sleep, irritability, restlessness, difficulty concentrating, etc. The focus of the worry is often about some future event that the person predicts will go badly, and over which they have little or no control. Common themes of these worries include fears of: illness and death related to self and family; inability to cope; loss of control; financial and relationship difficulties.

The patient with GAD is likely to overestimate the potential threat or danger of a given situation and underestimate their ability to cope with it. The anxiety and worry are not confined to one specific catastrophe, as in a Specific Phobia (e.g. worry about being bitten by a dog), or fear of having a panic attack, as in Panic Disorder, but they are far more pervasive; hence the term 'generalized' anxiety.

Patients with GAD just cannot seem to put aside their worries and concerns, despite often realizing that their level of worry outweighs the amount warranted by their life situation. The sense of worry and anxiety can feel almost constant and can lead to panic attacks.

Unlike patients suffering from other anxiety disorders such as phobias, patients with GAD do not tend to avoid specific situations, although some might.

Prevalence

GAD is one of the most common anxiety disorders. During the course of a year, approximately 5% of adults will suffer from GAD. About 55% to 60% of those suffering from GAD are female. Ninety per cent of people suffering from GAD will also have another psychiatric disorder, most commonly depression.

Prognosis

GAD is a chronic disorder that usually develops gradually and fluctuates in severity over time. The course of the disorder can be either constant, or waxing and waning in nature. Although most patients with GAD appear to be symptomatic for the majority of the time since onset, about 25% of patients with GAD do experience periods of remission (three months or longer symptom-free). Stress has been found to make the worry and anxiety associated with GAD worse.

Diagnostic criteria

For a diagnosis of GAD to be made, the patient must exhibit excessive anxiety and worry with

Emotional, physical, cognitive and behavioural symptoms of Generalized Anxiety Disorder (GAD)

Emotional symptoms	Anxiety Low mood Irritability Nervousness Feeling on edge		Dry mouth Nausea Diarrhoea Increased need to urinate Lightheadedness Palpitations Shortness of breath
Physical symptoms	Muscle tension Pain in the back of the neck Fatigue Numbness Pins and needles Pains running up and down the arm Trouble falling or staying asleep Dizziness Headaches Difficulty swallowing Trembling Stomach pains Twitching Sweating Hot flushes Clammy hands	Cognitive symptoms	Poor concentration Unrealistic assessment of problems Excessive worries Worries about the future Worrying about worrying Mind going blank Procrastination Lack of ability to problem- solve difficulties Hypervigilance Underestimation of ability to cope
		Behavioural symptoms	Fidgeting Restlessness Inability to relax

significant social, occupational and functional impairment that has persisted for a minimum of several weeks, but usually for a period of six months. The patient must have been troubled by symptoms of anxiety on most days over that period. These anxiety symptoms are:

- Apprehension (e.g. worry about the future, feeling 'on edge', difficulty concentrating)
- Motor tension (restlessness, headaches, trembling, inability to relax)
- Other symptoms of high arousal (e.g. sweating, accelerated heart rate, dry mouth, stomach upsets, dizziness, lightheadedness)

For more detailed information on diagnosis see ICD-10 (International Classification of Diseases) or DSM-IV-TR (Diagnostic and Statistical Manual of Mental Disorders).

Worrying about worrying

Patients with GAD, in addition to their worries (e.g. 'I will die young and not see my children grow up', 'my son will not pass all the exams he needs to get into university'), tend to worry about the act of worrying itself. They are concerned that they experience all these worrying thoughts and what this must mean, and are frequently concerned that they cannot seem to stop the thoughts.

Patients with GAD are usually very insightful and know that they are worrying excessively about things that they can do nothing about. For

Meet Julie

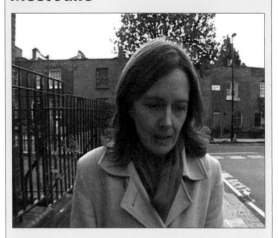

Julie is a 47-year-old married woman with two children. She describes herself as always having been a worrier. However, she has found that her symptoms have deteriorated over the last eight months, which has been triggered by her husband's job being under threat and her mother's diagnosis of bone metastases after having been in remission from breast cancer for the last four years. Her oldest child, Colin, 25, is about to get married, and her youngest child, Claire, 18, has recently moved out of town to go to university. She worries about her mother, who lives alone, her husband's job, her children and her own health, which is actually fine. She also worries about the fact that she is a worrier and the effect this is likely to be having on her mental health. She mentions worries that she may be 'going mad'. She experiences a range of physical symptoms when anxious, including muscle tension, headaches, muscle aches, difficulty swallowing, stomach pains and palpitations. She also experiences difficulty concentrating and lacks the ability to problem-solve.

 A video clip in which Julie introduces herself and discusses her anxiety is included on CD-ROM 3, and a transcript of the clip follows.

example, a healthy young man may be tortured by worrying thoughts about ill-health, or a person of relative wealth may worry about money.

When distanced somewhat from the situation, the GAD patient can often see that their worries do not make sense, but this has little effect on the frequency, intensity and duration of their worries.

Psychosocial assessment of Generalised Anxiety Disorder

In addition to the diagnostic symptoms, patients with Generalised Anxiety Disorder can report a wide range of disturbance. As well as confirming diagnosis using the diagnostic criteria from ICD-10 or DSM-IV-TR, it is helpful to group symptoms into four areas and identify the connections between these symptom areas. This information can then be used to help guide treatment. The model presented on page 143 can be used to help us understand the connections between symptoms presented by a client with Generalized Anxiety Disorder. These four areas are emotional, physical, cognitive and behavioural symptoms.

Video: Introducing Julie (Generalized Anxiety Disorder)

Julie: I suppose I've always been a worrier. I think I got it from my Mum but it's got worse over the last few months. David, that's my husband, might be getting made redundant, and my Mum has just been diagnosed with secondaries to breast cancer. As if that wasn't enough, my son Colin's about to get married and my daughter Claire has just left home to start at university. I do worry about her. She says she's loving it, but I'm not so sure that she doesn't just put a brave face on for me, as she knows how much I worry.
The latest thing is that the dog's unwell. I do hope that he gets better, the vet seems to think he will, but he is 16, which is old for a dog. I can't bear the thought of losing him.

You know, sometimes I worry that I'm going mad; all this worry can't be good for me. I never feel relaxed, just this on-edge way all the time. I sometimes can't sleep for worrying. It's exhausting. I'll end up being carted away one of these days. I can feel myself getting all tense and my neck is beginning to ache, and I can feel my heart going 10 to the dozen, just thinking about all this stuff. Oh no, I've got one of my headaches coming on now as well. Sometimes I get a sore stomach too, but that doesn't seem too bad at the moment, though I can feel the butterflies starting. Sometimes I get the runs, you know. Look, my hands have gone all clammy.

It's really getting me down, I hope seeing someone at the practice will help. They'll probably commit me!

Exercise

Watch the video clip about Julie, or read the transcript.
- Using the Emotional, Physical, Cognitive and Behavioural Symptoms of Generalized Anxiety Disorder list, consider which of the symptoms in the list Julie presents with.
- Then use the model on page 143 as a guide to help you demonstrate these links in a diagrammatic form.

Section summary

- GAD is one of the most common anxiety disorders
- The key characteristic of GAD is excessive worry
- In addition to worrying about events, etc., patients with GAD tend to worry about worrying
- Patients with GAD tend to overestimate the potential threat or danger of a given situation and underestimate their ability to cope with it
- Patients with GAD do not tend to avoid specific situations, although some might

References

American Psychiatric Association (2000). *Diagnostic and Statistical Manual of Mental Disorders: DSM-IV-TR: Fourth Edition Text Revision*. Washington DC: American Psychiatric Association. www.psych.org.

World Health Organisation (1994). *ICD-10 International Statistical Classification of Diseases and Related Health Problems*. Geneva: World Health Organisation. www.who.int.

Recommended reading

Kennerley, H. (1997). *Overcoming Anxiety. A self-help guide using Cognitive Behavioural Techniques*. London: Robinson.

National Institute for Health and Clinical Excellence (2004b). *Anxiety: Management of anxiety (panic disorder, with or without agoraphobia, and generalised anxiety disorder) in adults in primary, secondary and community care*. London: National Institute for Health and Clinical Excellence. www.nice.org.uk.

Test yourself

 To check your progress, locate this section on CD-ROM 3 and work through the interactive questions at the end.

Section 3: Other difficulties

The problems covered in this section do not fall under the categories of either depression or anxiety disorders. None the less, these problems are commonly encountered in the primary care setting, and are covered here for that reason.

Section 3a: Stress

Introduction

Stress is an extremely common problem for most of us at some time in our lives. Stress is the term used to describe the symptoms a person experiences when they perceive the demands made of them are being outweighed by their ability to fulfil them.

When a person feels that they have insufficient time, experience and resources to deal with their current circumstances, they are likely to feel stressed. It is not necessarily that the events are themselves stressful but that they are perceived by the person as such. The experience of stress is therefore determined by the person's appraisal of the demand and of the resources available to meet that demand. Inability to cope with these demands results in a variety of emotional, physical, cognitive and behavioural symptoms.

Often, stress occurs due to work overload, conflict with others, financial difficulties, and/or tight deadlines, etc. Loss, such as bereavement, divorce or separation, causes stress, as can long-term illness or disability. In addition, events that can be perceived as positive can cause stress (e.g. getting married, a new job, going on holiday and moving house, etc.).

The effects of stress are that it reduces performance and can lead to a vicious circle of high levels of stress and underperformance. As a consequence of stress, some people drink more heavily, smoke more, and may not take time to eat properly.

Stress can lead to serious health problems: there is a link between stress and heart disease. It can also affect the immune system and, therefore, people under stress can be more prone to infections (e.g. colds). It can also lead to an increase in headaches and aggravate irritable bowel syndrome.

Prevalence

There are limited studies on the prevalence of stress, probably due to the fact that it is not a diagnosable disorder. However, some data are available. The 2001/2 survey of Self-reported Work-related Illness (SWI01/02) estimate of prevalence indicated that over half a million people in the UK believed that they were experiencing work-related stress to a point where it was making them ill. This would indicate that work-related stress is the second biggest occupational health problem in the UK, second only to back problems. In addi-

tion, the Stress and Health at Work Study (SHAW) indicated that nearly one in five of all working people considered their job to be very or extremely stressful.

Prognosis

Many stressful experiences may be short-lived and the person will make a spontaneous recovery (e.g. moving house, preparing to go on holiday, etc.). If left untreated, long-term stress can cause or exacerbate many physical problems, including heart attacks, asthma, ulcers, irritable bowel syndrome, colitis, spots, eczema, dermatitis, alopecia, dandruff, herpes, shingles, high blood pressure, strokes, colds, pneumonia, bronchitis and influenza. In addition, according to some researchers, prolonged stress can contribute to the development of diabetes, autoimmune disorders and cancer. Psychological disorders caused by long-term stress include depression, panic attacks and phobias. Stress tends to respond well to psychological interventions such as lifestyle strategies, increasing relaxing activities, problem-solving and some CBT approaches.

Diagnostic criteria

Stress is not officially recognized in the ICD-10 (International Classification of Diseases) or DSM-IV-TR (Diagnostic and Statistical Manual of Mental Disorders) as a psychological disorder. When considering whether a patient is suffering from stress, check the 'Psychosocial Assessment of Stress' for a list of common symptoms of stress and rule out depression and anxiety disorders.

Stress in the workplace

The workplace is commonly where people undergo stress. Some of the common stressors at work include:

- Difficult relationships with work colleagues
- A critical or unsupportive boss
- Poor communication
- Work life interfering with home life

Emotional, physical, cognitive and behavioural symptoms of Stress

Emotional symptoms	Anxiety Low mood Irritability Apathy Low self-esteem Feeling tearful		Indigestion Hyperventilation Shaking Chest tightness Diarrhoea Increased frequency of urination
Physical symptoms	Headaches including migraine Muscle tension or pain Difficulty sleeping (getting off to sleep and early morning wakening) High blood pressure Stomach problems Ulcers Sweating Dizziness Bowel or bladder problems, including Irritable Bowel Syndrome Breathlessness or palpitations Dry mouth Sexual difficulties, including loss of sex drive	Cognitive symptoms Behavioural symptoms	Nausea and vomiting Increased vulnerability to illness Upsetting thoughts (e.g. 'I can't cope') Forgetfulness Poor concentration Increased sensitivity to criticism Difficulty making decisions Increased drinking or smoking Changes in eating habits Withdrawing from usual hobbies and pleasurable activities

- Feeling that there is too much to do in too little time
- Being faced with deadlines that cannot be realistically met
- Work that is just too difficult for one's capabilities
- Lack of say over how work is to be done
- Poor work conditions
- Feeling undervalued
- Threat of redundancy

When people are feeling under pressure at work, there is a tendency to work all the harder in an attempt to meet the tasks that are expected of them. In doing so, the person may stop taking breaks and begin to lose perspective of their own needs.

When a person feels that demands are too high, this will directly affect their level of performance. The graph in Figure 7 (see page 166) shows the effects of demand on performance. The left-hand axis of the graph shows that, when there is minimal demand on us, there is little incentive for us to focus our energy on it.

This is particularly the case when there are other, more urgent or more engaging tasks to complete. When demand is increased, we can reach our optimum level of performance, are able to focus our energy on the task, and perform well but without excessive demand. The right-hand side of the graph shows that when demand is too high, the person will underperform. As the person becomes more stressed, they perceive that the demands placed on them exceed their ability and they will suffer stress. Symptoms may include difficulty concentrating, feeling overloaded, feelings of inability to think and focus, difficulty making decisions, being overwhelmed with negative thoughts and anxieties.

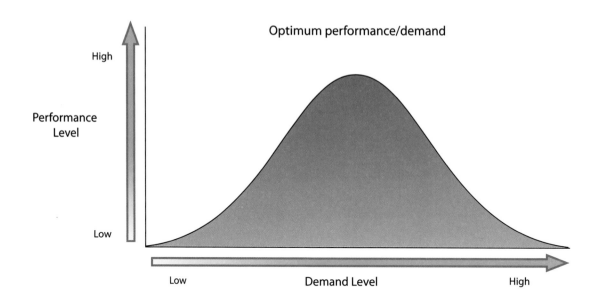

Figure 7: The effects of demand upon performance

Exercise

Northumberland, Tyne and Wear NHS Trust have produced a self-help stress booklet, which is available online at www.nnt.nhs.uk/mh/leaflets/stress%20A5.pdf. The booklet contains a quiz which will help to decide which personality type a person belongs to. A copy of the quiz can be found in the Appendix to this book, and is also included in PDF format on CD-ROM 3.
- Complete the quiz and find out what personality type you have.
- You can also use this quiz with your patients.

People who experience stress

Research has shown that some people are more likely to experience high levels of stress than others. These people are known as 'Type A' personalities. They have a tendency to be more competitive and to function at full speed, compared to 'Type B' personalities who have a more laid-back attitude to life.

Psychosocial assessment of stress

Patients with stress can report a wide range of disturbance. It is helpful to group symptoms into four areas and identify the connections between these symptom areas. This information can then be used to help guide treatment. The model presented on page 143 can be used to help us understand the connections between symptoms presented by a client with Stress. These four areas are emotional, physical, cognitive and behavioural symptoms.

If a patient is presenting with some of these symptoms, they may be experiencing stress. It is important to remember that stress has long-term health risks that include heart disease, high blood pressure, depression, stroke, migraine headaches, anxiety, asthma, reduced immunity to infection, bowel complaints, stomach problems (especially ulcers), fatigue and sleep difficulties.

Revisiting Tim

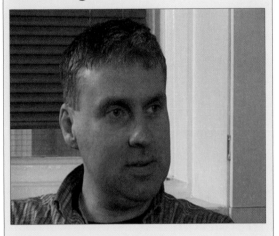

Tim was introduced in Part 2. Age 46, Tim works for an IT company as a website designer and, although his job is not under immediate threat, he has seen a marked increase in his workload following the redundancy of a number of his close colleagues. He works long hours and has little time for anything other than work, which is even interfering with his weekends; and he smokes heavily, has a high caffeine intake, and lives on junk food as he lacks the energy to cook a meal and rarely has the time to go food shopping.

 A video clip in which Tim introduces himself and discusses his feelings of being under stress is included on CD-ROM 3, and a transcript of the clip follows.

Video: Introducing Tim (Stress)

Tim: My main problem is stress at work. I'm a web designer. Used to think I was quite good at it, thrived on the stress, but now I feel so anxious all the time, I seem to keep working to try and get it all right, but it just doesn't help. To be honest, even though I'm putting in all the hours that I can in, I think I'm underperforming. I find it hard to concentrate and I keep forgetting what I need to do, where I need to be, where I put things. My job has always been stressful, but now things are different because the company has been going through some financial difficulties, and some people have ended up losing their jobs. I've been lucky so far, although sometimes I wonder if I am that lucky, what with all this stress.

I find it so hard to switch off when I do eventually get home and I'm not sleeping that well, especially getting off to sleep and sometimes I wake up in the middle of the night and I can't get back off to sleep. I'm smoking like a chimney too which isn't helping.

My eating has all gone to pot. I tend to skip lunch and then just survive on coffee all day, and get a takeaway on the way home or see what John's left for me but whichever, it still means I end up eating late, and then I end up with indigestion and that doesn't help my sleep. It's a vicious circle, and I've also got this permanent headache that I just can't shift.

I've had to cancel arrangements to see friends at the weekend because I had to work part of the time, then I was just so exhausted I couldn't face going for a game of squash then drinks.

And John is getting fed up with not seeing me, and when we do have any time together, well, I have no desire at all to have sex. He seems to think I don't love him anymore but that just isn't true, I'm just so stressed out that it's the last thing on my mind.

Dr Mehra took my blood pressure and told me it was a bit high, which is a bit of a worry, and he thinks the stress I'm under is making me susceptible to these colds and stuff I've been getting lately. He thinks I should consider a holiday. I nearly laughed when he said that. How am I going to find time to take a holiday when I can't even find time to get down the gym for an hour?

Anyway, it's all come to a head, and I'm

feeling so low, I'm even tearful at times, and I just don't think I can cope anymore, so I've come to the practice for some help and I have been seeing the mental health worker, and my GP. I haven't been prescribed any tablets from the GP though.

Exercise

Watch the video clip about Tim, or read the transcript.
- Using the Emotional, Physical, Cognitive and Behavioural Symptoms of Stress list, consider which of the symptoms in the list Tim presents with.
- Then use the model on page 143 as a guide to help you demonstrate these links in a diagrammatic form.

Section summary

- Stress is an extremely common problem that affects most of us at some time in our lives
- There is a link between stress and serious health problems
- Type A personalities are more prone to stress

References

Jones, J.R., Huxtable, C.S., Hodgson, J.T. and Price, M.J. (2003). *Self-reported work-related illness in 2001/02.* Caerphilly: Health and Safety Executive. www.hse.gov.uk.

Smith, A.P., Wadsworth, E., Johal, S.S., Davey Smith, G. and Peters, T. (2000). *The scale of occupational stress: The Bristol Stress and Health at Work Study.* Caerphilly: Health and Safety Executive.

Recommended reading

Looker, T. and Gregson, O. (2003). *Managing Stress.* London: Teach Yourself Books.

Palmer, S. (2003). Whistle-stop tour of the theory and practice of stress management and prevention: Its possible role in postgraduate health promotion. *Health Education Journal*, 62 (2), 133–142.

Smith, A.P., Brice, C., Collins, A., Matthews, V. and

McNamara, R. (2000). *The scale of occupational stress: A further analysis of the impact of demographic factors and type of job.* Caerphilly: Health and Safety Executive.

Test yourself

 To check your progress, locate this section on CD-ROM 3 and work through the interactive questions at the end.

Section 3b: Sleep problems

Introduction

Insomnia is the most common of all sleep problems and can be extremely distressing for the sufferer. It is characterized by both lack of sleep and excessive worry about sleep disturbance. Insomnia can often be a symptom of other problems (e.g. depression, pain, etc.). Sleeplessness can be extremely distressing for the person and can often be helped with the introduction of sleep hygiene techniques, lifestyle and environmental changes.

Prevalence

Sleep difficulties are one of the most common problems in both the general health and mental health settings. It has been estimated that over 20% of the adult population suffers from some degree of lasting insomnia at some time in their lives.

Prognosis

Untreated sleep problems can result in a chronic course of ongoing difficulties with sleep. Insomnia is highly treatable and responds extremely well to psycho-education, establishing good sleep hygiene and making lifestyle and environmental changes. When assessing a patient's sleep problems, it is vital that their problem is examined in context and that other psychological, social or medical factors are considered for their role in the onset or maintenance of the sleep problem.

If there is evidence that a physical or mental

Sleep problems checklist

Always check for Depression/Stressful situations/ Anxiety

		Yes
A	Have you had any problems with sleep?	☐
B	Difficulty falling asleep?	☐
C	Restless or unrefreshing sleep?	☐
D	Early morning wakening?	☐
E	Frequent or long periods of being awake?	☐

If YES to any of the above, continue below

1 Do you have any medical problems or physical pains? ☐
2 Are you taking any medication? ☐
3 Do any of the following apply?
   Drink alcohol, coffee, tea or eat before sleep ☐
   Take daytime naps? ☐
   Experienced changes to your routine? ☐
   Disruptive noises during the night ☐
4 Do you have problems at least three times a week? ☐
5 Has anyone told you that your snoring is loud and disruptive? ☐
6 Do you get sudden uncontrollable sleep attacks during the day? ☐
7 Low mood or loss of interest or pleasure? ☐

		Yes
8	Worried, anxious or tense?	☐

How much alcohol do you drink in a typical week (number of standard drinks/week)?
Men (more than 21?) ☐
Women (more than 14?) ☐

Summing up

Positive to any of 1, 2, or 3: Consider management of the underlying problem
Positive to 4: indication of **sleep problem**
Positive to 5: consider **sleep apnoea**
Positive to 6: consider **narcolepsy**
Positive to 7: consider **depression**
Positive to 8: consider **anxiety**

Weekly drinking more than 21 standard drinks for men and more than 14 for women: Consider **alcohol use problems**

Reference

World Health Organisation (2000). *WHO Guide to Mental Health in Primary Care.* The Royal Society of Medicine Press. Reproduced with permission.

disorder, or a drug or alcohol problem are contributing to insomnia, then these conditions should be prioritized for intervention first. If medication appears to be contributing to the insomnia, it may be useful to talk to the patient's GP to see whether the type of medication or the dosage could be altered.

Diagnostic criteria

For the diagnosis of insomnia to be made, the patient must exhibit certain symptoms.

In summary, the key symptoms that must be met for a diagnosis of insomnia are the following:

*   The person complains of difficulty falling asleep, difficulty maintaining sleep, or poor quality of sleep
*   The person's sleep has been disturbed at least three days per week for at least a month
*   The person is preoccupied with their lack of sleep and shows excessive concern, day and night, over the consequences of this lack of sleep
*   The sleep disturbance causes marked personal distress or interferes with social and occupational functioning
*   There is no evidence that the disturbance is caused by an organic factor (e.g. a neurological or other medical condition), a

psychoactive substance use disorder or medication

For more detailed information on diagnosis see ICD-10 (International Classification of Diseases) or DSM-IV-TR (Diagnostic and Statistical Manual of Mental Disorders).

The Sleep Problems checklist can also be used as a handy tool for diagnosing and measuring sleep difficulties. The checklist is also included in PDF format on CD-ROM 3.

Common complaints made by people with insomnia

- Difficulty falling asleep
- Difficulty staying asleep
- Early wakening at the end of the sleep period
- Feeling anxious, worried, depressed or irritable, especially at bedtime
- Racing thoughts at sleep onset or during night-time wakenings
- Feeling physically or mentally tired during the day

Insomnia often begins during periods of increased stress. The person may lie awake at night thinking about personal problems, work, relationship difficulties, financial worries or the death of a loved one, etc. By the time the stressor is no longer an issue, the person may be preoccupied by their inability to get to sleep. In this way a vicious circle has been set up because worrying about not sleeping keeps the person awake.

How much sleep do we need?

Insomnia is not defined by amount of sleep per se. Some people can become very upset when they think they are not getting a good night's sleep, which in turn can make it harder to get off to sleep. The amount of sleep people need varies immensely. Most adults sleep from 7 to 8 hours a night. However, in some cases, people require only 3–4 hours sleep while others can need 10 hours or more. In addition, the amount of sleep a person needs varies throughout life. Newborn babies will sleep 16–17 hours a day, a

child of five years will need about 11 hours, and teenagers about 8–9 hours. By the time we get to our thirties, we may need less than eight hours and, as the years pass, the amount of sleep needed reduces further. Many people in their seventies need less than six hours sleep. It is not uncommon for people over 60 to complain of sleeping problems that are part of the natural aging process.

Another factor affecting how much sleep we need is our level of activity. People who are less active require less sleep, while someone who is on the go all the time will need more sleep.

Ultimately, it is really not important how much the person sleeps; what matters is how well the person feels both physically and mentally as a result of their sleep pattern.

Stages of sleep

There are a number of stages of sleep, varying from light to deep. Broadly speaking, sleep is divided into REM (rapid eye movement) and non-REM sleep. REM sleep occurs several times throughout the night and is when most dreaming takes place. Non-REM sleep is divided into four stages, from drowsiness through to our deepest sleep. During sleep, we go through each of the stages several times and wake up several times too, though most of us do not remember the waking periods. About 25% of a normal young adult's sleep will be spent in REM sleep. Older people will tend to have lighter and more broken sleep, with more frequent waking.

Medication for sleep problems

Medication is not a long-term answer for insomnia. Long-term use can lead to dependence and can result in increased difficulty in sleeping on stopping medication. That is why only short-term or intermittent use of sleep medication is recommended. A situation where short-term use of medication may be appropriate is if someone is extremely distressed following a bereavement.

Factors that may cause or maintain sleep problems

There are many possible factors contributing to sleep problems, including the aging process, physical factors, emotional issues, lifestyle (e.g. caffeine intake), environmental factors (e.g. noisy neighbourhood).

The aging process

When we get older we need less sleep and sleep less deeply. It is also not unusual for people to catnap during the day, which again reduces the need for sleep at night. In addition, the need to go to the toilet during the night occurs more in later life, with approximately 60% of women and 70% of men aged over 65 finding that they need to get up to go to the toilet at least once a night. It can be helpful to normalize reduced sleep in older adults, thereby reducing any distress it may be causing.

Physical factors

Physical illness and medication can have a significant impact on sleep. Pain can also affect a person's ability to sleep. If the patient you see has any physical factors relating to their sleeplessness, it may be appropriate to have their symptoms reviewed by their GP to see if there are any better ways to manage symptoms so that they are less disruptive to the person. Always ensure that you ask whether physical factors are interfering with the patient's sleep.

Emotional issues

It is not uncommon to experience sleep problems when depressed, anxious, angry or stressed. It is important to ask patients if they are feeling stressed, worried, tense, anxious, depressed or angry, and to use some of the strategies demonstrated in this book. You may find it helpful to ask patients, 'Is sleeping your main problem, or is there something else which may be causing you to have problems sleeping?'

Lifestyle factors

It is very common for a person's lifestyle to be a major contributory factor to sleep difficulties. Here is a list of some of the most common lifestyle factors which are worth asking patients about:

- Caffeine intake (e.g. coffee, tea, cola and chocolate drinks)
- Alcohol consumption, especially late at night
- Eating late at night
- Smoking excessively
- Strenuous physical activity just prior to sleep
- Very little exercise earlier in the day
- Working shifts, especially night shift
- Napping through the day
- Irregular going to sleep and waking times
- Intense intellectual activity just prior to sleep

Environmental factors

Sometimes it can be aspects of a person's environment that are the main contributing factors to their sleep difficulties, including a noisy sleeping environment, temperature (too hot or too cold), too much light, etc. Sleeping in a strange place can also affect someone's sleep. Make sure you ask patients about environmental factors when assessing their sleep problems.

Psychosocial assessment of Insomnia

In addition to the diagnostic symptoms, patients with insomnia can report a wide range of disturbance. As well as confirming diagnosis using the diagnostic criteria, it is helpful to group symptoms into four areas and identify the connections between these symptom areas. This information can then be used to help guide treatment. The model presented on page 143 can be used to help us understand the connections between symptoms presented by a client with Sleep Problems. These four areas are emotional, physical, cognitive and behavioural symptoms.

Meet Roger

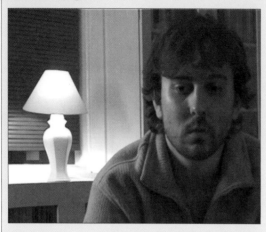

Roger is a 39-year-old married man. He has been having problems getting off to sleep for the past seven years, but this has been particularly problematic for the past seven months. For the past seven years Roger has worked shifts and always put his difficulty getting off to sleep down to his irregular work pattern. Now he no longer works nightshifts, and seven months ago started working regular 9–5 days. He had hoped that he would naturally settle into a regular, healthy sleep pattern. However, he has continued to have difficulty sleeping most nights, which is getting him down and affecting his ability to concentrate at work as he is so tired. Roger drinks tea at work throughout the day and generally has three cups of tea in the evening. He frequently doses in the chair for 1–1½ hours most evenings from around 7pm. When unable to sleep, Roger will read or watch television in bed. If he is still awake by around 1am (most nights), he will get up and make a cup of tea which he brings back to bed. He has got to the stage where he dreads bedtime as it has become a source of anxiety for him, always anticipating a poor night's sleep and worrying about his productivity the next day.

 A video clip in which Roger introduces himself is included on CD-ROM 3, and a transcript of the clip follows.

Emotional, physical, cognitive and behavioural symptoms of Insomnia

Emotional symptoms	Anxiety Low mood Irritability Frustration
Physical symptoms	Headaches Feeling tired a good part of the time Tension Restless sleeping Feeling unrefreshed after sleep Feelings of restlessness as bedtime approaches
Cognitive symptoms	Poor concentration Memory problems Difficulty making decisions Anxious thoughts as bedtime approaches Worrying about lack of sleep
Behavioural symptoms	Increased risk of accidents and injury Nodding off to sleep during the day Napping during the day Engaging in behaviours non-conducive to sleep

Video: Introducing Roger (Insomnia)

Roger: I've had problems getting off to sleep for about seven years now, but I always just put it down to the erratic shifts I've worked; but I've had a day job for the past seven months now, and I thought it would sort itself out, but it hasn't. It's really starting to get me down now. It's affecting my ability to concentrate at work, plus feeling exhausted all the time.

I've taken to having a doze in the chair most nights about 7 o'clock. I don't sleep long, you know, just an hour or so. I tried to stop doing that in case it wasn't doing me any good but to be honest I'm just so tired, and besides, I can be watching telly, something really interesting, and the next thing I know I'm waking up at half past eight. I just can't help it. It's my body telling me I need to sleep.

I've taken a TV into the bedroom now, and if Mary doesn't mind, I'll sometimes put that on. I've got headphones so the noise doesn't disturb her, and she just covers her eyes. She's off to sleep anyway before her head hits the pillows. I wish I was like that.

Sometimes I get so frustrated, I just get up and make myself a cup of tea, and maybe I'll stay downstairs or I'll bring it back to the bedroom and maybe watch telly some more, or maybe read. I do like my tea. Mary tells me I should cut down, but I'm not that sure that it contains that much caffeine. I mean, she seems to drink plenty of coffee and she still goes out like a light. I don't really see how it's going to make a difference really.

You know, it's got to the stage that I actually dread going to bed, because I just know I'm going to have problems getting to sleep, and I just end up getting all worked up about it. Even when I do get to sleep, I don't feel particularly refreshed in the morning anyway.

I asked Dr Hall if he would prescribe me some sleeping tablets but he said no. He said he wants me to see somebody instead. I don't know why; I thought that sleeping tablets would help me, but he seems to think that they're not the answer for my kind of sleep problem. I was really looking forward to a good night's sleep.

Section summary

- The most common sleep problem is insomnia
- Most adults require from 7 to 8 hours sleep a night, though this can vary from 3 to 10 hours or more
- Medication is not a long-term solution for insomnia

Exercise

Watch the video clip about Roger, or read the transcript.
- Using the Emotional, Physical, Cognitive and Behavioural Symptoms of Insomnia list, consider which of the symptoms in the list Roger presents with.
- Then use the model on page 143 as a guide to help you demonstrate these links in a diagrammatic form.

References

American Psychiatric Association (2000). *Diagnostic and Statistical Manual of Mental Disorders: DSM-IV-TR: Fourth Edition Text Revision*. Washington DC: American Psychiatric Association. www.psych.org.

World Health Organisation (1994). *ICD-10 International Statistical Classification of Diseases and Related Health Problems*. Geneva: World Health Organisation. www.who.int.

World Health Organisation (2000). *WHO Guide to Mental Health in Primary Care*. London: The Royal Society of Medicine Press Ltd.

Recommended reading

Bearpark, H. (1994). *Overcoming insomnia*. Rushcutters Bay, Sydney: Gore and Osment Publications.

Bootzin, R.R. and Perlis, M.L (1992). Non-pharmacological treatments of insomnia. *Journal of Clinical Psychiatry*, 53 (Suppl.) 37–41.

Lacks, P. (1987). *Behavioural treatment for persistent insomnia*. Oxford: Pergamon Press.

Lacks, P. and Morin, C.M. (1992). Recent advances in the assessment and treatment of insomnia. *Journal of Consulting and Clinical Psychology*, 60, 586–594.

Reite, M.L., Ruddy, J.R. and Nagel, K.E. (1990). *Concise Guide to the Evaluation and Management of Sleep Disorders*. Washington: American Psychiatric Press.

Test yourself

 To check your progress, locate this section on CD-ROM 3 and work through the interactive questions at the end.

Section 3c: Anger problems

Introduction

Anger is an emotion that we have all experienced, whether as a momentary annoyance or as an all-out rage. Anger can range from mild irritability to outbursts of intense rage, which can lead to violence. Sometimes getting angry can be appropriate and is clearly justified, but when anger is too frequent, too intense or lasts too long, is disproportionate to the situation or leads to violence, then there is a problem. Sometimes people can feel fully justified for their level of irritability or anger at the time and it is only later, on reflection, that they can see that it was excessive. Anger can be a particularly difficult problem to live with for others close to the angry person, as well as for the person themselves.

Anger is a completely normal emotion. However, when it is out of control it can have a negative impact on work, personal relationships and a person's overall quality of life. People with anger problems can sometimes feel that they are completely at the mercy of a highly unpredictable and destructive emotion.

Prevalence

There are limited studies on the prevalence of anger problems in the general population, probably due to the fact that it is not a diagnosable disorder.

Researchers have tended to focus on prevalence of violence, rather than anger problems which have not resulted in criminal charges. It is not appropriate for the mental health worker in primary care to be working with patients who are known to be physically violent.

Prognosis

Patients with anger problems can respond well to anger management treatment which combines behavioural and cognitive approaches. Patients whose anger problems have resulted in police bringing charges against them clearly have severe anger difficulties and under these circumstances should be referred to the forensic services.

Diagnostic criteria

Anger problems are not officially recognized in the ICD-10 (International Classification of Diseases) or DSM-IV-TR (Diagnostic and Statistical Manual of Mental Disorders) as a psychological disorder. When considering whether a patient is suffering from anger problems, check the 'Psychosocial Assessment of Anger' for a list of common symptoms of stress and rule out depression and anxiety disorders.

Triggers for anger

Anger can be triggered by both external and internal events. For example, a person may be angry with someone in particular (e.g. a colleague or partner) or because of an event (e.g. being stuck in a traffic jam or a meeting being cancelled at short notice); these are external events. Internal events that may trigger an anger episode might be ruminating over problems, or thinking over a past event that made the person angry in the first place and, in their mind, has not been resolved.

Some people tend to be more angry than others and seem to have a low tolerance of frustration ('a short fuse'). These people are unable to brush irritations off or just take things in their stride. People who come from families that are poor in dealing with and communicating emotions, and where high levels of anger are expressed, are more likely to have problems with anger.

Purposes of anger

There is a natural instinct for us to respond aggressively when experiencing anger. It is an adaptive response to threat which enables us to defend ourselves if we are under attack and, therefore, it is an essential emotion which ensures our survival. However, it is obviously inappropriate (and illegal) to be physically aggressive to everyone who annoys us. One purpose of anger is to try to discourage others from behaving in a way we don't want them to.

However, we are more likely to get the result we want from encouraging good behaviour than from discouraging bad behaviour. Too much anger is almost always counterproductive.

Expressing anger

Expressing anger in an assertive, non-aggressive way is clearly the most functional way to express anger. In doing this, the person makes clear what their needs are and how to meet them, without the need to hurt others, either emotionally or physically. However, when someone has a problem with anger, it is unlikely that they can express it in this way. Patients who have asked for help with anger problems are likely to have difficulty expressing their annoyance in an assertive way, and instead have little control over their anger. They might end up shouting and may resort to violence towards objects or people. It may not always be the subject of the evoked anger who has the aggressive response directed towards them; it may be delayed, and someone else might receive the person's wrath (e.g. being angered by a work colleague and taking it out on a partner on returning home).

Factors that can lower a person's threshold for anger

Certain physical conditions can lead to anger. These include:
- Being overtired
- Feeling hungry
- Sexual frustration
- Hormonal changes (e.g. premenstrual syndrome (PMS), menopause)
- Withdrawal from addictive substances, leading to cravings for nicotine, alcohol, caffeine, illicit drugs, etc.)
- Being drunk or under the influence of

other substances
- Feeling ill
- Being in pain, whether chronic or acute

Note: Not everyone experiencing these factors will respond in an angry way, and therefore it is not the factors in themselves that are directly anger provoking. Otherwise, everyone in these circumstances would respond in the same way. However, people under these circumstances may blame their inability to control their anger on any one of the above factors, but the reality is that many people do succeed in controlling their anger despite experiencing stressors such as these.

Key areas to ask the angry patient about

When assessing a patient's anger problems, it can be useful to establish whether they have a tendency to:
- shout at people and use violent language
- brood over episodes of anger with people
- be unable to deal with trying situations without getting angry
- become violent, perhaps with legal repercussions
- get angry about situations rather than finding solutions to problems or learning to accept it
- experience physical health problems associated with anger (e.g. hypertension or problems with indigestion)
- be seen by others as an 'angry person' and appeased or feared because of this
- have a strong dislike for strangers because of a characteristic of theirs (e.g. ethnicity, gender, etc.)
- avoid situations because of a fear of getting angry

Psychosocial assessment of anger problems

Patients with anger problems can report a wide range of disturbance. It is helpful to group symptoms into four areas and identify the connections between these symptom areas.

Meet Ben

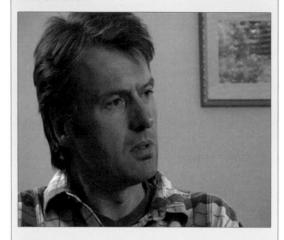

Ben is a 27-year-old male who has been living with his partner, Sue, for the past two years. He has recently changed jobs and has to travel greater distances on a daily basis. He frequently gets caught up in rush-hour traffic, which he finds extremely irritating and frequently gets him very angry. He has experienced a couple of 'road-rage' incidents where he drove in an aggressive manner and shouted obscenities at the offending drivers who had cut in front of him. Sue is finding it increasingly difficult to cope with Ben when he comes home in the evening from work in a rage. He frequently takes his anger out on Sue and will be irritable with her and shout at her. On occasions, he has stayed angry for the entire evening and been uncommunicative and snappy with her. He has never been physically violent towards her, but he has punched walls and broken ornaments in rages, and this has frightened her. Sue is expecting their first baby in four months time. They are both excited about the arrival of their first child. However, they are both concerned about the new stresses a baby will bring and the effect that this will have on Ben's temper. Ben realizes his anger is out of control at times.

 A video clip in which Ben introduces himself is included on CD-ROM 3, and a transcript of the clip follows.

This information can then be used to help guide treatment. The model presented on page 143 can be used to help us understand the connections between symptoms presented by a client with anger difficulties. These four areas are emotional, physical, cognitive and behavioural symptoms.

Video: Introducing Ben (Anger)

Ben: I wouldn't really describe myself as an aggressive person, but I think that's exactly what I'm becoming. I suppose I've never been one to suffer fools gladly, but it's just the way I was brought up. I mean, my Dad is a real grumpy old bugger, always has been.

Anyway, I suppose I only really noticed my temper recently. I've just got a new job in town, so I get stuck in these horrendous car journeys to and from work every day.

You should see how some of these crazy people drive. Honestly, they shouldn't be on the roads. Sometimes I wonder how I manage to get home in one piece. What really riles me is when people cut right in front of me, forcing me to brake. I just think to myself, 'how dare you do that to me, who the hell do you think you are?' I swear, some people just do it on purpose to be annoying. I must admit, I have lost control a couple of times, and have driven right up to their bumper just to show them that I'm no pushover, and have driven alongside them and wound down the window and given them a piece of my mind.

It's usually worse driving home than on the way to work, maybe because I'm tired and I just want to get home and have my tea and relax. Sue's getting fed up of me coming home in a foul temper. I can't blame her, I suppose, but she doesn't know what it's like, and as soon as I get in the door she's rabbiting on about something mundane like her mum coming over, or something like that. I've taken it out on her a few times by saying some pretty nasty

Emotional, physical, cognitive and behavioural symptoms of Anger Problems

Emotional symptoms	Anger Rage Irritability
Physical symptoms	Increase in heart rate Increase in blood pressure Increase in energy hormones (adrenaline and noradrenaline) Tight chest Breathing heightened Stomach churning Tense muscles Feeling hot Urge to go to the toilet Sweating Headache Increased cholesterol levels Increased susceptibility to infection due to depressed immune system Increased supply of testosterone (men only) Eyes widening and pupils dilated Flushing Indigestion

Cognitive symptoms	Thoughts that people are trying to annoy on purpose Poor concentration Mind going blank when angry Thinking the worst of people Seeing everything as a big problem Seeing others' actions as unjust and unfair
Behavioural symptoms	Snapping at people Shouting and arguing Lashing out at others or objects Stamping around Banging doors Throwing things Leaving situations Saying hurtful things to people Physically attacking others Urge to shout and to move limbs quickly and forcefully Voice gets louder Speech quickens Clenching of fists

things, and it isn't even her fault. I've never been violent, though, she'll tell you that. It's just, by the time I get home, I've usually got a raging headache, I'm as tense as anything and feeling absolutely knackered. Sometimes I've got a right sweat on and my chest feels really tight, and my face is bright red by the time I get in. I just don't want to talk, and she sometimes pushes me to my limit with her chatter, and I just give her a mouthful and storm off, slamming the door behind me. I damaged it the other day. I felt pretty awful about that when I calmed down.

Sometimes just thinking about things gets me annoyed. I can be sitting quite relaxed and then I'll start thinking about it, and I can get all worked up again. It's really stupid.

We've got a baby on the way, and I really need to sort myself out before he or she arrives, because that's going to be stressful in itself, let's face it.

Exercise

Watch the video clip about Ben, or read the transcript.
- Using the Emotional, Physical, Cognitive and Behavioural Symptoms of Anger list, consider which of the symptoms in the list Ben presents with.
- Then use the model on page 143 as a guide to help you demonstrate these links in a diagrammatic form.

Section summary

- Anger is a normal emotion
- Anger is a problem when it is too frequent, too intense or lasts too long, is disproportionate to the situation or leads to violence
- Practising new skills learned to deal with anger is crucial

Recommended reading

Davies, W. (2000). *Overcoming Anger and Irritability. A self-help guide using Cognitive Behavioural Techniques.* London: Robinson.

Dryden, W. (1996). *Overcoming Anger.* London: Sheldon Press.

Harbin, T.J. (2000). *Beyond Anger: a Guide for Men: How to Free Yourself from the Grip of Anger and Get More Out of Life.* New York: Marlowe and Co.

Test yourself

 To check your progress, locate this section on CD-ROM 3 and work through the interactive questions at the end.

Chapter 3.2
Active listening and engagement skills

Aim

To outline the essential interpersonal skills necessary for engaging and working with patients in primary care.

Learning outcomes

By the end of this Chapter, the reader will be able to:
- Understand the importance of active listening and engagement skills
- Use these skills in interactions with patients
- Identify and effectively use verbal and non-verbal communication skills
- Apply appropriate communication skills in face-to-face and telephone interactions with patients
- Understand the importance of maintaining patient confidentiality
- Critically evaluate the importance of setting appropriate clinical boundaries

Introduction

It cannot be over-estimated how important our natural intuitive response is in our interactions with others. Some people find that they are sought out by friends and family who have a problem they want to discuss. This is no accident; these people have qualities that make others feel safe and comfortable enough to confide in them about their problems. This ability to help others in distress is a quality that many people in the helping professions already possess. The aim here is to improve mental health workers' effectiveness in dealing with others, by combining these intuitive responses with some practical therapeutic techniques to benefit patients. We can all learn how to listen and communicate effectively, which forms the basis for effective therapeutic skills.

Some readers may find it to be of interest and of benefit to consult the various theoretical models of therapeutic engagement that are available. Authors to look out for include Barker, Egan, Heron and Wilber. Some of their work is included in the recommended reading for this Chapter. Rather than follow any particular theoretical model, we focus here on the practical skills to enhance therapeutic engagement with patients.

The communication skills covered within this Chapter are as follows:
1 Core therapeutic skills
2 Non-verbal communication
3 Verbal skills
4 Core attitudes and values
5 Confidentiality
6 Setting appropriate clinical boundaries
7 Telephone contact skills

Recommended reading

Barker, P. (1997). *Assessment in psychiatric and mental health nursing: In search of the whole person.* Cheltenham: Stanley Thornes.

Egan, G. (2001). *The Skilled Helper: A systematic approach to effective helping* (seventh edition). California: Brooks/Cole.

Heron, J. (2000). *Helping the client: A creative practical guide* (fifth edition). London: Sage.

Norman, I. and Ryrie, I. (eds) 2004. *The Art and Science of Mental Health Nursing.* Maidenhead: Open University Press.

Wilber, K. (2000). *Sex, Ecology and Spirituality: The spirit of evolution.* Boston MA: Shambhala.

Section 1: Core skills for mental health workers

The following skills are central to our ability to communicate effectively with patients.

Introductions

Introductions constitute the opening to any contact with patients and are therefore crucial to get right. The first few minutes of an interview with a patient, whether it be face-to-face or by telephone, set the scene for the rest of the session.

The five stages of introductions are:

1 Checking the patient's name
2 Introducing the mental health worker's name
3 Stating the mental health worker's role
4 Stating the purpose of the session
5 Stating the time allocated for the session

1 Checking the patient's name

It is important that we know from the outset that we are talking to the right person, which will obviously be apparent with ongoing face-to-face contact but should always be clarified before anything else is said in every telephone contact. At the first contact, it is important to clarify what the patient prefers to be called. Some people prefer to use a shortened form of their first name or to use a middle name; others prefer to be addressed by their title and surname. Patients can feel uncomfortable if addressed in a way that they do not like, so it should always be established at the very start and adhered to thenceforth.

2 and 3 Introducing the mental health worker's name and role

Next, we introduce ourselves, with both first name and surname. In the first face-to-face contact and in every telephone contact we should state our full name and role (e.g. 'I'm Waseem Malik and I'm a Graduate Mental Health Worker').

4 and 5 Stating the purpose and time allocated for the session

The next stage is to describe the purpose of the interview (e.g. 'I'd like to find out how you have been getting on with the medication that Dr Rushforth prescribed. I'd also like to find out how you've been getting on with the self-help booklet I sent to you').

The time allocated to the interview is also clearly stated (e.g. 'We've got 20 minutes'). By doing this, an agenda is being set for the session which provides structure to how the conversation will proceed. The patient should also be asked if they would like to add anything to this agenda so that any issues they bring are not addressed merely as an afterthought at the end of the session, or, worse still, are not addressed at all.

Content of sessions

This will be discussed in Chapter 3.3 for assessment (page 193) and Chapter 3.4 for specific interventions (page 224); therefore, content of sessions will not be covered here.

Endings

Patients tend to remember the beginning and end of a session best. Therefore, like introductions, it is important that the session ends correctly. A final summary of what has been agreed in the session is fed back to the patient and their understanding is checked. Often this is done by asking the patient to say what they plan to do between this and the following contact. This is important, as the patient may go away with the wrong idea of what is expected of them. Feedback can by elicited from the patient by asking a question like 'Is there anything that you feel unsure about and would like me to explain further?'.

In addition, asking patients a question like 'Is there anything important that we haven't discussed today?' helps to ensure that nothing important is missed that the patient would like to have discussed.

Finally, the next appointment is agreed, with

the patient being clear about the time and place of the next contact; if this is arranged during a face-to-face contact, it can be written down on an appointment card; if by telephone, the patient can be asked to make a note.

Note-taking

Taking notes is an important part of the mental health worker's interview tasks. It is a vital skill to learn, as it is impossible to remember all the important points from each interaction. With this in mind, it is easy to see why patients may forget important parts of sessions too, so it can be helpful for patients to keep a note of the important aspects of each session as well, particularly any activities that they have agreed to do prior to the next session.

Note-taking should be as unobtrusive as possible, to ensure that we can communicate that we are listening attentively to the patient while making notes of pertinent points. Before an assessment interview, it can sometimes be helpful to write the various topics to be covered with the appropriate headings on the notepad.

However, although this can be a useful prompt, it must be kept in mind that an assessment is not a linear process and there must remain a degree of flexibility; the headings just ensure that each topic is covered. In addition, some mental health workers find it helpful to mark dots several times down the left hand side of each page as a reminder to use empathic statements; these dots can also be used as a prompt to summarize.

Special circumstances

Certain situations require special consideration. For example, providing telephone sessions rather than face-to-face sessions requires particularly good communication skills. Telephone contact skills are addressed in Section 7 (see page 190).

Cultural and ethnicity issues can emerge from time to time. When there is a language difficullty, it is important to ensure that there is an interpreter present, or perhaps a family member who is aware of the patient's problem can take this role. If a patient comes from a different culture, whether they speak English or not, it can be helpful to get some degree of understanding of this culture prior to seeing the patient, to ensure that the patient is not inadvertently offended by something we say or do.

If working with patients who have impaired hearing, it is crucial to know how that person communicates. For example, it may be necessary to include someone in the session who can translate what the mental health worker is saying using sign language. However, not every deaf or hard-of-hearing person will communicate using sign language. Some may actually prefer to lip read or have any information given in written form. When working with a patient who lip reads, it is important to speak clearly and always to have one's lips visible. This may seem simplistic advice, but it is important, as it is not unusual to turn away when writing a note or even to cover one's mouth inadvertently. Attention to small details such as these can make a big difference to effective communication.

Part 2.1, Section 2 will also be of relevance to the reader, in respect of issues related to ethnicity and patients who are hard of hearing.

Negotiating end of contact

For some patients, ending contact can seem as difficult as starting it; however, the end should not come as a surprise to the patient. Right from the start, the patient knows that contact will not go on indefinitely. The mental health worker provides guidance and support to the patient and works together with them, so that ultimately they can work on their problems alone. Clear goals are negotiated at the outset and, when these goals are met, contact can be discontinued, unless it is appropriate to set new goals. However, it is not in the best interests of the patient to keep them in therapeutic contact indefinitely.

If the contact has gone well and the patient has gone a long way to overcoming their problems, it is likely that they will have some warm feelings for the mental health worker as they may well have confided to them information that they have not told anyone else. However, if the patient is having severe difficulty in terminating contact, then we must ask ourselves about whether we maintained professional boundaries or whether the patient has become a 'friend'. If the patient has confided information solely to us, then part of the contact should have been to encourage the patient to start sharing these things with the people in their life. In this way, by the time termination of contact has been reached, the patient will be experiencing the type of closeness with a partner, friend or family member that they were previously only able to experience with the mental health worker.

If you experience difficulties in negotiating end of contact with a patient, you should seek guidance from your supervisor.

Dealing with a patient's concerns about end of contact

Towards the end of therapeutic contact, it is important to examine the patient's concerns about the contact coming to an end. Most patients will be happy about how they have improved but perhaps be a little apprehensive about relapse or their ability to cope without any contact with the mental health worker.

It is important to acknowledge the patient's feelings and to evaluate their thoughts in the same way as any other negative thoughts (e.g. evidence for and against, which is covered in Part 3.4, Section 4e).

Section summary

- Introductions are an important start to any contact with a patient
- Sessions should end with a summary of what is to be tackled before the next contact
- Note-taking is an important skill that should be as unobtrusive as possible
- Cultural and ethnicity issues should be addressed appropriately when they arise
- Any concerns a patient has about end of contact should be addressed

Test yourself

 To check your progress, locate this section on CD-ROM 3 and work through the interactive questions at the end.

Section 2: Non-verbal communication

The following non-verbal communication skills are central to our ability to relate effectively to patients.

Non-verbal communication

It is important to develop skills to communicate to patients that we are listening and attending to what is being said without having to verbalize this. Non-verbal communication often speaks louder than any words. Attentive listening encourages patients to trust us, thereby encouraging them to open up and share their problems. If a patient detects only half-hearted attending or that the mental health worker is not interested at all, then they may be reluctant to reveal their problems as it will not feel safe to do so. It is important to develop an awareness of how we use our bodies to communicate with others and to become aware of the messages we are sending out. Although it is vital to develop an awareness of non-verbal behaviour, it is also important not to become consumed with our body language to the point where we are completely preoccupied by it.

There are three main ways of demonstrating our attention to patients non-verbally:
1 Eye contact
2 Facial expression
3 Posture

Eye contact

It is important to maintain good eye contact but not to stare. If you watch two people in deep conversation you will see that there will be a great deal of direct eye contact between them. However, it is acceptable to look away and, as you are likely to be taking notes during the contact, this will be necessary at times anyway. However, looking away too frequently can make the patient feel uncomfortable.

Exercise

Next time you are in a social situation (e.g. pub, café, restaurant), look around you and observe eye contact between people in conversation. What do you notice?

Facial expression

It is important that what the patient says is responded to with appropriate facial expression. Interest in what the patient is saying can be communicated by use of facial expression (including lip movements and eyebrow lifts to demonstrate understanding).

Exercise

When in conversation with a family member, friend or colleague, observe their facial expressions in response to what you are saying. Note how they communicate using facial expression. Then repeat the exercise and ask the other person to use no facial expression and only respond verbally. Notice what it feels like when no facial expression is given in response to what you say.

Posture

Posture should be open, as crossing arms and legs can indicate a barrier to others. Leaning on the arm of a chair with one's head propped up by a hand can indicate that we are a little weary or bored. An open posture indicates to the patient that we are open and receptive to what they are saying. Leaning forward can show attentiveness, but doing this too often or leaning too far forward can feel threatening. It is, therefore, important to get the balance right. Be sure to watch out for fidgeting, as this can come across as a sign of being nervous or uncomfortable.

As well as attending to our own non-verbal behaviour, it is crucial to attend to patients' body language too. A skilled mental health worker will learn to read:

1 Body language (i.e. posture, movements and other gestures)
2 Facial expressions (i.e. frowns, eyebrow lifts, lip movements)
3 Voice (e.g. tone, pitch, emphasis, etc.)
4 Physiological reactions (i.e. increase in breathing, blushing, etc.)

Seating arrangements

Seating should be slightly off-square, so that chairs are at slight angles to each other. The distance should be far enough apart for the patient to move their legs comfortably without worrying about touching the mental health worker, but close enough so that if something is to be shared in the session (e.g. a diary or some written information relevant to the patient's problem) both parties can lean forward and read whatever it is together without discomfort.

Verbally encouraging people to talk

Using brief responses to patients can convey the message that we are listening attentively. If we intersperse utterances such as 'yes', 'uh-ummm', 'I see', 'carry on', etc., in our communication, this helps encourage patients to talk and tells them that we are actively listening.

Listening skills

What makes a good listener? It seems that there are a number of qualities that can be identified in a good listener.

A good listener:
• does not interrupt
• gives their full attention
• is non-judgemental
• is accepting of others
• does not give direct advice
• clarifies any vagueness or anything that may be misunderstood

- gives adequate time for the person to talk
- does not undervalue what someone's problem is by telling them about an even worse problem

Section summary

- Attention to patients can be demonstrated non-verbally, using eye contact, facial expression and posture
- A skilled mental health worker will be able to read a patient's body language, facial expressions, voice and physiological reactions

Test yourself

 To check your progress, locate this section on CD-ROM 3 and work through the interactive questions at the end.

Section 3: Verbal skills

There are a number of core techniques that are present during a therapeutic relationship. These include the following:
- Paraphrasing
- Reflection
- Empathic responses
- Summarizing

The core techniques

Paraphrasing

Paraphrasing involves repeating back to a patient what they have said, in their own words, but not parrot-fashion.

For example:

Nigel: Since Jenny left, I've been at home most of the time and just been brooding over things. I've not been able to face going to work and bills are piling up. I've just ended up putting them in a drawer until I feel I can deal with them.

Mental health worker (Waseem): So it sounds like your time to brood over the breakdown of your marriage has ended up making it difficult for you to keep on top of things.

Reflection of feelings

This involves acknowledging the feelings that the patient is telling us about or demonstrating to us throughout their communication, even if this is implicit rather than actually being verbalized by the patient (e.g. 'I can see that this is upsetting for you to talk about'). The patient may not have said 'This is upsetting for me to talk about', but because they are tearful, say, or in some other way overtly distressed, we can acknowledge these feelings.

Empathic responses

Empathy should not be confused with sympathy. Sympathy is about conveying our understanding as we are experiencing the same distress as the person involved, while empathy is about entering that person's world to understand what they are experiencing without having to actually experience it ourselves. It is empathy that we want to convey to patients.

Empathy involves being sensitive to the experience of the other person. If we fail to communicate empathy to the patient, they will feel that we have not understood them and that we are uncaring. It is helpful to use the same language as the patient, or at least to use non-contentious language.

Note: We should never say 'I understand', as this can feel patronizing to the patient and may result in the retort, 'How can you possibly understand when you haven't gone through what I've gone through?' Appropriate statements include 'It sounds like you've had a difficult time recently', 'Things certainly haven't been easy of late, from what you're saying', or other similar statements that demonstrate empathic understanding.

Summarizing

Frequent summarizing throughout the session shows that we have been listening to the patient and understand what they are saying, and it demonstrates warmth. It is similar to paraphrasing, but done in bigger chunks over longer periods, often identifying themes.

For example:

Mental health worker (Waseem): From what you've said about your friends and family, it seems that over recent weeks you feel that no-one is very interested in your problems and this has resulted in you seeing yourself as unimportant and feeling more depressed.

Julian: Yes that's right.

Summarizing should be done frequently to clarify a shared understanding. Many novice mental health workers do not summarize often enough.

Emphasizing the patient's personal strengths and competencies

Patients have strengths and competencies that we should build on. It is important for the patient to feel that they are using their own skills, despite requiring some help from a mental health worker. By asking questions similar to the following, we can emphasize the patient's personal strengths and competencies: 'How have you handled difficult situations in the past?', 'Can you tell me a bit about how you managed to do that?', 'Do you think that what you did could be useful in addressing other difficulties?'.

Developing rapport

The working relationship between patient and mental health worker, as in all therapeutic contacts, is crucial. Attempts are made to build rapport by using active listening skills, by making frequent summaries of what the patient says to communicate understanding, and by showing genuine warmth and empathy.

Useful questions to ask

- How did you know that something was wrong?
- When you got to the stage when you realized you were experiencing difficulties, who did you talk to about it?
- Was there anything they said that you found helpful?
- Did that help to change anything for you?
- Of all the times you have talked this problem over with people, which has been the most useful?
- What is going to be the most important thing for us to talk about today?

 CD-ROM 3 includes a video clip showing the interaction between mental health worker, Katie, and her patient, Andrew, whom we met earlier. In this clip, Katie demonstrates some good verbal communication skills. A transcript of the clip is given below.

Video: Active listening and engagement skills (good)

Mental health worker (Katie): It sounds like the party last week didn't go too well for you. Can you tell me a little bit about what happened?

Andrew: Yes, my friend introduced me to a woman, then just left me to it. I was mortified. I didn't know what to say. I got all tongue-tied and I went bright red, and I came over all sweaty. I guess I panicked a bit, so then I mumbled something and dashed off to the loo, and I tried to compose myself. Then I left and I called my friend on the way home, and said that I was feeling ill and that was why I left the party. I still get upset when I talk about it now.

Katie: That does sound upsetting for you, and I can see that it's quite uncomfortable for you to talk about it. It sounds to me like you found yourself in a situation that you didn't feel prepared for and, because you got so anxious and upset, you felt that your only option was to leave.

Andrew: Yes, that's exactly it.

Section summary

- Basic verbal skills involve: paraphrasing, reflection, empathic responses and summarizing
- All these verbal skills should be used frequently during contacts with patients

Test yourself

 To check your progress, locate this section on CD-ROM 3 and work through the interactive questions at the end.

Section 4: Core attitudes and values

The following attitudes and values are central to our ability to communicate effectively with patients.

Communicating respect

It is important that we convey our respect for the patient, demonstrating that we think the patient is worthwhile and the information that he or she is giving is considered valuable. We do that by using the verbal and non-verbal techniques described earlier, as well as being well prepared for the session and starting and finishing on time.

Communicating empathy

Demonstrating empathy is about showing we understand the other person's world as they understand it themselves. This is predominantly a verbal skill. The verbal techniques already mentioned help us demonstrate empathy. In addition, we can convey empathy by reflecting back what patients have said to us and by frequently checking back with the patient that we have understood what they have said. We must always try to see things from the patient's point of view and try to imagine how we might feel if we were experiencing the same circumstances.

Communicating genuineness

It is important that we come across to patients as genuine and open. We do this by responding in a natural way, and by not pretending that we are something that we are not. We must always remember that the patient will have their own strengths and will be the expert on their own problem, and that we are working in partnership with them to help them overcome their difficulties rather than being the fount of all knowledge.

There will always be a power differential in this type of relationship and this should be recognized, so that the mental health worker and patient work in partnership to share decision-making about the help required to best address the patient's particular needs. Both will bring different qualities to the relationship: the patient brings their experience of the problem, while the mental health worker brings knowledge in the most appropriate strategies to address the patient's difficulties. The relationship should always be maintained on a professional footing, with clear boundaries, and using a patient-centred approach (see Section 6, page 188, on setting appropriate clinical boundaries). A relationship that has progressed into a friendship will be confusing and unhelpful for the patient. A friendly and genuine manner is called for without the over-familiarity that can lead to confusion of the relationship boundaries.

Our own personal beliefs and attitudes

Our own attitudes and beliefs can hinder our ability to relate to some patients and, therefore, it is imperative that we are aware of our own prejudices and that we can suspend them to enable us to communicate effectively with patients without our own belief system getting in the way. For example, it is unhelpful if: a mental health worker who feels strongly that children should be born within a marital relationship makes this known to a patient who is a single parent; or a mental health worker who holds strong homophobic beliefs makes value judgements about gay or lesbian patients they are working with. Prejudicial beliefs have no place in the helping professions and it is our responsibility to challenge and change our own thinking. Any issues surrounding conflict between the patient's and your own personal beliefs should be discussed with your supervisor.

Section summary

- The mental health worker should communicate respect, empathy and genuineness to the patient
- Personal attitudes and beliefs should not get in the way of the therapeutic alliance

Test yourself

 To check your progress, locate this section on CD-ROM 3 and work through the interactive questions at the end.

Section 5: Confidentiality

Introduction

Patient confidentiality is an important issue. It is imperative that we know what we can and cannot do with private, and at times very sensitive information given by patients. The mental health worker must learn under what circumstances they should disclose information and who they can disclose this information to. Patients trust health practitioners with confidential information which should be respected at all times. In this section, some of the common issues arising from confidential information are addressed.

As a mental health worker you must protect confidential information

Confidential information should only be used for the purposes it has been given, namely to inform the patient's care. This information can be shared with other members of the care team who are involved with the patient, but the patient has a right to know who will have access to this information. Improper disclosure of confidential information must be avoided; therefore, no-one outside the care team should learn about this information.

Never assume that patients want members of their family to have access to confidential information

We must always check with patients to ensure that it is acceptable to them for confidential information to be shared with their family.

When is it appropriate to disclose confidential information without the consent of the patient?

Confidential information can be disclosed without the patient's consent when:
- it is within the interest of the patient or the public to do so (i.e. when the patient is at risk of harming themselves or someone else). The decision to disclose this information is usually made by the GP. The patient's history of risk and other relevant information is taken into consideration when this is an issue. It is essential that, if any confidential information is disclosed, it be clearly documented and the accountable practitioner must be able to justify their actions.
- there are child protection issues. It is best to check with Department of Health guidelines for what action should be taken if child protection issues arise (www.dh.gov.uk).

Note: the information in this section is based on the Nursing and Midwifery Council's Code of Professional Conduct. More detailed information about confidentiality can be found in Chapter 1.2, Section 9 .

Section summary

- Mental health workers must protect confidential information
- One should never assume that patients want family members to have access to confidential information
- Confidential information can be disclosed without the patient's consent when the patient is at risk of harming themselves or someone else, or when there are child protection issues

Reference

Nursing and Midwifery Council (2004). Too much information: When to tell and what not to tell about your patients. *NMC News,* July 2004.

Test yourself

 To check your progress, locate this section on CD-ROM 3 and work through the interactive questions at the end.

Section 6: Setting appropriate clinical boundaries

Introduction

'Clinical boundaries' refers to the behaviours, language, space, time, touch and levels of self-disclosure demonstrated in the clinical setting to patients. For appropriate therapeutic intervention, it is essential that clinical boundaries are not breached. It is important to note that it is not only the mental health worker who may cross these boundaries but that patients, too, may do so. However, the responsibility for maintaining appropriate professional boundaries rests with the mental health worker.

Behaviours

Giving presents to patients, sexual physical contact or communication, highly personal self-disclosure and meeting outside the clinical environment for personal reasons are clear breaches of clinical boundaries. Receiving gifts or favours (e.g. financial advice, providing lunch, discounts, etc.) are exploitative and destroy the therapeutic alliance.

Language

We should always use language appropriate to the patient; however, swearing and crude language should never be used. If a patient is using such language, we should advise them that we would prefer it if they refrained from using this during our contacts.

Space

Contact will generally take place in the mental health worker's office or by telephone. Any exception to this may represent a boundary crossing, although there may be times when it is appropriate to make a home visit or to accompany a patient to a hospital appointment, etc. Seeing a patient who is housebound at home is clearly appropriate. There may be times when a mental health worker is helping a patient with phobic anxiety that they might accompany the patient in a car, lift, on public transport, etc.; but this is rare, as exposure (see Chapter 3.4, Section 4d) is usually carried out by the patient outside sessions. Whenever a patient is seen outside of the healthcare setting it is imperative that personal safety issues are considered. The mental health worker's personal safety should clearly never be put at risk. Advice should be sought on Trust policy about seeing patients outside of the health centre or surgery setting.

Time

The mental health worker and patient will negotiate scheduled contacts, and it is important that the time allocated is adhered to, rather than allowing the session repeatedly to run over time. The contact should start and finish on time and the patient should be aware of clear beginning and end times. However, it maybe necessary to extend a contact if an emergency arises. Note that this is very different to just running over time because the mental health worker is a poor timekeeper.

Time boundaries provide structure for patients and can help reassure them that they only have to endure (as that may well be what it feels like) the stress of the contact for a set time. Patients should never be rescheduled to the end of the day to avoid interruption by the next patient's arrival if the session overruns. If this is a continuing problem with certain, or all, patients, it should be discussed in supervision and advice sought.

Touch

The use of touch can cause a great deal of confusion. In times past, hugs were seen as an appropriate way of using physical contact with patients. This would be seen as highly inappropriate nowadays and be open to suspicion about the sexual connotations, and, therefore, should not be encouraged. A handshake on first meeting a patient is appropriate and desirable but, apart from that, touch should generally be avoided. Always bear in mind that most of your interaction with patients will take place behind closed doors; therefore, limiting physical contact is prudent advice.

Self-disclosure

It is important not to burden a patient with personal information about ourselves. Some information may hinder a patient from being able to disclose further information about themselves (e.g. perhaps a mental health worker feels strongly that people should not have children outside of marriage, but must accept that others will have different views).

Even information about social plans, holiday arrangements, expected births in the family, etc., are irrelevant for the patient to know. Whatever moral codes we hold about ourselves and our families, we should not share these with patients, nor judge patients by our own personal beliefs. Any issues such as these that arise should be raised in supervision.

Sometimes we can really connect with a patient and feel that, if it were not for the situation, this person could be a friend. It is vital to remember that this person is NOT a friend. The mental health worker is someone the patient is coming to see for professional help. Friends share lots of personal information about themselves. We should not share intimate details about our lives, nor should we seek any advice about anything at all from the patient.

Dealing with personal questions

Sometimes patients ask personal questions. It is important to deal with such questions sensitively, but without self-disclosure. Responses such as 'Yes, like many people, I have had bereavements too – but we're here to talk about you ...', or 'Yes, I think we all get stressed from time to time, but what I'm really interested in is hearing about how stress is affecting you right now', 'Thank you for asking, but lets remember this is about you' are all appropriate responses to patients who prompt us for self-disclosure.

Section summary

- 'Appropriate clinical boundaries' refers to behaviours, language, space, time, touch and levels of self-disclosure in the clinical setting
- Sessions should always start and finish on time
- Apart from a handshake on first meeting, physical contact should be avoided
- Self-disclosure should always be avoided

Recommended reading

Epstein, R.S. (1994). Keeping *boundaries – Maintaining safety and integrity in the psychotherapeutic process*. Arlington, VA: American Psychiatric Publishing Inc.

Gutheil, T.G. and Gabbard, G.O. (1993). The concept of boundaries in clinical practice: theoretical and risk-management dimensions. *American Journal of Psychiatry*, 150 (2), 188–196.

Test yourself

 To check your progress, locate this section on CD-ROM 3 and work through the interactive questions at the end.

Section 7: Telephone contact skills

Introduction

The skills that have been described and illustrated so far have been referred to, in the main, in the context of seeing the patient face-to-face. These communication skills remain highly relevant to telephone contact. However, there are some additional considerations that need to be made regarding our communications with patients over the telephone. Obviously, the main issue is that neither person can see the other, so communication is based purely on the person's voice, their inflection and the content of what they are saying.

As the patient cannot be seen, it is all the more important to be aware of vocal tones and communication habits that may lead to misunderstandings. Communication should be clear, audible and flow easily. Good listening skills, as described in Section 2, are essential. We should be prepared to listen and not to rush to fill any gaps in communication that the patient would fill if given a little more time. Instead of the non-verbal cues such as nods to encourage patients to continue, verbal prompts are used more often (e.g. 'yes', 'uh-ummm', 'I see', 'carry on', etc.). As with any communication, paraphrasing, reflection and summarizing should be used, as they would in a face-to-face contact, to clarify understanding as described in Section 3. Empathy should be demonstrated throughout. It is up to the mental health worker to start and end the call; this should be done in a professional manner.

Stages of a telephone contact

1   Check that you are speaking to the right person.

2   We should always introduce ourselves by name and organization. If the person answering the telephone is not the patient, then issues of confidentiality must be considered (see Section 5).

3   The format for the call will follow the protocols of the approaches used (e.g. Case Management, Medication Management, Behavioural Activation, Problem Solving, or any of the other self-help approaches covered in Chapter 2.4).

4.   Clarify that both parties have a shared understanding of the action plan arising from the call. Often it is best to get the patient to tell you their understanding of what the plan is, so that any misunderstandings can be clarified.

5.   Ending the call. As the mental health worker initiated the call, it is their role to end it. This should be done following the agreement of the action plan and having asked if the patient has any further questions. Clear and specific follow-up plans should then be arranged (e.g. next phone call).

Examples CD-ROM 3 includes two video clips in which Katie, the mental health worker, initiates and concludes telephone contacts. Transcripts of the contacts are shown below.

Video: How to start a telephone call

Tim: Hello.
Mental health worker (Katie): Hello, is that Tim Dawson?
Tim: Yes, speaking.
Katie: Hi Tim, it's Katie Walsh here from Cochrane Park Health Centre. We agreed that I'd call today.
Tim: Yes, I was waiting for your call.
Katie: That's great. Tim, there are a few things I'd like to discuss with you during the call and I know that you'll probably have some things you'd like to talk about too. Perhaps it would be helpful to decide how

we're going to spend our time from the start. We've got up to 15 minutes. How does that sound?

Tim: That sounds fine.

Video: Correct use of summarizing and ending a telephone call

Mental health worker (Katie): Okay, that's good. Well, we seem to have covered everything we set out to cover. Can I just check with you that we're both clear about what you plan to do until we speak again next week?

Sarah: Yes. I said I would continue to take the medication Dr Mehra prescribed and maybe I'll get some boiled sweets to help with my dry mouth, and I'm going to start taking the tablets just before I eat something. I'm going to read the leaflet on antidepressants and try to fill in the activity diary you gave me.

Katie: Yes, that's right. Do you think anything might get in the way of you being able to do any of these things?

Sarah: I don't think so, although my concentration isn't great at the moment for reading, and the diary sounds like a big job; but I'm willing to give them a try.

Katie: That's what it's about, giving things a try. You might find it helpful to read the leaflet in small chunks if you find your concentration starts to flag. Please don't worry too much about the diary. Any information is useful, so if you feel that you can only fill it in part of the time then that's okay. Having some information about what you are doing at the moment would be really helpful in guiding us as to where best to start on getting you more active.

Sarah: Yes, okay. I'll give it a go.

Katie: Great. Now, is there anything important that we haven't discussed today?

Sarah: No, I don't think so.

Katie: Okay. Do you have anything you want to ask me before we come to a close?

Sarah: No.

Katie: Right, well, let's arrange a time to speak again. How would next week at the same time suit you?

Sarah: Yes, that's fine.

Katie: Great. Okay, well, I'll speak to you next Thursday at 1 o'clock.

Sarah: Okay, thanks. Bye.

Katie: Bye.

Note how, as she begins her contact with Tim, Katie makes certain that she is talking to the right person before saying who she is and where she is calling from, in case any confidentiality issues are breached. Then, as she prepares to end her telephone contact with Sarah, Katie confirms that a shared understanding of the action plan has been reached.

Exercise

Practise a telephone contact with a colleague.

- Ask your colleague to take the role of someone who is depressed.
- Go through the stages of a telephone contact.
- Get feedback on your performance (e.g. accuracy, empathy, summarising, etc.).
- Repeat the exercise, with your colleague taking the role of a patient with an anxiety disorder.

Section summary

- When talking to a patient on the telephone, we must pay special attention to our voice, inflection and the clarity of the content of what we are saying
- Communication should be clear, audible and flow easily
- Instead of the non-verbal cues, such as nods, to encourage patients to continue, liberal use of verbal prompts should be used
- Paraphrasing, reflection, empathic statements and summarizing should be used, as they would in a face-to-face contact

- The stages of a telephone contact are: checking that you are speaking to the right person; introducing yourself; contact content; clarification of the action plan; ending the call

Test yourself

 To check your progress, locate this section on CD-ROM 3 and work through the interactive questions at the end.

Chapter 3.3
Assessment

Aim

To enhance mental health worker skills in patient-centred interviewing and assessment.

Learning outcomes

By the end of this Chapter, the reader will be able to:

- Effectively assess patient problems using a patient-centred interview model
- Safely determine patients' level of risk to themselves or others
- Summarize patients' problems using concise problem statements
- Collaboratively agree appropriate goals for intervention
- Evaluate the progress of interventions using patient-centred and standardized measures of clinical outcomes

Introduction

Any clinical intervention will only be as good as the assessment information it is based on. Therefore, for any clinical intervention to be successful, an accurate assessment is vital. The interventions included in this programme have proven effectiveness, but careful assessment is essential to ensure that they are used appropriately. It is crucial that an accurate assessment of the patient's problems takes place prior to consideration of any intervention.

The assessment is likely to be the main source of information about the patient, though some information is also likely to have been obtained from the referrer (in the main, this will be the GP). The assessment interview is also an opportunity to begin establishing rapport with the patient, which is essential for any clinical intervention to be successful.

Although the main focus of the assessment is on the gathering of information, assessment continues throughout the whole of the contact with the patient. A number of sources can be used to gain information, including the interview itself, validated questionnaires, case-specific measures and monitoring diaries.

Patient-centred interviewing

Mental health workers must try to see the mental health problems that patients present with as they are experienced by them. It is vital to view the patient as a whole person, not just as a set of symptoms; and therefore both the social and psychological aspects of patients' lives must be taken into consideration in the assessment. In doing this, the chances of building a good therapeutic alliance are increased. There is a power imbalance between the mental health worker and the patient, and this needs to be recognized so that power is shared and the patient becomes a partner in making decisions about what is most likely to meet their needs. Both parties bring different aspects to the therapeutic relationship: the patient brings their experience of living with their problem, and the mental health worker brings their expertise in organizing information, together with technical knowledge of evidence-based strategies that are likely to help the patient to overcome such difficulties.

The mental health worker needs to be realistic about the limitations of what they can do in the time available and with the resources at hand. Therefore, the patient is encouraged to learn how to use self-help strategies to tackle their difficulties.

Aims of the assessment

The aim of assessment is to get an understanding of the patient's problems, including the main emotional, physical, cognitive and behavioural symptoms. Information is also sought on what areas of the patient's life are affected (e.g. work, relationships, etc.). The patient is asked to describe the current problems in the context of the last month or so.

The mental health worker is interested in how the problems started, their duration and any factors which make the problems better or worse (e.g. being accompanied). The patient is asked if there is anything that they avoid because of the problems, including more subtle avoidances or 'safety behaviours'. Information on past history is only elicited if it is of direct relevance to the problems, their development and maintenance, though it is unlikely that much will be learned about the patient's early life in the first interview if at all.

The first session gives the patient a flavour of what future sessions will be like, the agenda is negotiated, there is a focus on problems, a collaborative approach is used, and feedback is sought. From the first session, self-help activities are negotiated. This might be to complete questionnaires, read some literature relevant to the patient's difficulties, or use a diary to monitor symptoms (e.g. activity levels).

It is important that the patient feels safe to disclose information about their problems. Therefore the mental health worker must demonstrate warmth and empathy, and communicate to the patient genuine interest in understanding what problems they are experiencing. In this way, a strong therapeutic alliance is nurtured.

A patient is more likely to feel motivated to work on their problems if they believe that they are competent and possess the ability to overcome their difficulties themselves. Therefore, the patient's strengths (e.g. determination) are elicited, and positive aspects of their lives (e.g. a supportive partner) identified. There will also be times when the problem has not always been there, and acknowledging this can help foster hope.

Interpersonal skills

The mental health worker should come across as warm and empathic to the patient. Statements such as 'I realize that this is very distressing for you' and 'I can see that this is upsetting for you to talk about' are good empathic statements which demonstrate warmth and understanding. Warmth is not only demonstrated verbally, but also non-verbally with attentive eye contact, open posture, appropriate facial expression and nodding. Paraphrasing and reflection are used to acknowledge the patient's problems and to elicit further information (e.g. 'So you felt like you were about to collapse when you were standing in the supermarket queue.').

Summarizing should also be used frequently throughout, as this helps clarify understanding and elicit further information (e.g. 'You woke up very early and were unable to get back to sleep, you felt very low in mood and unable to go to work that day, is that right?').

Note-taking

Accurate note-taking during the interview is essential. Inexperienced mental health workers sometimes find it difficult to take notes and at the same time continue to demonstrate they are paying attention to the patient. This is an important skill to learn as, even with the best of memories, it is impossible to remember all the important parts of the interview. Checking later in the interview can be used to ascertain that key issues have been correctly identified. It is therefore necessary to learn how to take notes in as non-intrusive a way as possible. Some mental health workers find that they can use abbreviations or key words as reminders; it is certainly no use if they keep their head down, writing everything verbatim. If this were the case, the patient would be likely to feel that they are not receiving any attention and that the mental health worker is uninterested and cold.

Interview format

As it is likely that the session will be reasonably short (e.g. 30–45 minutes), it is imperative that the time is used efficiently and that the session is appropriately paced, starting and finishing on time. There should be a clear beginning, middle and end, with a shared decision of where to go next, rather than the session drifting and ending abruptly. The aims of the session should be stated clearly at the beginning in the form of an agenda, and adhered to throughout. However, it is equally important to have a degree of flexibility, so that the order in which items are addressed are changed in response to the patient's needs and that the interview is short-circuited if concerns regarding suicidality or other safety issues emerge.

Phase 1: Introductions

Phase 2: Content of the assessment including additional information

Phase 3: Problem summaries and goals are agreed

Phase 4: A shared decision is made about what strategies should be used to tackle the patient's difficulties, and clinical measurement tools are determined

Following these four phases ensures a clear beginning, middle and end to the session. Each of the four phases will be elaborated on in detail throughout this Chapter.

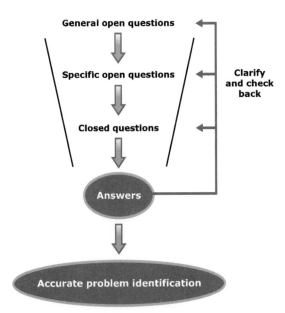

Figure. 8: The question funnel

Assessment information-gathering

The quality of the questions asked will directly determine the quality of the information received, therefore it is important to develop good questioning skills. Any question asked should be clear and easy to understand. Only ask one question at a time rather than asking two or three rolled into one ('What did you do and what were you thinking and feeling at the time?' are three separate questions).

The question funnel

It is useful to use a kind of funnel approach to questioning, as shown in Figure 8. The mental health worker should start with general, open questions which help to get the patient beginning to talk about their problems (e.g. 'What problems are you experiencing that have led you to seek help?'). The 'what', 'where', 'whom', 'when' questions, elaborated on later, are used to elicit this information about the patient's problems.

The next step involves asking more specific questions but continuing to keep them open (e.g. 'Can you tell me a bit more about how your low mood has been affecting you?'). The patient has already chosen the focus of the questioning and they are now being encouraged to talk about it in more detail.

Continuing down the funnel, closed questions are then used to clinch details. Closed questions such as 'How often do these panic attacks happen?' or 'How often do you wake during the night?' result in specific answers to questioning around a problem already being focused on. We must be careful not to use too many closed questions early in the interview, as important information will not be gleaned. However, clinching specific detail about patients' problems is vital. The 'frequency', 'intensity' and 'duration' questions, elaborated on later, are examples of closed questions used to clinch details.

Summarizing

Frequent summarizing will help check that we have an accurate understanding of the patient's difficulties. It can sometimes feel a little unnatural doing this, but it really does help with clarification and also facilitates the disclosure of further information. Summarizing should occur frequently throughout the interview, reflecting back what the patient has said, showing that they are understood and demonstrating warmth and empathy. Correctly feeding back information that has been given shows the patient that we have an understanding of their problems, and rapport is thereby strengthened. However, if we are not on the right track, the patient has the opportunity to correct us before proceeding any further. A final summary takes place towards the end of the interview; this is an extended clarification and an opportunity to check that a shared understanding of the patient's problems has been reached.

Phase 1: Structure of the assessment interview

Introductions

The first few minutes of an interview set the scene, so it is crucial to get this right. The mental health worker should introduce themselves with both first name and surname, and then clarify the patient's full name and find out what they prefer to be called. Next, the mental health worker should state their role clearly (e.g. 'I'm a Graduate Mental Health Worker'). They then go on to explain the purpose of the interview (e.g. 'I'll be asking you to describe what has been happening to you recently that has brought you here today. We'll then go on to look at what we can do to help with this.'). The time allocated to the meeting is also stated clearly (e.g. 'We have 45 minutes'). Setting the agenda for the session like this helps to keep the interview focused. For example, telling the patient that you want to find out about their problems especially over the last month or so will guide the patient to concentrate on more recent events. Confidentiality (Chapter 3.2, Section 5) should be explained to the patient at this stage.

CD-ROM 3 includes a video clip in which Waseem, the mental health worker, starts an assessment session with Nigel. A transcript of the clip is given below.

Video: Starting an assessment

Mental health worker (Waseem): My name's Waseem Malik and I'm a Graduate Mental Health Worker, and I know that you're Nigel McCann; but how do you like to be known?

Nigel: Nigel is fine.

Waseem: Okay, nice to meet you, Nigel. I'd like to try and get a picture of the type of problems you've been facing, Nigel, so we can try and decide what the best way of helping you is. We've got around about 40 minutes or so. In particular, I'd like to try and discuss the problems you've had over the last month or so. The sort of things that have prompted you to seek help. Would that be okay?

Nigel: Yes, that's fine.

Waseem: Before we start, we need to discuss one or two things about confidentiality. Anything you tell me will be kept confidential with those involved in your care, so that's Dr Rushforth and myself; but should there be a referral to anyone else at some point, important information will be shared with them too. Does that sound reasonable?

Nigel: Yes, but my work or family wouldn't … ?

Waseem: Oh no, no, absolutely not, I can assure you of that. It's only people directly involved in your care.

Nigel: That's fine.

Waseem: I'll take notes throughout, so we make sure we've got all the important points, and then we can make sure we help you in the best possible way. What I'd like to know, Nigel, is what has been the main aspect of the problem that has prompted you to seek help?

Nigel: I've been feeling pretty low over the last four months now, since my wife Jenny left me. I was devastated when it happened, and I am still devastated now. I can't seem to shake it off, and the last few weeks I've not even been able to get into work, I just can't face it.

Waseem: It sounds like it has been quite a tough time for you recently.

Note how Waseem introduces himself, sets the scene for the session and explains confidentiality, before proceeding to ask Nigel about his current difficulties.

Phase 2: Content of the assessment

Assessment questions

Once the scene has been set with introductions, etc., the mental health worker attempts to elicit as much information as possible about the problems the patient is presenting with.

Questions to start with

What is the problem?

The mental health worker might have a good idea from the referrer about the patient's problems, but this is not as important as the patient's own account of exactly what their difficulties are. A useful question to start off with might be 'Can you tell me a bit about the main problems which led to you asking for help?'

Where does the problem occur?

The problem may not be present all the time, but only occur in certain situations, particularly in the case of anxiety problems. A list can be made of all the situations where the problem occurs, and then an attempt made to see what these situations have in common. A useful question to ask might be 'Where does 'the problem' happen?' (e.g. 'Where do these panic attacks happen?').

With whom is the problem better or worse?

It is not uncommon for a problem to be better in the company of certain others (e.g. 'I'm less panicky in the supermarket if my partner is with me'), or indeed it can sometimes be worse (e.g. 'I find that when my sister is around I am more on edge, as she is so critical', or 'When I'm in the company of strangers I get really uptight').

When does the problem happen?

It is useful to find out if the problem happens in a predictable way (e.g. 'Do you find that your mood is lower at any particular time of day?', 'When do these panic attacks occur?', 'Do you find that some days are better than others?').

These four key question areas enable a fairly detailed description of the patient's problems to be ascertained. If there is more than one problem area, then the process can be gone through again for each area.

To elicit more details, the following questions can be helpful:

Frequency

These questions centre around how often the problems occur (e.g. 'How often do you have anger outbursts?', 'How many days a week do you find that you wake up early and are unable to get back off to sleep?', 'How often do you find that your mood is so low that you stay in bed all day?').

Intensity

Questions around the intensity of the problem can help ascertain how upsetting the problem is to the patient and whether the problem fluctuates or has improved/deteriorated over recent times. It can sometimes be helpful to use a scale of 0–100 when asking about intensity. An example of questioning a patient with anger difficulties might be 'Using a scale of 0–100, where 100 is the angriest you could possibly ever be, how angry can you get in these situations?', 'Do you always get as angry as that?', 'Has it always been as intense as it is now?'

Duration

It is helpful to find out the duration of a problem. In anxiety problems it is important to find out how long the patient tends to tolerate symptoms before doing something to reduce the anxiety (e.g. 'How long do panic attacks tend to last?', 'How long do you tend to stay in the supermarket once the anxiety symptoms come on?'). In the case of anger, the question might be 'How long does an anger episode tend to last?'

Severity of the problem

It is useful to ask the patient how severe or distressing they consider their problems to be. In the case of a patient who presents with more than one problem, doing this can help prioritize the problem needing to be addressed first as it causes the most distress to the patient. A scale of 0–100 can be used to do this, with 0 representing no problem and 100 representing the most severe the problem could possibly be. This scale can be used to rate the problem throughout contact to ascertain whether the intervention is having any effect.

Examples CD-ROM 3 includes two video clips in which mental health workers Samantha and Katie use skills in problem identification. Note the questions that Samantha and Katie ask, their use of paraphrasing and summarizing, and their use of empathy. Transcripts of the clips are given below.

Video: Problem identification (1)

Mental health worker (Samantha): Can you start by telling me a bit about the problems that have brought you here today?

Julie: It's all the worrying that I'm doing, you know, I'm worrying all the time. I just can't relax. I have all these dreadful thoughts about my husband being made redundant, my Mum dying, my son's leaving and getting married, my daughter's off to university, and the dog's sick. I'm just overwhelmed with worrying really.

Samantha: It sounds like you've got a lot on your mind. There's the worries about your family and the worries about the pet dog as well. Can you tell me a bit more about these worries?

Julie: Well, my husband may be made redun-

dant from his job, and obviously that may mean that we might lose the house, you know. I'm really worried, obviously, and then I don't want to move, of course. And then my Mum's really sick with breast cancer, she's got secondaries in her bones now, and she's very sick, and maybe she'll need to come and live with us. Colin, that's my son, he's going to get married very soon and I don't know whether it's the right girl, you know, whether it will work out; and then my daughter Claire, she's just gone to university and that's a long way away, about a hundred miles away, you know, and I don't know whether that's really going alright; and then obviously the dog is really sick, you know. The vet says he might pull through, but he's 16 you know, so I'm really worried about all that really. I'm sure there will be something else to worry about.

Samantha: So a lot then, isn't there? So there's the worries about David losing his job and the implications about losing the house, there's your Mum having been diagnosed with secondaries, it sounds like she's really poorly, there's Colin getting married and you're worried about the girl he's getting married to, there's Claire being away from home at university, and your dog doesn't sound too well either, and there's all this worrying about the worrying itself.

Julie: Yes.

Samantha: Yes. So there's quite a lot, isn't there, that's on your mind. Okay, can you tell me, do these worries happen anytime, or are there particular times of the day that are worse than others?

Julie: You know, it can happen anytime, you know, worrying, and it especially gets bad when I'm going to bed and I start worrying about the worrying, and it's just very difficult to get to sleep.

Samantha: Right, okay, so being in bed is a bad time and nighttime in general, by the sounds of it. Are there any other times when you are prone to worrying?

Julie: Well, it gets worse, you know, like when David came home and said he might lose his job, that obviously got me all churned up.

Samantha: I can see why that would worry you. Does it make a difference where you are?

Julie: Well, when we went on holiday, actually I was still worrying then, because I was worried about the house, you know, whether it might be burgled, who was looking after Mum, you know, so I still worry wherever I am.

Samantha: Okay, alright then. What about if anyone else is around, does that make a difference at all?

Julie: That can help, actually. Yes, it does help, maybe to get distracted. When people are around I can talk and do other things.

Samantha: How intense does it get? If we were to use a 0–100 scale, 100 being the most intense, how intense can the worrying get?

Julie: Oh, up to 100.

Samantha: Really. Is it always as intense as that?

Julie: Not always, it does go down a little bit sometimes, yes.

Samantha: Okay, so, it's every day, and the worrying can be really intense too. How long do these worry periods last?

Julie: They seem to last most of the day, especially when I'm on my own.

Samantha: Okay, so they can last a long time; they can last for hours and hours from what you've said. How do they tend to pass?

Julie: Well, I think when I do some housework, you know, do some chores, I get distracted and that helps, and also if I've got someone else to share the worry with. David's quite good. They'll listen and perhaps they'll calm me down and say 'Don't worry it'll be alright', you know, that helps.

Samantha: It really does seem to help if there is someone else around, doesn't it?

Julie: Yes, that's right.

Samantha: Okay.

Video: Problem identification (2)

Mental health worker (Katie): A good place to start might be for you to tell me a little bit about the problem that's made you seek help and why you're here. So, can you tell me a little bit about it and how it has been affecting you recently?

Andrew: Yes, it's that I feel very uncomfortable around people, especially strangers.

Katie: In what way are you uncomfortable with people?

Andrew: Well, I keep getting worried about what they think of me and I feel that I am making a fool of myself in front of them.

Katie: So, you're uncomfortable with people and you worry what they think of you. Can you tell me a little bit more about it? Is it any particular kind of people?

Andrew: It's strangers in the main, sometimes with people that I know just a bit, but mostly strangers.

Katie: Okay, so it's mostly strangers. Does this happen anywhere in particular?

Andrew: No, it can happen anywhere, but it's mainly parties and restaurants I don't like because, anywhere where you have to eat and drink in front of people I find very difficult and I'm not too keen on meeting new people; so parties, I don't like them.

Katie: So, restaurants and parties are difficult, particularly if there's any expectation that you are going to have to eat or drink anything, and meeting new people is especially difficult, is that right?

Andrew: Yes, that's what makes me really uncomfortable, so I don't like that.

Katie: I can see that it's really getting you down. It must be quite restricting. What is it that you dislike about these particular situations?

Andrew: Well, I get very nervous and people can see that I am, and I never know what to say so I get all tongue-tied and my mind goes completely blank. I end up making a fool of myself.

Katie: So, you feel that you get anxious and nervous, and that you might make a fool of yourself, and that people will think less of you because of it?

Andrew: Yes. I mean, that's exactly what I think.

Katie: Well, I think maybe that's something that we can discuss at a later stage. I think it might be quite an important thing to talk about, actually. It can't be very nice for you, feeling that people will think less of you. But before we do that, I'd just like to learn a little bit more about the problem. Does it make any difference if you are with someone you know?

Andrew: If it's just my mates and my immediate family, it's okay. If there are strangers there and I have to speak to them, then it doesn't really make any difference. Like the other week, I was at a family do and my immediate family were there, but so were some that I hadn't seen for years, so I was dead nervous.

Katie: So, if you are on your own with people close to you, then you're okay, but whether they're there or not, meeting people is always difficult. Is that right?

Andrew: Yes, that's right.

Katie: Are there certain times when the problem is worse?

Andrew: It's actually worse in the winter, would you believe? It's because it's hot in the summer and, you know, you can have a sweat on and it doesn't look so unusual, but when it's cold, it's not the case.

Katie: I think that's quite interesting. So, when it's the summer you feel it's okay because, although you might be sweating, other people are too.

Andrew: That's right, yes.

Katie: I can see how that makes sense. You said a little while ago that the problem happens most days. How severe can the anxiety get?

Andrew: Well, sometimes it's quite mild and then other times I go completely bright red and I start to shake.

Katie: How often is it as bad as that?

Andrew: Not very often. It's like when there's a real biggy, like that family do that I mentioned; and if I have to go to a meeting and my boss will be there, but that doesn't happen too often.

Katie: I'd like to understand how severe the anxiety gets, so if we use a scale of say 0–100, where 0 is not a problem and 100 is really, really severe anxiety, where would you say you are on that scale at the moment?

Andrew: It's pretty bad, it's really getting me down. It's probably 70.

Katie: So you've given it a 70, which I think reflects quite how much it's getting you down. Maybe what we can do is, we can come back to this scale at a later stage and

then see whether anything has changed if we re-rate it, and then we can see whether any of the things we do are helping.

Andrew: Yes, I hope so.

Katie: Okay, good. Well, first I'd like to just get a little bit more detail on the problem.

Exercise

Ask a colleague to play the role of Deborah, the patient with agoraphobia we met in Chapter 3.2.

- Ask 'Deborah' questions to gain an understanding of her problems.
- Use the question list and ensure that you move from open to more closed questions to clinch details.
- Try to paraphrase and summarize frequently.
- Use empathic statements throughout.
- Ask your colleague to give feedback to how it felt to be interviewed

---

Triggers

Triggers to the problem are important to ascertain. For example, a patient with anger problems may find that anger is triggered by certain situations at work. Some anxious patients may find that entering certain situations triggers panic symptoms. These are examples of external cues, but some triggers may be internal (e.g. mulling over negative and distressing events, worrying thoughts popping into one's mind, or noticing unpleasant or unusual bodily sensations).

Finding out more about a recent problem

One of the best ways to elicit detailed information about a problem is to ask about a time when the problem occurred recently (e.g. 'Can you describe what happened the last time you felt really down?/had a panic attack?/got really angry?/felt really stressed?/had problems getting off to sleep?', etc.). The mental health

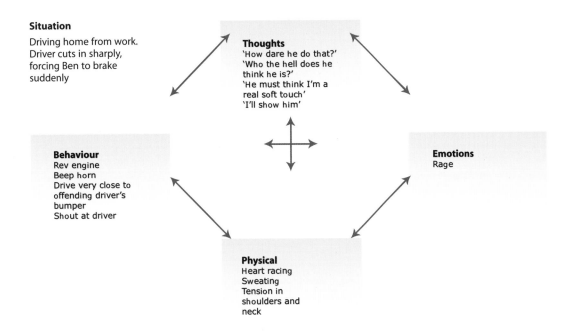

Figure 9: Ben's triggers

Situation
Driving home from work. Driver cuts in sharply, forcing Ben to brake suddenly

Thoughts
'How dare he do that?'
'Who the hell does he think he is?'
'He must think I'm a real soft touch'
'I'll show him'

Emotions
Rage

Behaviour
Rev engine
Beep horn
Drive very close to offending driver's bumper
Shout at driver

Physical
Heart racing
Sweating
Tension in shoulders and neck

worker can then enter the patient's world and follow up with questions to obtain important detail about the problem. This gives far more concrete information about the problem than a basic description by the patient, and is also likely to reveal information about maintenance factors. While the patient is describing the incident, the mental health worker can ask about emotional, physical, cognitive and behavioural symptoms.

It is at this stage that the mental health worker can share the model first shown in Part 3.1, and use this to analyse in detail the symptoms experienced by the patient at the specific time when the problem occurred.

Both parties can then see how different problem areas are linked and how one area can have a knock-on effect on another. For example, Ben's angry thoughts led to him getting angry and tense, resulting in his aggressive behaviour, each area feeding into the other.

Examples

Ben

Situation: Driving home from work. Driver pulls in sharply, forcing Ben to brake suddenly (see Figure 9).

Julie

Situation: Son Colin talking about forthcoming wedding. Start thinking about all that needs to be done for the big day (see Figure 10).

Immediate impact of the problem

It is useful to illicit the immediate impact the problem is having on the patient. For example, one patient might be constantly on edge, wondering when they will have another panic attack, another may feel exhausted most of the time due to lack of sleep, yet another may be frequently troubled by tension headaches due to ongoing stress and worrying, etc.

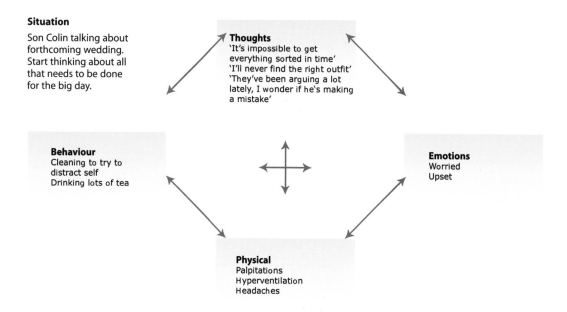

Situation
Son Colin talking about forthcoming wedding. Start thinking about all that needs to be done for the big day.

Thoughts
'It's impossible to get everything sorted in time'
'I'll never find the right outfit'
'They've been arguing a lot lately, I wonder if he's making a mistake'

Behaviour
Cleaning to try to distract self
Drinking lots of tea

Emotions
Worried
Upset

Physical
Palpitations
Hyperventilation
Headaches

Figure 10: Julie's triggers

CD-ROM 3 includes two video clips in which mental health workers Waseem and Samantha ask their clients Alison and Roger to describe recent instances of their respective problems and their immediate impact. Notice how the mental health workers ask questions around the four common symptom areas. Transcripts of the clips follow.

Video: Triggers through to immediate impact (1)

Mental health worker (Waseem): Alison, can you tell me a little bit more about what triggers your panic attacks?

Alison: They seem to come out of the blue. I don't seem to know when they are going to happen. That really bothers me about them.

Waseem: So there is no real pattern to them, they are fairly unpredictable. That must make life quite difficult for you.

Alison: Yes, they are very unpredictable, yes.

Waseem: Okay, well, what we'll try to do today is we'll try to examine your panic attacks to see whether there is any sort of pattern that goes on whilst you are having a panic attack.

I'll write things down as we go along, and then we can see what we make of it then.

Alison: Okay, that sounds helpful.

Waseem: Can you tell me what happened the last time you had a panic attack?

Alison: The last time it happened was Tuesday, and I was in a meeting at work, and it finished late, and so I was late leaving work. I had to pick up Chloe, my daughter, she was at the after-school club, and I was worried that I wasn't going to get there in time. I got in the car and there was lots of traffic, so I was getting really flustered about getting there. I managed to get there and then we get in the car to go home, and I realize that we've got nothing for tea, so we're going to have to go to the supermarket.

Waseem: Okay, I've written this down under 'situation' and, as you said, you were late leaving work, you were picking up your daughter, Chloe, you got stuck in traffic so that made you even more flustered. You realized you had nothing in for tea so you had to go to the supermarket.

Alison: That's right.

Waseem: What happened then?

Alison: Well, we got to the supermarket. Chloe

was really hyper, she was running around, I was having real difficulty keeping control of her, and I started to feel really hot and I was having difficulty breathing, I felt that I was really out of breath and my heart was pounding, and then I started to get these pains in my chest and I had this tingling going on in my arm, right down my arm.

Waseem: So, very uncomfortable for you.

Alison: I was very frightened. I was scared.

Waseem: I'll write this down under physical symptoms, so, you were hot, you felt out of breath, you said your heart was pounding, you had these chest pains and you had tingling down your arm.

Alison: Yes, that's right.

Waseem: What did you think was going to happen, Alison?

Alison: Well, I thought I was going to die. I thought I was having a heart attack. I was really, really frightened, really scared.

Waseem: It must have been very difficult. Okay, I'll write this down under 'thoughts' and 'emotions'. You thought you were going to have a heart attack, and you felt very scared.

Alison: Yes, I thought I was going to die.

Waseem: It must have been very difficult. So, what did you do?

Alison: Well, I'd lost Chloe so I had to find her. I abandoned my trolley, I just left it in one of the aisles, and I managed to find her and then I just grabbed her and we left, just straight for the nearest exit. I just had to get out of there.

Waseem: (writes under 'behaviour') When you left the supermarket, did you go and sit in the car to calm down, or did things calm down by themselves quite quickly?

Alison: Once I found Chloe and I got out, it was straight to the car. Once we got in the car and we started to drive off, I started to feel calmer. I felt, as we were driving along, I was starting to feel more calm, and by the time we got home I felt a lot calmer, yes.

Waseem: It sounds like quite a day, doesn't it? Now, let's just see what we've got then from what you've said. I'll just go through it again. You said that you were late leaving work and late to pick up Chloe. You got stuck in traffic and you were flustered and you had to go to the supermarket because you had nothing in for your tea, and that's the situation you found yourself in. Soon after you got there, you felt these physical symptoms. You said you were hot, felt out of breath, your heart was pounding, you had chest pains, you had tingling down your arm. It made you feel very scared; if you had to describe your emotions, you said you were scared.

Alison: I was scared.

Waseem: In fact, you thought you were going to die. It must have been very, very scary for you. So of course, the thing you did was abandon your trolley and just left the supermarket. Do you see how all these things are connected from what you've told me?

Alison: Yes, I've never really thought about it like that before, but yes, I can see what you mean.

Waseem: It's a very useful way for us to see what is going on during a panic attack and then work out what the best way is to help you. We'll talk more about this a little bit later on. Now, you've said one or two things about how this is affecting you in your day-to-day life. Any other problems that it's causing?

Alison: Well, I avoid Sainsbury's now. It's the closest supermarket to home, it's where I want to go, but I can't go there anymore because as soon as I get close to there, I think about these things that have happened in there, so I'm ending up going further afield to Tescos. So it takes me more time, it's a real pain to do that.

Waseem: So it's having a direct impact on your day-to-day life.

Alison: Yes, it is.

Video: Triggers through to immediate impact (2)

Mental health worker (Samantha): Okay, Roger, do you find that there is anything in particular that can lead to a bad night's sleep?

Roger: I'm not sure, really; maybe if I've had a stressful day at work, that can be a problem, or it might be that maybe I've napped too long in front of the TV in the evening.

Otherwise it might just be that I've got something on my mind, you know, thoughts running round in my mind and I just can't switch off.

Samantha: Okay, if you've had a particularly stressful day at work then, napping too long in the evenings, and if there's something on your mind, all those things can lead to a bad night's sleep.

Roger: Yes.

Samantha: Well, that's been really useful getting that information about the problem, but one of the things that can really help can be to look at a recent incident of the problem actually occurring, so one of the best ways is to find a recent time, say in the last week, when it's happened. Has it happened at all?

Roger: Yes, no problem, it happened last night actually. It was a bad night.

Samantha: Right, well the good thing about that is, that it's going to be really clear in your mind, so that is a good one to go for. Okay, can you tell me a bit about what happened last night then; but it would be more helpful if you put it into context of the whole day, and what I'm going to do is I'm going to write down what you tell me.

Roger: Okay. Well, it wasn't anything out of the ordinary, the day. Work was a standard day at the office. I got home at my normal time, about 6 o'clock, and Mary had the dinner on. Dinner was ready about 10 minutes later, I think. So, we sat down to dinner, I had a couple of cups of tea and then we went and sat down in front of the telly. I think I dozed off in front of the telly about 7 o'clock, I tend to do that most nights, only for about an hour, and then I woke up and carried on watching TV with Mary.

Samantha: Right, so nothing out of the ordinary happened yesterday, it was work as usual, back at 6 o'clock, had dinner, a couple of cups of tea, watched a bit of telly, had a doze in the chair for about an hour and then carried on watching TV. I've written that under 'situation'. What happened next?

Roger: I think we just carried on watching telly. I think the last thing we watched was Newsnight, and when that finished it was

about 11.15. Mary wanted to go up to bed, she was pretty shattered. I was pretty tired as well but, at the same time, I was starting to get worked up at that point.

Samantha: When you say 'worked up', what do you mean?

Roger: Just sort of worried about the night ahead, worried that I was going to lie there tossing and turning and not sleeping.

Samantha: Okay. So 'I'll lie there, tossing and turning and not sleeping'. I'm writing that under 'thoughts'. How did that thought make you feel?

Roger: Worried; I worried about it. I guess agitated is the best way to describe it.

Samantha: Okay, worried and agitated, I'm writing that under 'emotions' here. Did you feel sleepy?

Roger: I didn't really feel sleepy, I felt tired but at the same time, in my head if you like, I was feeling restless and also, it sometimes happens, and it happened last night, I was feeling churning around in my stomach as well.

Samantha: Okay, 'churning around in your stomach', I'm going to write that under 'physical symptoms'. What happened next?

Roger: Mary went up, so I made another cup of tea and then I went up to bed and followed Mary. She went out like a light and, as predicted, I just lay there getting more and more worked up that I wasn't sleeping.

Samantha: Right, so after your cup of tea you headed upstairs after Mary. Mary went to sleep right away as usual, and you lay awake. I'm going to write that under 'behaviour' and then I'm going to write 'worked up' under 'emotion'.

Roger: I guess I lay there for about a good hour, hour-and-a-half. Eventually, I just got up and made myself another drink and then I took that back to bed and read for a while. I think, in the end, I probably just finally dropped off about two or three hours later, so it's not surprising that I feel so old at the moment.

Samantha: I can see how it's really getting you down. You had a real problem last night though, didn't you? Is that a typical night for you?

Roger: Yes, unfortunately it is.

Samantha: Okay, can you see how I've written these things down? There's the situation, the thoughts, the emotions, the behaviours and the physical symptoms. Is there anything else that you notice?

Roger: Well, you've drawn arrows connecting them up.

Samantha: Yes, this is because they are all connected to each other and one affects the other. Like worrying about getting to sleep made you feel more tense and agitated, and then you ended up lying awake. Does this diagram make sense?

Roger: Yes. I'd never thought of it like that, but yes, it does make sense.

Samantha: Okay, good. This can be a really helpful way of looking at problems. When we come to talking about what you can be doing to work on the problem, we can look to see how intervening in any one of those areas helps the problem or not. So we can use this diagram in treatment; but before all that, I'd really like to know how this insomnia is affecting your life.

Roger: Well, obviously I'm exhausted all the time and, also because of it, I think it's making me a bit more clumsy. I'm certainly more accident-prone than I used to be; and also I think it makes me more ratty. I can sense that, especially in the morning when I wake up and I still feel tired.

Samantha: Okay, so it's affecting you by making you feel exhausted a lot of the time, and you're that bit more accident-prone too, and the rattiness particularly in the morning.

Roger: Yes.

Notice how, in both interviews, the mental health workers ask questions around the four common symptom areas and share the model with their patients.

Risk

In the case of primary care, patients will usually remain the primary responsibility of their GP, and only patients who are considered to be of no safety risk will be seen on the GP's behalf by

Exercise

Ask a colleague to play the role of Nigel while you take the role of the mental health worker. Ask Nigel questions about triggers to his problems, a recent incident when he felt particularly low, and the impact it is having on his life. Ensure you ask questions around the four symptom areas, as well as getting information about the situation where these symptoms occurred. Present to him the model as demonstrated in the two video transcripts. Ask your colleague for feedback when you have finished the role-play.

the mental health worker. Patients who are considered to be at risk should not be referred to a primary care mental health worker, and should instead be referred to secondary services.

However, it is essential that every mental health worker is able to determine whether a patient is suicidal or likely to self-harm. If the patient is suicidal, then the GP must be contacted immediately. It is important to err on the side of caution, so that if there is any doubt in the mental health worker's mind, they should advise the GP as soon as possible.

Sometimes mental health workers worry that, if they ask a patient directly if they have suicidal thoughts, this will somehow plant that idea in their minds when it was not there in the first place. This is not the case, and asking direct questions is always the best way. Questions such as 'Do you ever get so low that you feel you just can't

Factors indicating high risk of suicide

- Recent marital conflict
- Currently untreated severe mental illness
- Alcohol abuse
- Previous suicide attempts
- Recent suicide attempts
- Age group 18–29-year-old (increased risk)

Categorizing risk

Risk	Description	Action
Low risk	No current thoughts, or infrequent thoughts	Continue follow-up contacts and monitor. Normalize thoughts and differentiate between thoughts and actions
Intermediate risk	Frequent current thoughts but no plans or intent	Assess risk carefully at each contact. Liaise with specialist mental health services. Ensure the patient knows how to access services.
High risk	Current thoughts with plans and preparations	Stay with patient until GP arrives. The patient is then referred to specialist mental health services and engaged in a collaborative approach to treatment and monitoring

carry on?' and 'When you feel that way, do you ever have thoughts of taking your own life?' are appropriate. If the patient responds with a 'yes' to these questions, the mental health worker then ascertains intent by asking about plans (e.g. 'Have you given any thought to how you might end your own life?' and 'Have you gone any way towards that?').

For example, the patient may have been stocking up on painkillers, or have bought a rope recently, or written notes to leave to loved ones, etc.

The mental health worker should also ask if the patient has made any previous attempts at suicide or self-harm, but should not necessarily be reassured if they have not, as this may be the first and only time. Next, the patient should be asked about factors that would stop them from following through with a suicide attempt (e.g. the patient's partner, elderly parent, children, religion, etc.). Factors such as hopefulness, responsibility for children and strong social support are protective factors that have been found to reduce the risk of suicide. A patient with no protective factors or ones that are weak (e.g. 'I haven't killed myself so far because of my 10-year-old son, but now I think he'd be better off without me. Besides, he'll get over it in time') would be a concern and require further investigation.

The following list of questions is useful when assessing suicide risk. The mental health worker only carries on down the list of questions until they receive a 'no' response from the patient. For example, if the patient responds with a 'no' to the question, 'Do things ever feel so bad that you think about harming or killing yourself?', there is little point in asking them 'What is stopping you killing or harming yourself at the moment?'

Key questions

Intention – thoughts

'Do things ever feel so bad that you think about harming or killing yourself?'
'Do you ever feel that life is not worth living?'

Plans

'Have you made plans to end your life?'
'Do you know how you would kill yourself?'

Actions

'Have you made any actual preparations to kill yourself?'
'Have you ever attempted suicide in the past?'

Prevention

'How likely is it that you will act on such thoughts and plans?'

'What is stopping you killing or harming yourself at the moment?'

It is also important to ask about risk to others, especially where patients are not known to the primary care practice or if the patient is being seen for problems related to anger. An example question might be, 'Have you ever been in trouble with the police?'

Risk assessment examples

CD-ROM 3 includes three video clips in which mental health workers perform risk assessments with Nigel, Sarah and Julian. Transcripts of the clips follow.

Video: Assessing risk (Nigel)

Mental health worker (Waseem): Nigel, do things ever feel so bad that you think about harming or killing yourself?

Nigel: Yes, occasionally I feel like life isn't worth living anymore.

Waseem: Have you actually made any plans to end your life?

Nigel: No, it's never gone that far. I wouldn't be able to do that to the children.

Waseem: Good I'm glad to hear that. I'd like to keep a check on these thoughts though, so I'll ask you about them every time we meet up or talk on the phone if that's okay?

Nigel: That's fine, but I'd never do anything suicidal.

Video: Assessing risk (Sarah)

Mental health worker (Katie): Do you ever feel that life isn't worth living?

Sarah: Yes, sometimes.

Katie: Have you thought of ending your own life?

Sarah: Sometimes.

Katie: Have you made any plans?

Sarah: Not exactly, but I think I'd probably take tablets.

Katie: Have you made any preparations to kill yourself?

Sarah: No, nothing like that. I've just thought about it sometimes, but I wouldn't really do it. Mum and Karen would be too upset.

Video: Assessing risk (Julian)

Waseem: Do things ever feel so bad that you think about harming or killing yourself?

Julian: Yes, all the time.

Waseem: Have you made any plans to end your life?

Julian: Recently, I've been thinking about it, yes.

Waseem: Do you know how you would kill yourself?

Julian: Probably I'd go into town and jump off a bridge, or I might hang myself.

Waseem: Julian, have you made any actual preparations to end your life?

Julian: Yes, I wrote my wife a note, sorted out my papers and things like that. Why am I telling you this anyway? I should just go ahead and do it.

Waseem: Well, I'm glad you are telling me, I'd like to help you. You're obviously feeling quite low at the moment that you're even considering this to be an option. Have you ever attempted suicide in the past?

Julian: No, the last time I felt this way I thought about it but I didn't. It's just this time it seems far worse.

Waseem: And how likely do you think it is that you will act on these plans?

Julian: Well, I'm not sure. I'm not sure that I'd tell you anyway, because you'd just try and stop me, wouldn't you?

Waseem: Well, you're right there, I would try and stop you. What's stopping you killing yourself at the moment?

Julian: Yesterday I had my will sorted out. I saw my solicitor about that. Nothing.

Waseem: Julian, I think it may be helpful if we can get your GP, Dr Attenborough, to come in and have a couple of words. I know she's on the premises and she'd like to talk to you.

Julian: I don't want to see her. I want to go.

Waseem: Please just stay, just for a moment, just at least to hear what she's got to say. I'll just ring her to see if she's free. (dials phone) Hello Rebecca, is Dr Attenborough there, please? Could you put me through please? Thank you. Dr Attenborough, hello, it's Waseem here, I'm with Julian Williams and we've been talking about suicide risk, and I'm a little bit concerned. I just wondered if you could come in and have a few words with him? Okay, good, thank you. (puts phone down) She'll be over in just a couple of moments.

Julian: No, I don't want to see her. I just want to go.

Waseem: Please, Julian, let's at least hear what she's got to say.

Julian: Okay.

Notice how the mental health workers stop asking questions only when they receive a negative response to one of their questions.

Exercise

In your opinion, having read the transcripts, at what level of risk were each of the three patients?

Additional information

How the problems started, their course thenceforth, and their long-term impact on the person, are all useful information to be collected during assessment.

Onset of problems (how and when they started)

The patient should be asked how the problems started. It might be that the problems started suddenly (e.g. a dog phobia developing after being bitten by a dog, depression followed the death of a loved one), or it may have been a gradual onset.

Progress of the problems (fluctuations)

Symptoms may have changed over time and it may be that they went away for a while and came back again. If this is the case, then it is helpful to find out what the triggers were to these fluctuations.

Factors that bring about an improvement

There may be some factors, that have not been elicited earlier in the interview, that bring about relief from the problems, so it is worth specifically asking about these. Some of these behaviours may be desirable (e.g. a patient with low mood might find that when they have been for a walk they feel a little brighter). On the other hand, some behaviours may actually help to maintain the problem (e.g. a patient who gets anxious when in the supermarket might find that carrying a mobile phone in case of emergency helps them to feel more able to cope). Therefore, in addition to finding out what helpful behaviours the patient is engaging in, it is also a good opportunity to elicit safety behaviours, which may be helping to maintain the problem (e.g. the patient who clutches the handles on a pushchair until symptoms of light-headedness pass, in the belief that this will stop them from collapsing).

Factors that make the problems worse

In addition to the factors that might appear to make a problem better there may be some factors, that have not been elicited earlier in the interview, that make the problem worse. Therefore, it is worth asking questions specifically about these as well. For example, a patient might find that their mood is lower if it is a rainy day, or a patient with anxiety about using public transport may find it more difficult if the bus/train is busy, etc.

Past treatment (what helped and for how long, what didn't help or made the problem worse)

It is always useful to know what help the patient has had in the past for their problems. If they have had a negative experience when seeing a mental health worker in the past, then they may have reservations about entering into contact again. It may be that they have tried using self-help materials which brought about some benefits, but these were limited due to the difficulties of maintaining the momentum alone. This is something that can be built on, by offering encouragement and support.

Are there any other problems causing the patient distress that haven't been discussed already?

It is worth checking with the patient that the main problems have all been discussed. It may be that the patient has another problem that they were too embarrassed to mention at the beginning of the session, but now that a rapport has been built they might feel more confident in discussing it.

Prescribed medication, illicit drugs, alcohol and caffeine

Substances such as these can have a significant impact on a person's functioning. The mental health worker may already be aware of the prescribed medication that the patient is taking, but it is still necessary to confirm that this is the case. It is also important to ask about 'over-the-counter' drugs. It is questionable whether anyone will tell a relative stranger that they are taking illicit drugs, but it is still worth asking. It is important to ask about alcohol consumption (e.g. total intake, frequency, type of drink, etc.). Excessive alcohol consumption may be aggravating the problems. Caffeine is a strong and long-lasting stimulant, therefore it is particularly important to ask patients presenting with sleep difficulties and those with anxiety problems about their consumption of coffee, tea and cola drinks.

What would the patient like to change about their problems?

This is a key question to find out exactly what the patient wants from the contact and the mental health worker. This introduces the idea of treatment goals. A good question to ask is 'What would you like to be able to do that you can't do now because of your problems?'

What has led the patient to seek help now?

It might seem obvious that, due to the distress the problems are causing, the patient would naturally seek help. However, if problems have been around for many years, then it is especially important to ask this question. A patient's reasons for seeking help at this point in time may affect how much they wish to engage with the mental health worker. For instance, a patient whose reason is 'I've had enough of being restricted by my problem so I asked the GP for help' may be more likely to engage readily in guided self-help activities than a patient whose reason is 'My partner nagged me to do something about it, but I don't really want to.' As the therapeutic approaches used will place a great deal of emphasis on the patient taking control of working on their problems with guidance and support, assessing a patient's readiness for change could be crucial when seeking to engage patients in guided self-help work.

Wide-ranging consequences

The presenting problems may have an impact on several areas of the patient's life (e.g. work, home, social, leisure, relationships with partners, family, friends, work colleagues, etc.). Therefore the patient is asked how the problems affect different areas of their lives (e.g. 'Has your irritability at work had any impact on your relationships with colleagues?', 'Has your anxiety about being in crowded places had any impact on your relationships with your family?', 'Has your low mood and poor concentration affected your ability to work?', etc.).

CD-ROM 3 includes two video clips in which mental health workers Waseem and Katie interview their patients Lorraine and Tim about the wide-ranging consequences their respective problems are having on their lives. Transcripts of the clips follow.

Video: Onset through to long-term consequences (1)

Mental health worker (Waseem): Lorraine, you've told me quite a lot about how your phobia is affecting you on a day-to-day basis. I'm interested to know how it started.

Lorraine: Okay, well, I had a car accident about six months ago and it wasn't that serious or anything. I mean, nobody was hurt. The car wasn't even very badly damaged. I was at a roundabout and I should have gone because there were no cars coming, but I stalled. Anyway, the bloke in the car behind me, he wasn't really paying attention to what I was doing. As the exit was clear, he must have thought I had gone, and he bumped into the back of me.

Waseem: It must have been quite a fright for you at the time.

Lorraine: Yes it was. I do feel that I'm over that now. though; it's just the driving that I have an issue with.

Waseem: So would you say that things are getting better than they were six months ago?

Lorraine: Well yes, they are better, things were a lot worse then. I was pretty nervous even as a passenger in the car for the first few days, so in some ways things are a lot better. It's just the actual driving.

Waseem: It's good to hear that things appear to be getting better. Your problem appears to be very specific to the driving; would that be fair to say?

Lorraine: Yes.

Waseem: At least we can concentrate on that aspect of the problem then. Can you think of anything that makes the problem better or worse?

Lorraine: I can't think of anything that makes it better but the weather can definitely make it worse. If it's icy out, I feel pretty scared as a passenger and I certainly wouldn't dream of going behind the wheel.

Waseem: Really. So icy weather makes the problem worse. Anything else?

Lorraine: I do feel pretty wary as well if it's dark out, but apart from that, I can't really think of anything.

Waseem: Okay, so icy weather and darkness make the situation worse. Have you had any treatment at all for this over the last six months?

Lorraine: No, this is the first time. I did think it would get better itself but obviously it's been six months now since the accident, so I thought I'd better do something about it.

Waseem: Well, I'm glad you have. We'll do our best to help. Your GP, Dr Attenborough, said that you're not on any medication at all; is that right?

Lorraine: Yes, that's right. I would be though if I had my way.

Waseem: Is that right? Has somebody mentioned something to you?

Lorraine: Yes, I did hear about beta-blockers. Somebody said that they might help for me.

Waseem: Yes, people do say this, but what we tend to find is that beta-blockers are very much a short-term measure. I think it's probably better for you if we did something longer-term and developed a strategy for your improvement. We'll talk more about this a bit later on, but I just wanted to ask you one or two more questions. Are you taking any sort of drugs at all, whether prescribed or even illegal?

Lorraine: No, paracetamols, that's it. I take the odd paracetamol for a headache but even that's very rare.

Waseem: What about caffeine: tea, coffee, fizzy drinks?

Lorraine: I do drink coffee. I'd say I have about four cups a day, but I don't drink tea and I don't drink coke either; I don't drink fizzy drinks.

Waseem: Tell me, what would you like to be able to do that you can't do because of your problem?

Lorraine: I'd just like to be able to go anywhere in my car, like I was able to do six months ago.

Waseem: I think that seems like quite a reasonable goal.

Lorraine: Yes.

Waseem: Now, you've told me a little bit about how the problem is affecting you directly in terms of the driving, but do you think it is having any wider effect on your life?

Lorraine: Yes, I think it's affecting my ability to be independent, I suppose. I'm usually free to come and go whenever I like, but at the moment I'm quite dependent on my Mum for lifts, that's if I don't use the bus.

Waseem: Right, and do you think your Mum minds? Is this having any effect on your relationship you have with your Mum?

Lorraine: No, I don't think it's having an effect, but it's obviously a pain for her at times.

Waseem: Any other aspects of your life that you think have been affected by this? Can you think of anything at the moment?

Lorraine: Not that I can think of, no.

Waseem: Okay.

Video: Onset through to long-term consequences (2)

Mental health worker (Katie): This problem with stress sounds really draining for you. When did it all start?

Tim: A few weeks ago. The company I work for started to get into a bit of financial difficulty, and that kind of put some stress on me.

Katie: And what's it been like since then?

Tim: Well, it was alright at the start, I kind of like stress, I thrive on it, but recently it's been getting beyond a joke.

Katie: Is there anything that makes it better at the moment?

Tim: No, not really.

Katie: And is there anything that makes it worse for you?

Tim: Well, when my boss is on my back, then it's worse.

Katie: So when your boss is around, you feel like you're under more pressure?

Tim: Yes. It's not his fault really; he's under a lot of pressure too, but he does make things worse.

Katie: Have you tried anything to help with this problem?

Tim: That's ironic really. I bought a book on stress management and I haven't had time to read it.

Katie: I can see the irony, but you are going to have to make time to test out some of the strategies that we discuss. You do realize that?

Tim: Yes, I know I'm going to have to give this some time, or else something's going to give.

Katie: Good, because it does sound to me like you might be putting your health at risk.

Tim: Yes, Dr Mehra took my blood pressure last time I saw him, and told me it was high, which was concerning.

Katie: That is worrying. Well one of the first things we can do is look at what steps we can take to get that down. Are you having any other difficulties that we haven't discussed?

Tim: No, I don't think so.

Katie: Okay. Right, are you taking any medication, prescribed or over-the-counter?

Tim: Just regular painkillers. I've got a headache I can't shift at the moment.

Katie: And any other drugs?

Tim: You mean like illegal drugs?

Katie: Yes.

Tim: No, I'm not; and I'm not sure I'd tell you if I were.

Katie: No, I realize that, but you do understand I do have to ask. What about your alcohol intake?

Tim: I have a couple of beers when I get in of a night, but that's about all. It just helps me to unstress.

Katie: And your caffeine intake?

Tim: Oh God, yes, that is too high. I drink, I suppose, it must be about 30 cups of filter coffee a day.

Katie: Right, that is quite high. I think maybe that's something we can come back to later because I think it possibly might not be helping.

Tim: No, I'm sure you're right.

Katie: What would you like to be able to do that you feel you can't do now, because of the problem?

Tim: Oh, that's pretty easy. I'd like to work shorter hours, I'd like to go to the gym five times a week, I'd like to see friends a couple of times a week, I'd like to spend more time with John, and go out with him a couple of times a week too. I'd like to sleep every night like a log, I'd like to buy fresh food from the supermarket rather than just living on takeaways and whatever John's got left, yes.

Katie: Okay, all those things sound reasonable. I'm writing them down because I think they may be useful as specific goals. So, you'd like to work shorter hours, you'd like to go to the gym five times a week, you'd like to see friends maybe twice a week, you'd like to spend time with John, who is your partner, a couple of times a week, you'd like to sleep like a log and you'd like to have time to go to the supermarket to buy fresh food rather than living on take-aways. Is that right?

Tim: Yes that's right, except I think we'd better up the number of times I see John a week. If I'm seeing my friends twice, I'd better see him three times, or go out three times.

Katie: Okay. What made you seek help now?

Tim: When Dr Mehra told me my blood pressure was up, it did give me a bit of a fright.

Katie: Yes, that is worrying, but it's good that it's prompted you to address the problem now. It does sound like this stress is having quite a wide-ranging impact on your life, including on your physical well-being; and you mentioned earlier the effect it is having on your performance at work. Is it affecting important relationships in your life in any way?

Tim: Well, I must admit, I think if I was actually married, then me and John would be divorced by now.

Katie: So it's affecting your relationships too.

Tim: Yes, definitely, and friends are getting tired of me cancelling on them all the time.

Katie: Do you think there's any other way in which it is impacting on your life?

Tim: Isn't that enough? No I think we've just about covered it.

Katie: Yes, you're right, but you see, it is having a really wide-ranging impact.

Exercise

Ask a colleague to take the role of Andrew, the patient with Social Phobia in Part 3.2, while you take the role of a mental health worker.
- Role-play the interview from impact of the problem on Andrew through to the long-term and wider consequences for him of living with his problem.
- Take notes, and feedback what you have learned from playing the role.

Any relevant further information

Always take the opportunity to ask the patient if there is anything else they feel is relevant to their current difficulties that they think the mental health worker should know.

Phase 3: Problem summaries and goals

Problem summaries

Patients sometimes present with one problem and at other times present with several. The mental health worker aims to assess all the presenting problems and the connections between them, break them down into problem summaries, then, with the patient, prioritize which problem should be addressed first.

Problems are usually prioritized according to the level of associated distress. Problems with the highest levels of distress, or sometimes with the widest impact, are tackled first.

By the end of the assessment session, the mental health worker needs to have elicited enough information about the patient's difficulties to be able to share a brief summary with them. This summary includes a description of problems, triggers, presenting symptoms (emotional, physical, cognitive and behavioural) and consequences.

For example:
- 'Avoidance of leaving home alone, due to symptoms of anxiety and fear of collapse, leading to becoming increasingly housebound'
- 'Distress and suicidal thoughts when alone, following breakdown of relationship, leading to concerns about personal safety'
- 'Difficulty dealing with stressful situations, due to low threshold to frustration, leading to outbursts of anger and irritability'
- 'Difficulty facing social situations, due to fear of negative evaluation by others, leading to drinking alcohol before going out'

These problem summaries can be rated by the patient on a 0–100 scale, then returned to periodically throughout the therapeutic contact to review progress.

Goal setting

Goals are agreed which are then used to structure the therapeutic contact. Setting goals can help to iron out any issues regarding unrealistic expectations of the help the patient is to receive. For example, it is unreasonable to expect never to feel anxious again, but it is reasonable to expect to be able to go to the local supermarket without anxiety. Equally, it is unrealistic to expect never to have a bad night's sleep, but it is reasonable to expect a restful sleep most nights.

Sometimes a patient suggests goals such as 'to feel better'. In this case, the mental health worker might ask the patient 'If you were feeling better,

what would you be able to do that you can't do now?' Goals should never be vague but always explicit, realistic, concrete and achievable. This means that goals are best set in behavioural terms, ensuring that it is evident when they are achieved (e.g. 'go to the cinema once a week with friends' rather than 'do normal things').

Goals should be written positively so that it is clear what the patient is working towards, rather than what they are expected to stop doing (e.g. 'to go to the supermarket twice a week for an hour, alone, at busy times with minimal anxiety' rather than 'to stop asking my husband to accompany me to the supermarket' or 'to stop leaving the supermarket when I feel anxious').

CD-ROM 3 includes two video clips in which Deborah and Ben, with their respective mental health workers, Waseem and Samantha, make problem summaries and set goals. Transcripts of the clips are given below.

Video: Problem summary and goal setting (Part 1)

(Mental health worker) Waseem: Is there anything else that you want to talk about, anything that perhaps we haven't touched on?

Deborah: No, I can't think of any.

Waseem: Okay. Well, you've given me a lot of information about your problem and about how you're avoiding going out to busy places because you're feeling very anxious. I think it might be worth our while trying to perhaps summarize this so that we can work our way through it; try to sort of put the problem in a nutshell if you like. What do you think?

Deborah: Okay, okay that's fine.

Waseem: Okay. What would you say is the main aspect of the problem as far as you're concerned?

Deborah: I would say the main part of the problem is my fear of going out on my own and particularly my fear of fainting.

Waseem: Right, not going out because of your anxiety?

Deborah: Yes.

Waseem: I'll just write it down. So your 'Avoidance of leaving home' shall we say?

Deborah: Yes, okay.

Waseem: 'Avoidance of leaving home' by your-self, I assume. Does it happen when you are with somebody else, or is it more of a problem if you are by yourself?

Deborah: It's not as bad when I'm with Paul, but, as you know, at the moment I'm not going out at all really.

Waseem: Alright, okay. So, well, let's add that on to here then. So we'll have 'Avoidance of leaving home alone due to symptoms of anxiety and fear of fainting' as you mentioned, and you said you're not going out as much so it is 'leading to becoming increasingly housebound'.

Deborah: Yes, I am really housebound at the moment.

Waseem: Do you think this summarizes it? I'll just read it out to you again. 'Avoidance of leaving home alone due to symptoms of anxiety and fear of fainting, leading to becoming increasingly housebound'. Is anything missing?

Deborah: I think that is it, except the other thing that's happened since I've stopped going out is that I rely on Paul an awful lot, you know, my husband, because he's doing everything for me. So I think one of the other issues is that I'm very dependent on him.

Waseem: I think that's important. I think we should add that on here. So if we were trying to summarize your problem we'd say you have an 'Avoidance of leaving home alone due to symptoms of anxiety and fear of fainting, leading to becoming increasingly housebound and dependent on Paul'.

Deborah: Yes, I think that's it. That's it in a nutshell.

Waseem: Okay, it's really important that we have an idea what the problem is so that we can then try to sort out how we are going to tackle it. It must be quite distressing for you, this. If you had to rate it on a scale of say 0–100, where about would you put it?

Deborah: I think I'd put it at about 90.

Waseem: 90; so it's obviously quite distressing for you then.

Deborah: It is, yes.

Waseem: I'll make a note of that, and perhaps we can come back to it in a few weeks time to see whether there is any change to that.

Deborah: Okay.

Waseem: Right, now that we know what the problem is, let's see what we can do to help you tackle it. Perhaps we should set some goals to the treatment. What is it that you can't do at the moment, because of the problem, that you would like to be able to do?

Deborah: I suppose I'd really, really like to be able to go shopping.

Waseem: And how often would you like to be able to do this?

Deborah: Well, at least once a week.

Waseem: Okay. Should we say something about how busy it is at the time?

Deborah: Well, I'd like to be able to go out when it's reasonably busy, but I'd really like to be able to go out on my own.

Waseem: Okay, let's just take a moment to write that down, then. So, as a goal you'd like to be able 'To go out shopping alone at busy times' we said, didn't we?

Deborah: Yes.

Waseem: 'To go out shopping alone at busy times with minimal anxiety'?

Deborah: Yes, that sounds more realistic.

Waseem: Yes, I think so. Okay. 'To go out shopping alone at busy times with minimal anxiety, at least once a week'?

Deborah: Yes.

Waseem: Okay, good. Now we know what the problem is and we know what the goal is, perhaps we can talk about what actually happens.

Deborah: Right.

Waseem: I'm just going to draw you this graph.

Deborah: Okay.

Waseem: (draws habituation graph) If you can imagine anxiety – and that's time, so it's starting from when you first enter the situation, or the supermarket in your case. Now, from what you are telling me, when you go into the supermarket, your anxiety level goes up.

Deborah: Yes.

Waseem: Right, so you get scared and you leave?

Deborah: Yes, and I get all these awful palpitations and dry mouth.

Waseem: Right. When you leave the supermarket do you feel less anxious?

Deborah: Oh yes, definitely.

Waseem: So if I was drawing it on my graph, your anxiety comes down like that, but the next time you go to the supermarket it goes up again, and it goes down because you leave. Do you see what's happening?

Deborah: Yes.

Waseem: All that's happening is that you are getting a series of peaks and then troughs, and then peaks and then troughs, but the situation itself isn't getting any better, it's just being repeated. If anything, it's probably getting worse because it's building up a barrier for you to go in.

Deborah: Yes.

Waseem: Deborah, what do you think would happen if, at that peak there, you didn't leave?

Deborah: It's a very scary thought, but I imagine I would probably faint. That's what feels like is going to happen, but certainly the palpitations and the dry mouth, and the difficulty I have with swallowing, I think they would probably get worse.

Waseem: And you think you would faint because you'd feel more anxious being there and staying there?

Deborah: Yes, I feel as if I'm going to faint and I really have to hold on to something or sit down. I just can't cope with it at all. The only thing that I can do is get out of there.

Waseem: Sure. So what you are telling me is that, if you stayed there, you think that this graph would go up like this, just keep going up and up and up, it would be over there in the corridor?

Deborah: Yes, yes.

Waseem: Actually what would happen, would you believe, is that it wouldn't go up, it would start to level off and then just slowly start to come down, and next time you went in the peak wouldn't be quite as high, and over a period of time it would start to come down, and the next time the peak would be lower.

Deborah: So that would happen gradually?

Waseem: Yes, gradually, over a period of time, we find that it doesn't peak as much.

Deborah: Okay. It's still a very scary thought, but I can see the logic of what you are saying.

Waseem: You said something about how you are afraid of fainting. Have you ever fainted?

Deborah: No, I haven't actually, but I feel faint and anxious whenever I'm in a busy place.

Waseem: But you always feel anxious when you go there.

Deborah: Yes.

Waseem: Do you know what happens to your blood pressure when you feel anxious?

Deborah: I did read something about this. Does it go up?

Waseem: Yes, it goes up. And do you know what happens to your blood pressure when you faint?

Deborah: I think it goes down, doesn't it?

Waseem: In fact it goes down quite quickly, so quickly in fact that you lose consciousness. So, you see what I'm getting at?

Deborah: It wouldn't actually be possible to faint because of anxiety.

Waseem: Right. Because anxiety causes blood pressure to go up and fainting causes blood pressure to go down, they are not really compatible.

Deborah: But then you still feel that way, don't you? Or, well, I do, anyway, as if I'm going to faint.

Waseem: You do feel that way. Have you ever heard of something called fight or flight?

Deborah: Yes, I think so.

Waseem: Well, when a person is faced with what they see as a dangerous situation, their bodies prepare them to deal with it. Blood goes to all the main muscle groups to prepare the person to fight or run away.

Deborah: Which is what I do.

Waseem: Right. Often people can feel lightheaded and dizzy as they try to take in more oxygen and end up breathing out too much carbon dioxide, and that can affect us in that way. Remember you said that your breathing is out of control?

Deborah: Yes, yes.

Waseem: You said that you were panting a little

bit. So basically what you are experiencing are completely normal symptoms that you would in a dangerous situation, but the only thing is, we don't really consider the supermarket to be a dangerous situation.

Deborah: Well, not to most people.

Waseem: Right, but what we need to do is teach your body and your mind that being in a supermarket isn't a dangerous situation and you'll start reacting differently to it.

Deborah: Okay. How would you do that?

Waseem: Well, I'm not going to ask you to leave now and go shopping in a busy store.

Deborah: No, I wouldn't be able to do that, I really wouldn't.

Waseem: That wouldn't work. One of the tried and tested ways of doing this is to get you to face your fears in a graded way. We can't expect you to go to the supermarket alone now, just from this session. We need to break it down into manageable steps towards your ultimate goal. You'll need to devote quite a lot of your time to it, even up to an hour a day. Do you think you have that type of time to devote?

Deborah: Yes, yes, I think so. I would have an hour a day.

Waseem: Good. It might be a bit scary at times and you will experience anxiety, but it's not going to be helpful to put you in such scary situations that you might dash out.

Deborah: Okay, and will it involve going out on my own?

Waseem: Slowly, yes, you'll go out by yourself, but we'll take things in bite-size chunks so you feel in complete control of it. Next time we meet up we'll do a hierarchy and get started. You've also told me a lot about these anxious thoughts you get about fainting. I think it might be a good idea to keep some diaries of them and any other anxious thoughts, so we can examine them and see whether they are maybe not helping matters. What do you think?

Deborah: That sounds fine. Actually, I have started to feel a lot better just being able to talk about it and understand it a bit more.

Waseem: Good. Well, we're coming towards the end of the session. It's just worth my while summarizing one or two things that we talked about today. Do you remember that we started off by trying to summarize what your problem was, and, as we've decided, the problem is 'Avoidance of leaving home alone due to symptoms of anxiety and fear of fainting, leading to becoming increasingly housebound and dependent on Paul'.

Deborah: Yes, that's it exactly. That is the problem.

Waseem: We set a goal, and the goal we set was 'To go shopping alone at busy times with minimal anxiety at least once a week'. We spoke a little bit about what actually happens if you stay in the anxious situation and how your anxiety wouldn't just keep going up and up and out off the graph and into the corridor, remember?

Deborah: Yes.

Waseem: We said that it would slowly start to get better over a period of time, and I spoke to you about what happens to your blood pressure when you are anxious and what happens when you faint, so those two things aren't really compatible. Okay?

Deborah: Yes.

Waseem: Good. Right, that's been a very productive session. What I'll do is make an appointment for you to come in next week, then perhaps see you again four weeks later; but we'll have telephone contact. We'll maybe have 8–10 contacts in total.

Deborah: Thanks, that feels really positive and hopeful, actually, because I was beginning to think that nothing could change; but that does seem very hopeful.

Waseem: I'm sure it will, and the fact that you're determined and enthusiastic will make a big difference to it. I'm going to give you this leaflet to read by the time you next come in, Deborah. This leaflet is about Agoraphobia. Have a bit of a look at it and if there's anything you see that you want to discuss with me next time, then just highlight it.

Deborah: Okay.

Waseem: Also by the time you next come in, if you could fill in these questionnaires. They're pretty self-explanatory; the details of how to fill them in are just at the top here, and then over a period of time we can compare the results, and see how things are improving.

Deborah: Okay, so there's two there.

Waseem: Yes, there's two here. Each explains how to fill it in at the top. I won't go through it with you now; it's fairly obvious, and if you find that there is anything that you want to highlight and discuss, then we will just do that. Or if you find that you want to change the goals, then give it some thought. Hang onto those.

Deborah: Thank you.

Waseem: Good. Let's arrange an appointment for you to come next week, shall we?

Deborah: Okay, thanks very much.

Video: Problem summary and goal setting (Part 2)

Mental health worker (Samantha): Is there anything we haven't discussed already that you think I should know?

Ben: No, I think we've covered everything, actually.

Samantha: Okay, well perhaps it might be useful to try and sum up the problem in some way, to put it in a kind of nutshell so we can rate it now, how severe it is at the moment, and then we can come back to it later, and we can see whether that's improved or not. I think it would be a good time to think of a couple of goals that we can work towards. How does that sound?

Ben: Yes, that sounds fine, yes.

Samantha: Okay, so if we were pulling it together what would you say the main points of the problem were?

Ben: Hmmm, I suppose getting angry when I shouldn't, and then taking it out on Sue, and I've also got a problem with frustration. I just get frustrated really easily.

Samantha: Okay. Are there any other things that you think we should have in the problem statement?

Ben: Yes, there's the thing about losing control when I'm driving the car and shouting at other drivers.

Samantha: Okay. How do you think this

sounds? 'Difficulty dealing with stressful situations, particularly traffic jams, due to low threshold of frustration, leading to outbursts of anger at the time and irritability when I get home, putting a strain on my relationship with Sue'.

Ben: Yes, I think that sums it up, yes.

Samantha: It's a bit wordy, but I think we need it to be to get everything in there. Okay, if you were to rate that on how severe it is as a problem now, what would you rate it as on a scale of 0–100, 0 being not a problem and 100 being its most severe?

Ben: I suppose about 80.

Samantha: 80, okay. Good, well we'll come back to that later and see whether we can get that down at all, but the next step is to think of a couple of goals that we can work towards. What would you like to be able to do that you can't do now?

Ben: Well, I suppose I'd like not to get so angry on the way home, and then not to get ratty with Sue.

Samantha: Okay, it sounds like you've got a couple of goals there. Let's separate them out. So, what about 'To be able to travel to and from work with minimal anger', as one of them?

Ben: Yes, that sounds fine.

Samantha: And then the one about Sue, 'To spend half an hour chatting with Sue about our respective days, with minimal irritability'?

Ben: Yes, that would be really good if I could do that. Yes.

Samantha: Yes, they sound okay?

Ben: Yes.

Samantha: Okay, the next step now is to start looking at how you can reach those goals here. Anger is a really common problem, actually. It's something that a lot of people are troubled with. Now, it can be useful to look at the physical symptoms of anger in particular and some of the angry thoughts that you are having. So what I think might be a good idea is to look at these physical symptoms and to see if we can use some relaxation strategies to help with them, and to start examining some of your thoughts to see whether we can work with some of the thoughts, and get them to be a bit less angry too. How does that sound?

Ben: Yes, I think if I could learn to relax and control the angry thoughts, that would be half the battle, actually.

Samantha: Okay, good. Well I think we should start the relaxation next week. I'd like to teach you how to use the relaxation strategies. It's not as easy as it sounds, to be honest, so I think we should practise it in session next week and then what we'll do is we'll develop it over a number of weeks, so you can transfer it to all sorts of different situations. I do think, as well, that we should start looking at your thoughts right away, so I've got an 'Anger Diary' here. I wonder if I can I give that to you? It's pretty straightforward; all you do is put in the day and the date, what's triggered the anger, your level of anger and how you responded. So, I'll give that to you; and I'd also like to give you a booklet on anger that maybe you could read between now and next session?

Ben: Sure, yes.

Samantha: After meeting up next week, I think we can do some of the contacts over the phone if that's going to be convenient for you. We'll need to meet up sometimes too, but we'll be able to do some telephone contacts. I would expect us to meet up or talk on the telephone about 8–10 times. How does that sound to you?

Ben: Yes, that sounds fine. I think talking on the phone might be a good idea. It's just I'll need to get out the back and find a quiet space, and as long as it doesn't take too long, because I can't leave my desk for a long time.

Samantha: Right. No, the telephone sessions are generally short, maximum 20 minutes, but probably about 10 on average.

Ben: Yes, that would be fine.

Samantha: Good. We've covered lots today, so I think it might be useful at this stage to just do a bit of a recap of the session if that's alright. You've told me a lot about the problems with anger and how it is affecting you and your relationship with Sue, and also about the baby being on the way, and I can understand that you want to get the problem sorted. We've come up with a really good problem statement, I think, that

sums it up in a nutshell. We've got 'Difficulty dealing with stressful situations, particularly traffic jams, due to low threshold of frustration, leading to outbursts of anger at the time and irritability when I get home, putting a strain on my relationship with Sue'. And then we came up with some goals for us to work towards, so that is 'To travel to and from work with minimal anger' and 'To spend half an hour chatting with Sue about our respective days, with minimal irritability'. Do they still sound okay?

Ben: Yes, that sounds fine, yes.

Samantha: And then we talked about the nature of anger and how the physical symptoms and the thoughts are contributing to the problem, and we've looked at ways of tackling that, mainly by using relaxation, which we're going to come onto next week, and also the working with thoughts, and you've got a diary to start working with them. Okay, is there anything that you feel confused about that you would like to discuss further, because we have covered a lot today?

Ben: No, I don't think so. I think we've covered everything, actually, yes.

Samantha: Okay. Is there anything that we haven't discussed today that you think would have been useful to cover?

Ben: No, I think we've covered all the main points. Yes, it's good.

Samantha: Okay, well, what I think we should do is arrange an appointment for next week at a convenient time.

Ben: Okay, fine.

Notice how the goals they arrive at together are positively stated, realistic, concrete, measurable and achievable. The Anger Diary mentioned in the above session between Ben and Samantha is 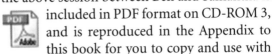 included in PDF format on CD-ROM 3, and is reproduced in the Appendix to this book for you to copy and use with your patients.

Educate the patient about the nature of contact

Most of us feel more confident when we know what to expect and what is expected of us. The

Exercise

Ask a colleague to play the part of Roger while you play the role of the mental health worker. Role-play agreeing a problem summary and two treatment goals. Ensure that your goals are positively stated, concrete, measurable and achievable.

patient entering into contact with a mental health worker is no different. The structure of therapeutic contact is explained, as is how long contact is likely to last, and how long a session lasts (e.g. 30 minutes). The patient learns from the outset that they will develop new skills to tackle their difficulties, which will enable them to take responsibility for their own improvement with the guidance and support of the mental health worker. The general approach used for the assessment is continued throughout the remainder of contact. The patient learns from the start that treatment is highly active and that they are effectively learning how to take control of their own problems. The patient also learns not only that will they develop skills to deal with their current problems, but also that the skills learned will be useful for similar problems that may be encountered in the future.

Phase 4: Shared decision-making

Agreed treatment plan

The mental health worker and the patient agree what will occur during their contact, how that will be structured, the frequency and type of contact, etc. The therapeutic contact may predominantly either be by telephone or face-to-face, or a mixture of both. A precise plan of what will occur during the contact helps to guide the intervention and keep it on track. Both parties are clear from the outset what the expectations are and how contact will then proceed. The problem summary agreed by the patient and mental health worker is used to set

goals and the treatment plan. The treatment plan will be determined by what advice the patient agrees they are likely to follow and by the services available.

Five main factors are used to inform the decision as to what interventions are appropriate:

1. Information about the problem
2. Level of risk
3. Agreed problem summaries and goals
4. The mental health worker's knowledge of available services and treatments
5. An estimation of the likelihood that the patient will follow advice

All these factors enable the mental health worker and the patient to reach a shared decision about what approaches will be appropriate at this time.

For example, there is little point in recommending the patient to make an appointment at the Citizens Advice Bureau if it is 40 miles away and they do not have a car, or to recommend antidepressants to a patient who is opposed to medication. Information about the choice of approaches are given to the patient, who will make the decision on how they want to take things forward.

Elicit feedback

The mental health worker makes a final summary of the interview and asks for feedback at the end, in case anything has been misunderstood. If this is not done, the patient may go away with the wrong idea and perhaps not return. Remember, misunderstandings are common in daily communication. The chance of what we say being misconstrued is increased when talking with depressed patients in particular, because of the negative interpretations they may be prone to making.

Useful questions used to elicit feedback include:

- 'Is there anything that I've said today that has bothered you?'
- 'Is there anything you feel confused about and would like me to explain further?'

- 'Is there anything important that we haven't discussed today?'

Measurement

Measurement is an important component of any therapeutic intervention, as it helps us evaluate whether the interventions we use with patients are being effective. Whether the interventions are going well or badly, good measurement enhances awareness of this and increases the likelihood that appropriate action will then be taken. Therefore it is important to establish how severe the patient's problems are in the first place (baseline), before they are introduced to any therapeutic intervention, so that a comparison can be made with later measurements. This means that any change can be evaluated and the effectiveness of interventions that have been used can be established. The assessment session is an ideal time to introduce measurement.

Why measure?

There are several reasons why measurement in clinical practice is important. These include:
- To establish a baseline
- To compare against benchmarks
- To change our practice
- To implement clinical governance
- To develop a body of knowledge

but most importantly…
- To give patients accurate feedback on progress

What kinds of measures can we use?

Three types are commonly used:
- Outcome measures
  a. Validated measures
  b. Case-specific measures
- Process measures
  c. Diaries

Validated measures

Completing validated questionnaires provides useful information about a patient's symptoms. There are many self-report instruments of this kind commonly used, including the Clinical Outcomes in Routine Evaluation Outcome Measure (CORE-OM), the Hospital Anxiety and Depression Scale (HADS), and the Beck Depression Inventory (BDI). There are also many other measures used for specific disorders. Questionnaires such as these are commonly used at the start of any therapeutic intervention, to monitor progress throughout, and at the end of the intervention to evaluate change. Some measures have a cost attached (e.g. the Beck Depression Inventory and the Hospital and Depression Scale). Check with your organization to find out what licences are held on what measures.

Permission has been granted for the use of the following self-report measures, which are well validated and easy to use. The CORE-OM (Evans et al, 2002), PHQ-9 (Kroenke et al, 2001) and WSAS (Mundt et al, 2002) can all be printed off and used. They are included in PDF format on CD-ROM 3 and can be freely used with patients.

Clinical Outcomes in Routine Evaluation – Outcome Measure (CORE–OM)

The CORE-OM (core-om.pdf) is one of the most widely used outcome measures in the psychological therapies within the UK. The CORE System Trustees own the copyright, which means that the measure cannot be changed in any way without their permission. However, its use is 'copyleft' – that is, it may be printed and photocopied freely provided it is not used for financial gain.

It comprises 34 items addressing domains of subjective well-being (4 items), problems (12 items), functioning (12 items) and risk (6 items: 4 risk-to-self items and 2 risk-to-others items). Within the problem domain, item 'clusters' focus on anxiety (4 items), depression (4 items), physical problems (2 items) and trauma (2 items). Within the functioning domain, item 'clusters' focus on general functioning (4 items), close relationships (4 items) and social relationships (4 items). Items are scored on a 5-point scale from 0 'Not at all' to 4 'All the time'. Half the items focus on low-intensity problems (e.g. 'I feel anxious/nervous') and half focus on high-intensity problems (e.g. 'I feel panic/terror'). Eight items are positively keyed.

Patient Health Questionnaire – 9 items (PHQ–9)

The PHQ-9 (screener_cover phq.pdf and screener_pad phq.pdf) can be used as a depression severity tool for monitoring treatment. With possible scores ranging from 0–27, higher scores are correlated with other measures of depression severity. Scoring is as follows: of the 9 items in question 1, count one point for each item checked several days, two points for items checked more than half the days, three points for items checked nearly every day, and sum the total for a severity score. This measure can be repeated to check on response to treatment. Its reproduction is with permission of Pfizer Inc.

Work and Social Adjustment Scale (WSAS)

This measure (work and social adjustment scale.pdf) uses a 0–8 scale to assess how five key areas in a patient's life are affected by their problems. These include: ability to work; home management (cleaning, tidying, shopping, cooking, looking after home or children, paying bills); social leisure activities (with other people, such as parties, bars, clubs, outings, visits, dating, home entertainment); private leisure activities (done alone, such as reading, gardening, collecting, sewing, walking alone); ability to form and maintain close relationships with others. The higher the scores, the more disabled the patient is by their problems. A WSAS score above 20 appears to suggest moderately severe psychopathology. Scores between 10 and 20 are associated with significant functional impairment but less severe clinical symptomatology. Scores below 10 are associated with sub-clinical populations (e.g. individuals who are not clinically depressed or anxious). Permission has been granted by Professor Isaac Marks to repro-

duce the WSAS.

Case-specific measures

Not everyone has ready access to validated questionnaires. Despite some validated questionnaires being available to administer freely, others can be expensive to use. It is also sometimes not appropriate to use questionnaires (e.g. if a patient has poor literacy or very poor concentration). In these circumstances it can be useful to record problem severity on an individualized scale (e.g. a scale of 0–100 of how depressed the patient feels, where 0 means not depressed at all, and 100 means the most depressed the patient has ever felt). The patient can think back over the last week and give a rating. This personalized scale can easily be used throughout treatment. These kinds of scales can generally be very helpful for the patient as they directly measure their problems. Like questionnaires, case-specific measures are commonly used at the start of treatment, for monitoring of progress throughout, and at the end of the intervention to evaluate change.

Diaries

Diaries are another useful measurement tool. They are commonly used to monitor behaviours and thoughts and also to measure change. A number of diaries will be presented in Chapter 3.4, and will be downloadable or copiable for you to use with your patients (e.g. activity schedule, thought diaries, sleep diary, anger diary, exposure diary, etc.). However, sometimes it can be particularly helpful to develop a personalized diary to record a specific problem. For example, a patient may be asked to record the frequency of a specific upsetting and intrusive thought at particular times of the day in a specially designed diary.

Note: It is important that the patient does not feel overwhelmed by being given too many measures to complete. Try to keep it simple, especially in the early stages of contact when patients are getting used to the self-help nature of the therapeutic intervention and may not have developed the necessary skills for good record keeping.

When should we measure?

Using the types of measures described above can help a great deal in the assessment of a patient's difficulties. As part of assessment, the patient is likely to be asked to fill in validated questionnaires relevant to their problem and rate their problem severity (case-specific measure).

The patient may then be asked to complete a diary over the next week to record a particular symptom (e.g. panic attacks or level of activity). Diaries are likely to continue to be used throughout the therapeutic intervention and offer a great deal of useful information, both to the mental health worker and to the patient, on progress and problems arising. At the end of the therapeutic contact, the validated questionnaires and case-specific measures can be repeated and will offer feedback on how successful the therapeutic interventions have been. In addition, it can often be appropriate to use validated questionnaires and case-specific measures at each session, depending on the severity of the problem (e.g. the PHQ-9 may be used at every session for a patient with moderate to severe depression).

Assessing your interview skills

Developing effective interviewing skills is vital for the mental health worker to function effectively. Professor David Richards from York University developed a useful tool for measuring competency of interviewing. This measure, the 'Assessment of Contact with Patients Tool' (ACPT), has been adapted to fit with the interview format described here. To use the ACPT appropriately, the mental health worker must either video-record their sessions with patients or ask their supervisor to sit in on the session to be assessed. **Remember: It is imperative to gain written consent from your patient when recording sessions.** This measure can be used for per-

sonal reflection on interviews, and for the purposes of supervision, whether this be for feedback on assessment interviews or any other face-to-face contact with patients.

Exercise

If possible, arrange to record an assessment interview with a patient. Obtain their written consent, making sure that you follow appropriate protocols in gaining this consent.
- Play the session back to yourself.
- Use the 'ACPT' to assess your level of skill.
- Take note of the skills you perform well and those that require more practice.
- Ask a colleague or your supervisor to role-play a patient so that you can practice developing those skills that you need to improve on.
- Get into a routine of regularly recording your contacts with patients for the purposes of self-reflection and supervision.

Section summary

- A thorough assessment is crucial for successful therapeutic intervention
- A patient-centred interviewing approach should be used
- The aim of assessment is to get an understanding of the patient's problems, including the main emotional, physical, cognitive and behavioural symptoms, and the areas of the patient's life which are affected
- A funnel approach to questioning should be used, leading from open questions to more closed questions
- A good way of eliciting information about a problem is to ask about a time when it has occurred recently, then making connections between symptoms
- If a mental health worker is concerned about risk, they should inform the patient's GP immediately
- Problems should be prioritized using

problem summaries
- Goals are agreed for each problem to be addressed
- The mental health worker and the patient agree a treatment plan
- Three types of measures are commonly used: self-report questionnaires; case-specific measures; and diaries
- Patients should not feel overwhelmed by being given too many measures to complete
- Measures that are free to download from CD-ROM 3 are CORE-OM, PHQ-9, and WSAS

References

Barkham M, Gilbert, N., Connell, J., Marshall, C. and Twigg, E. (2005). Suitability and utility of the CORE-OM and CORE-A for assessing severity of presenting problems in primary and secondary care based psychological therapy services. *British Journal of Psychiatry,* 186, 239–246.

Barkham, M., Margison, F., Leach, C., Lucock, M., Mellor-Clark, J., Evans, C., Benson, L., Connell, J., Audin, K. and McGrath, G. (2001). Service profiling and outcomes benchmarking using the CORE-OM: Towards practice-based evidence in the psychological therapies. *Journal of Consulting and Clinical Psychology,* 69, 184–196.

Evans, C., Connell, J., Barkham, M., Margison, F., Mellor-Clark, J., McGrath, G. and Audin, K. (2002). Towards a standardised brief outcome measure: Psychometric properties and utility of the CORE-OM. *British Journal of Psychiatry,* 180, 51–60.

Kroenke, K. and Spitzer, R.L (2002). The PHQ-9: A new depression and diagnostic severity measure. *Psychiatric Annals,* 32, 509–521.

Kroenke, K., Spitzer, R.L. and Williams, J.B. (2001). The PHQ-9: validity of a brief depression severity measure. *Journal of General Internal Medicine,* 16, 606–613.

Mundt, J.C., Marks, I.M., Greist, J.H. and Shear, K. (2002). The Work and Social Adjustment Scale: A simple accurate measure of impairment in functioning. *British Journal of Psychiatry,* 180, 461–464.

Recommended reading

Gamble, C. and Brimblecombe, N. (2005). *Key Skills in Community Mental Health Nursing.* London: Quay Books.

Mead, N. and Bower, P. (2000). Patient centredness: A conceptual framework and review of the empirical literature. *Social Science and Medication,* 51, 1087–1110.

Newell, R and Gourney, K. (2000). *Mental health nursing: An evidence-based approach.* London: Churchill Livingstone.

Norman, I. and Ryrie, I. (2004). *Art and Science of Mental Health Nursing: A textbook of principles.* Maidenhead: Open University Press.

Rollnick, S. (1999). *Health behaviour change: A guide for practitioners.* Edinburgh: Churchill Livingstone.

Test yourself

 To check your progress, locate this section on CD-ROM 3 and work through the interactive questions at the end.

Chapter 3.4
Clinical interventions

Aim

To enhance clinical skills in a range of therapeutic interventions suitable for people with common mental health problems in primary care.

Learning outcomes

By the end of this Chapter, the reader will be able to:
- Select appropriate therapeutic interventions, including: case management, medication management, psycho-education, behavioural activation, problem solving, working with thoughts, and other self-help approaches
- Collaboratively plan an intervention programme based on a patient-centred assessment of needs
- Deliver evidence-based, low-intensity, patient-centred intervention programmes for people with common mental health problems in primary care

Introduction

This Chapter covers a series of strategies that can be incorporated into a case management framework. Case management is not an intervention in itself; rather it is an organizational system used to support patients. Case management can include medication management or guided self-help, or a combination of the two. Case management may also include 'signposting' people to other services.

In primary care, medication management and guided self-help are embedded within a 'stepped care' framework. Firstly, therefore, the Stepped Care model will be described, to be followed by case management and medication management. A series of guided self-help strate-gies then follows. Everything the mental health worker does with the patient should be organized within a case management approach. Therefore this will be covered before the principles of medication management and the specific interventions used in guided self-help.

Assisting patients with medication management and guided self-help in a case management organizational system will allow the mental health worker in primary care to see many patients for brief periods of intervention. The role of the mental health worker in primary care is to provide a combination of pharmacological and psychological support to patients who are ultimately the experts on their own problems.

Chapter 3.4 content is as follows:

1   A Stepped Caremodel
2   Case management using scheduled contact
3   Medication management
4   The self-help framework
    4a Psycho-education
    4b Behavioural activation
    4c Problem-solving
    4d Graded exposure
    4e Working with thoughts
    4f Controlled breathing
    4g Relaxation
    4h Sleep hygiene and improving the sleep environment
    4i Lifestyle strategies, including:
- Healthy eating habits
- Physical exercise
- Controlled drinking
- Smoking cessation

Section 1: A Stepped Care model

Introduction

Stepped care, originally developed in the United States as a model of healthcare for guiding the pathway of treatment of alcohol problems, has been successfully applied to a variety of disorders. A number of attempts have been made to develop stepped care models in the UK. These include the NICE Guidelines for depression and anxiety, and the *Enhanced Service Specification for depression under the new GP contract* (2004). NICE Guidelines describe stepped care in the particular context of depression and anxiety (panic disorder, with or without agoraphobia, and generalized anxiety disorder), and use the stepped care framework to match the needs of patients to the most appropriate services, depending on the characteristics of their illness and their personal and social circumstances.

Features of stepped care

There are two main features of stepped care:
1   The first line treatments offered to the patient are the least intensive of those available, yet are still expected to bring about positive outcomes. More intensive interventions are kept for those patients who fail to benefit from these lower-intensity treatments. For example, a mental health worker in primary care may offer guided self-help materials and minimal support, then if this fails to bring about positive change for the patient, more formal Cognitive Behavioural Therapy (CBT) from a specialist practitioner is offered.
2   Second, the Stepped Care model means that the outcomes of interventions and decisions about treatment provision are monitored systematically, and changes are made (this is called 'stepping up') if the interventions the patient is currently receiving do not result in significant improvement.

How stepped care works

As already stated, stepped care means that the patient is offered the least intensive treatment that is still expected to bring about significant clinical improvement. There are a number of important issues to note. Watchful waiting is for patients with mild depression, who do not require or want a specific intervention. The other interventions and steps are for increasing levels of symptoms, distress and problem complexity. It is appropriate for patients to bypass previous steps if their symptoms are severe enough, or if they have previously tried a step but benefited little.

NICE Guidelines for depression

The National Institute for Health and Clinical Excellence (2004) gives an example of stepped care applied to depression (see Figure 4 on page 51).

Principles of the steps

The principles of the steps are as follows:
1   Each step offers options to the patient about what type of treatment would be most suited to them.
2   Shared decision-making between the patient and the healthcare professional should take place during all steps.
3   Step one is for recognition and diagnosis of the disorder.
4   Steps two to five represent the interventions offered to increasing complexity of problems.
5   Some patients may start with interventions at step 2, and if these fail to bring about improvement the patient then moves up to step 3, and so on.

Step 1: Recognition in primary care and general hospital settings

The NICE Guidelines for Depression (www.nice.org.uk) suggest that screening for depression should be carried out in primary care and in general hospital settings in high-risk groups (e.g. patients with a history of depression, significant physical illnesses causing disability, or other mental health problems such as dementia). Screening should include at least two questions related to mood and interest:

- 'During the last month, have you often been bothered by feeling down, depressed or hopeless?'
- 'During the last month, have you often been bothered by having little interest or pleasure in doing things?'

Severity of depression can be assessed with the help of the criteria shown in Chapter 3.1, Section 1.

Step 2: Treatment of mild depression in primary care

Over 80% of patients with depression are cared for solely in primary care, and most of the patients who use secondary care services continue to receive much of their treatment in primary care. Some patients may improve while being monitored without additional help (watchful waiting), while others often respond to low-intensity interventions such as those listed here:

- *Watchful waiting:* The NICE Guidelines suggest that watchful waiting should be used for patients with mild depression who do not want any intervention, or who, following assessment, are considered likely to recover without intervention. A further assessment should be arranged, normally within two weeks. Watchful waiting is usually carried out by the GP.
- *Guided self-help:* Patients at this level should be offered self-help, using brief CBT-based approaches (e.g. written literature) and with minimal support from a mental health worker who introduces the self-help and monitors progress. Guided self-help is covered in more depth later.
- *Computerized cognitive behavioural therapy (CCBT):* This involves supplying the patient with access to CD-ROM or internet-based materials. These packages require varying degrees of supervision from a mental health worker. Some organi-

zations will have access to this kind of intervention while others may not have this kind of provision available.

- *Sleep and anxiety management:* Patients with mild depression can benefit from advice on sleep hygiene and anxiety management (e.g. relaxation), both of which will be covered later.
- *Psycho-education:* This type of intervention can be done in a group or on a one-to-one basis, and involves providing information about depression and strategies for tackling the symptoms (e.g. behavioural activation, etc.). Psycho-education is discussed in more depth later.
- *Exercise:* Exercise has been shown to be helpful for patients with depression, as it can aid recovery. Some 'exercise on prescription' schemes have been successfully set up to enable patients to access facilities at local leisure centres where they can be offered regular advice from qualified professionals and their progress monitored. The mental health worker should check to see whether any such schemes are available in their area. An exercise programme of up to three sessions per week, each of around 45–60 minutes, for between 10 and 12 weeks is generally recommended.
- *Brief psychological interventions:* A patient may be offered one of a range of psychological interventions (e.g. CBT, problem-solving or counselling) over a recommended period of 10–12 weeks of 6–8 sessions). NICE Guidelines emphasize the importance of the therapeutic alliance, because it is associated with positive outcomes, regardless of the psychological intervention used.
- *Antidepressant medication:* Antidepressant medication is generally not recommended for mild depression. Treatment using antidepressant medication is only considered if the patient's mild depression persists after other interventions at this level have been ineffective and if the depression is associated with psychosocial and medical problems; or if the patient has a past history of moderate or severe depression.

Step 3: Treatment of moderate to severe depression in primary care

At this level, the choice of treatment will reflect patient preference, past experience of treatment and whether the patient has benefited from other interventions. Suicide risk must also be taken into consideration when choosing interventions. Assessment, degree of functional impairment and presence of significant co-morbidities or specific symptoms will determine whether referral to secondary services is appropriate, though the majority of patients with moderate or severe depression can be treated in primary care.

- *Antidepressant medication:* From step three onwards, antidepressant medication is generally offered before psychological interventions. NICE Guidelines recommend careful monitoring of symptoms, side-effects and suicide risk (particularly in those patients under the age of 30), especially in the early stages of taking antidepressant medication. Medication management will be covered in more depth in Section 3.
- *Psychological treatments:* Patients with more severe depression may require longer-term specialist psychological therapy, such as CBT or in some cases Interpersonal Therapy (IPT). The NICE Guidelines suggest a treatment period of 16–20 sessions over a period of six to nine months. A combination of CBT and anti-depressant medication is likely to be offered at this level.
- *Social support:* Patients with chronic depression who would benefit from additional social support may benefit from befriending in addition to medication and psychological treatments. Befriending is usually carried out by trained volunteers over a period of two to six months, and contacts occur at least weekly. A rehabilitation programme fostering a return to work can also be considered for patients with severe or chronic depression; work provides a number of protective factors against depression, including structure to the patient's day, social contact and self-esteem.

- *Enhanced care in primary care:* NICE Guidelines acknowledge that the effectiveness of treatments can be enhanced by the provision of telephone support by primary care mental health workers using clear treatment protocols, in particular for the monitoring of antidepressant medication regimes (see Medication Management in Section 3). It is also recommended that multifaceted care programmes integrate, through clearly specified protocols, the delivery and monitoring of appropriate psychological and pharmacological interventions for patients with depression (Section 2 on Case Management).

Step 4: Treatment of depression by mental health specialists

The focus of this step is on patients that present with treatment-resistant, recurrent, atypical and psychotic depression, and those at significant risk. These patients are generally treated by specialist mental health professionals, including GPs with a Special Interest in mental health, who will provide assessment, treatment and consultancy services. Crisis resolution and home treatment teams can be used to help manage crises for patients presenting as a significant risk. Patients may enter directly at this level if they are assessed as requiring specialist services. Medication in the secondary care setting is initiated under the supervision of a consultant psychiatrist. Psychological interventions (in particular, CBT) combined with medication may be offered. Mindfulness-based CBT may be offered to patients who are currently well but who have experienced three or more previous depressive episodes.

Step 5: Inpatient treatment for depression

A small number of patients may not improve from interventions provided at the lower levels, or perhaps the depression severity and/or a high degree of risk may make these earlier steps inappropriate. If this is the case, the recommendation would be referral by the GP to inpatient

Exercise

- From what you have learned so far about Nigel and his reluctance to take medication, his low level of risk of suicide, but moderate severity of depression, decide at which level of the Stepped Care model he should enter.
- From what you have learned about Sarah (video clips in Parts 3.1 and 3.3), and the fact that she is taking medication, that she is an intermediate suicide risk, and is moderately depressed, at which level of the Stepped Care model should she enter?
- From what you learned about Julian and his high suicide risk, at which level of the Stepped Care model should he enter?

In fact both Nigel and Sarah entered treatment at level 3. However, they receive different treatment approaches that are geared towards their own specific need. Nigel has refused anti-depressant medication which was offered as a first line treatment and is instead provided with psycho-education, dietary advice and brief CBT. Sarah is prescribed antidepressants and is provided with medication management, psycho-education, behavioural activation, signposting to a job club and guided self-help. Julian will not appear again until Chapter 3.5, as he was referred immediately to secondary care psychiatric services and was admitted to hospital that day for his own safety (entry at level 5). Chapter 3.5 contains a summary of Julian's and all other patients' courses of interventions and their outcomes.

psychiatric care to provide a place of sanctuary in a non-threatening environment, more complex psychological interventions, or perhaps electroconvulsive therapy (ECT) in exceptional circumstances.

 Note: A copy of *Depression: management of depression in primary and secondary care* (NICE, 2004a) is available in

PDF format on CD-ROM 3, and online at www.nice.org.uk/guidance/CG23/niceguidance/pdf/English/download.dspx.

NICE Guidelines for Anxiety

The National Institute for Health and Clinical Excellence gives an example of stepped care applied to anxiety (*NICE, 2004*).

General recommendations

Emphasis is placed on shared decision-making between the patient and the healthcare professional, during the diagnosis and at all levels of care. Information about the nature, course and treatments should be made available to patients, and where appropriate to family members and carers.

Step 1: Recognition and diagnosis
The NICE Guidelines for Anxiety (www.nice.org.uk) suggest a diagnostic process that includes the eliciting of necessary relevant information, such as personal history, any self-medication, and cultural or other individual characteristics that may be important considerations in subsequent care.

Step 2: Treatment in primary care
Primary care is considered to be the most appropriate service to provide interventions for patients with panic disorder or generalized anxiety disorder. Interventions include:
- *Psychological therapy:* CBT should be delivered in the optimal range of duration (7–14 hours in total for panic disorder, and 16–20 hours in total for generalized anxiety disorder), normally provided on a weekly basis over a maximum period of four months.
- *Pharmacological therapy:* Antidepressant medication with proven effectiveness in panic disorder and generalized anxiety disorder is the only pharmacological intervention that should be used in the longer-term management of either disorder.
- *Self-help:* Written materials based on CBT principles can be used to help patients

understand their psychological problems and learn ways to overcome them by changing their behaviour. Check to see if there is a book prescription scheme for common mental health problems in your area. Information about support groups should also be offered where available, and the general benefits of exercise as part of good general health can be discussed when appropriate.

Step 3: Review and consideration of alternative treatments

If, after an adequate course of one treatment from the above list, the healthcare practitioner and patient agree that there has been no improvement, then, after reassessment, consideration should be given to trying one of the other types of intervention.

Step 4: Review and referral to specialist mental health services

If the patient continues to present with significant symptoms after two of the above interventions have been provided, then, in most instances, the patient should be referred to specialist mental health services.

Step 5: Care in specialist mental health services

Following a thorough reassessment, the patient's care and management should be based on their individual circumstances and shared decision-making. Options include:

- Treatment of co-morbid conditions
- CBT with an experienced therapist if not offered already, including home-based CBT if attendance at clinic is difficult
- Structured problem-solving
- Full exploration of pharmacotherapy
- Day support to relieve carers and family members
- Referral for advice, assessment or management to tertiary centres

Note: A copy of *Anxiety: management of anxiety*

Exercise

- From what you have learned about Alison (video clips in Parts 3.1 and 3.3), and her presentation of panic disorder, identify the level of intervention using the stepped care framework.
- From what you have learned about Julie (video clips in Parts 3.1 and 3.3), and her presentation of generalized anxiety disorder, identify the level of intervention using the stepped care framework.

Follow Alison and Julie, who both entered at level 2, through treatment. See Chapter 3.5, Sections 4 and 8, for a summary of their individual treatment plans, interventions and outcomes.

(panic disorder, with or without agoraphobia, and generalized anxiety disorder) in adults in primary, secondary and community care (NICE, 2004b) is available in PDF format on CD-ROM 3, and online at www.nice.org.uk/ guidance/CG22/niceguidance/pdf/English/ download.dspx.

Each of the interventions from the Stepped Care model with relevance to the mental health worker in primary care is now covered in more depth. Stepped care is also referred to in Chapter 1.3, Section 3.

Section summary

- The first-line treatments offered to the patient are the least intensive of those available while still expected to bring about positive outcomes
- More intensive interventions are kept for those patients who fail to benefit from these lower-intensity treatments
- Outcomes of interventions and decisions about treatment are monitored, and changes made if interventions do not result in significant improvement
- The pathway of care is characterized by

five steps, each defined by a certain type of intervention of increasing intensity

References

National Institute for Health and Clinical Excellence (2004a). *Depression: management of depression in primary and secondary care.* London: National Institute for Health and Clinical Excellence. www.nice.org.uk.

National Institute for Health and Clinical Excellence (2004b). *Anxiety: management of anxiety (panic disorder, with or without agoraphobia, and generalised anxiety disorder) in adults in primary, secondary and community care.* London: National Institute for Health and Clinical Excellence.

National Institute for Mental Health in England North West Development Centre (2004). *Enhanced Services Specification for depression under the new GP contract.* Hyde, Cheshire: NIMHE North West Development Centre.

Test yourself

 To check your progress, locate this section on CD-ROM 3 and work through the interactive questions at the end.

Section 2: Case management using scheduled contact

Introduction

Case management has been shown to be particularly applicable to the management of depression in primary care. In this section, case management will be described in the context of depression, although it could also be applicable for the management of other conditions, such as Generalized Anxiety Disorder or Panic Disorder for example. Evidence shows that the best organizational approach to managing depression in primary care is multifaceted and includes collaboration between GPs, specialists and case managers. Mental health workers in the primary care setting are in an ideal position to provide case management to patients in primary care. There is strong evidence that case management, which includes telephone support, improves outcomes for patients with depression. Case management is also addressed in Chapter 1.3, Section 5.

Treatments offered to patients in primary care

Patients with common mental health problems, such as depression, are usually offered medication, encouraged to increase their physical activity, and are followed up by the GP. However, there is a wealth of evidence that patients do not always follow the advice they are given or take medication as prescribed. This offers an opportunity for the mental health worker in primary care to provide a case management role to help ensure patients receive the support they need to follow advice given.

What is case management?

Case managers work under supervision of the GP to improve quality of care for patients with depression. They do not work alone, but receive support from a specialist mental health professional, and share information with the GP. Case management involves providing telephone and face-to-face contact with patients following clear treatment protocols. This intervention is particularly relevant for monitoring and supporting those patients prescribed antidepressant medication. These interactions will include reviews of medication effect and side-effects (see Section 3), with accompanying support and the use of appropriate therapeutic interventions within a self-help framework. These interventions are evidence-based, low-intensity strategies such as problem-solving (see Section 4c) and behavioural activation (see Section 4b).

The primary care mental health worker provides information to the GP, reports on progress and gets supervision from the specialist mental health worker. This means that the primary care mental health worker can carry a large number of active cases.

Good case management

The five main components of case management are the following:

1   Assessment
2   Psycho-education
3   Shared decision-making
4   Feedback to the GP
5   Coordination of follow-up care and sign-posting

Assessment

A thorough and accurate assessment is vital for any clinical intervention to be successful. It is where rapport begins to be built with the patient, which is crucial for any therapeutic contact. Assessment is covered in detail in Chapter 3.3. Although assessment starts with the first contact, it continues through each therapeutic contact with the patient.

In addition to the information that is gained from talking to the patient, the mental health worker gains further information through the use of questionnaires, case-specific measures and monitoring diaries. You can find examples of all of these in other sections. The purpose of assessment is to gain a good understanding of what the patient is experiencing and to prioritize problems to work on. It is also an opportunity to assess risk (see Chapter 3.3). Assessment is made of the patient's clinical status and their adherence to treatment (both medication and psychosocial interventions).

Psycho-education

A major role for the mental health worker is to educate the patient about their disorder, medication and the strategies they can use to overcome their difficulties. Psycho-education can take many forms: about the disorder the patient has been diagnosed with; medication (its benefits and side-effects, and the time needed before improvements are likely to be shown); and therapeutic strategies (e.g. problem-solving, behavioural activation, working with thoughts, and lifestyle strategies such as healthy eating and controlled drinking, etc.). Mental health workers should learn about the disorders they are likely to encounter in the primary care setting, medications prescribed, their effects and side-effects, and the therapeutic strategies most likely to be of benefit to the patient. More is written about psycho-education in Section 4a.

Shared decision-making

In the main, patients prefer to be involved in making decisions about their treatment and to have a choice of how they are to be treated. Choices should be made available and the pros and cons of each should be discussed so that patients can make an informed choice of therapeutic interventions. Shared decision-making involves reviewing and summarizing a patient's problems and presenting a number of options from the resources available. The pros and cons of each option can then be discussed, which will help the patient decide on the best treatment option for them. Together, the patient and the mental health worker plan how to implement the option chosen and how to evaluate its success through follow-up.

CD-ROM 3 includes a video clip in which Nigel and his mental health worker, Waseem, use shared decision-making to arrive at the best treatment options for him. A transcript of the clip is given below.

Video: Case management – Shared decision-making

Mental health worker (Waseem): So, from what you are saying, you've been depressed over the last four months or so since the breakdown of your marriage. You've been low, you've been struggling with work and you've stopped doing a number of the things that you used to do, like playing badminton and going out with friends. You're also struggling with day-to-day stuff, just simple things like opening mail. You said you were finding it hard to sleep at nights, which is making you feel tired a lot of the time. Now I know that your GP has suggested that you try taking antidepressants, but you're not keen on the idea, is that right?

Nigel: Yes, you've pretty much summed up how I feel at the moment, and no, I'm not keen on taking tablets for this problem – but I am struggling, I admit that. There must be other ways to deal with this than tablets.

Waseem: Nigel, there are a number of ways of tackling depression. Antidepressants are only one of them. Some people do find that antidepressants are useful, but of course they can't take away the real-life problems that are causing you to feel like this. On the other hand, they may lift your mood sufficiently to allow you to make the changes that will make your life better. You're right, though, there are other approaches, and perhaps I can tell you about some of them.

Nigel: Yes, I'd like to hear about some of the other ways to deal with depression.

Waseem: Alright, well the things I'm going to tell you about are called self-help approaches. Having said that, we don't just leave you to it, we'll be there to support you and we'll have regular telephone contact.

Nigel: Okay.

Waseem: Now, as we know, one of the difficulties you're having is doing things, and you've lost a lot of your daily routine. So maybe we'll get you started, gradually introduce the things that you used to do, and build them up with time. The second thing we can do is talk to you about nutrition. There's a lot of evidence to connect depression with nutrition and in particular there is a lot of evidence to suggest that a lot of depressed people have low levels of something called Omega-3 and something else called Selenium. Now, as it happens, these things are readily available; Selenium is available in Brazil nuts, and Omega-3 you find in oily fish, so you can add these to your diet quite readily. There are other ways in which self-help can help you, but maybe we'll just discuss these two for now. What are your thoughts on this?

Nigel: Yes, I like the sound of that much more than tablets. I actually thought that you were just going to offer me tablets, so I'm pleased you've listened to me and offered me an alternative, and I like oily fish and Brazil nuts. I'm not really eating either at the moment, and I do really want some help getting my routine back and getting back to work.

Waseem: Good, it sounds really positive. There are different approaches we can take to tackle depression and not everybody wants to go down the medication route, and I respect your decision on that. I feel it would be beneficial for you to take some information on how nutrition is connected to mental health, if you get a chance to read this booklet.

Nigel: Yes, my concentration's not great at the moment, but I will try.

Waseem: Perhaps you could try reading it in small chunks and underline any parts that seem particularly relevant to you, and when we meet up next week, we can take it from there.

Nigel: Yes, that's a good idea.

Waseem: After that, we can try telephone sessions to save you coming in every time. I think the important point to remember, Nigel, is that we'll review your progress. If you find self-help isn't of benefit after a few weeks, then we'll look at different options, to see how else we can tackle your difficulties. Does that sound okay?

Nigel: Yes, that's okay. That sounds fine.

Notice how each option is considered, and Nigel's preferred option is then planned, with an agreement to review progress in a few weeks' time.

Feedback to the GP

A summary of every contact with the patient should be recorded and fed back to the GP using shared primary care records. It may be that something important has arisen from the contact (e.g. side-effects of medication resulting in the patient discontinuing treatment; or there may be concerns over a patient's risk of suicide) that needs to be dealt with directly by the GP.

Coordination of follow-up care and signposting

Part of the primary care mental health worker's role is to liaise with secondary services and to coordinate further support if needed. A patient may require more specialized treatment interventions (e.g. longer-term CBT) than the low-intensity strategies that the mental health worker has to offer. The primary care mental health worker can coordinate referrals to these services on behalf of the GP.

Signposting involves guiding the patient towards other services or agencies with more expertise than the mental health worker can provide. The patient is guided towards experts in the area they need help with but that the mental health worker may have limited knowledge of. This may mean suggesting a patient attends mental health support groups, smoking cessation groups, etc., or a gym to get advice about appropriate exercises for older people. To do a good job of signposting, the mental health worker must have an extensive knowledge of what is going on around them in the local community.

They should have a wealth of resources on tap to direct the patient to as appropriate, because, like coordination of follow-up care, signposting is an important aspect of the mental health worker's role.

> ## Exercise
>
> Consider each of the patients we have met so far in the programme, and allow yourself time to re-visit the video clips or transcripts. Taking into account your knowledge of what is going on around you in your community, think of at least one agency or organization to which it would be appropriate to signpost each of the patients.

Schedule of contacts

Normally, initial contact will occur within a few days of the GP identifying the patient as depressed. In the case of medication management (see Section 3), follow-up contact will then usually take place at 2 weeks, 4 weeks, 8 weeks, 12 weeks and 16 weeks after first contact (this is the minimum frequency of contact for medication management). Contacts may be more frequent. It is important to note that patients started on antidepressants who are considered to present a suicide risk (including all patients under the age of 30, as this age group has been found to be most at risk) should normally be seen after one week. The recommendations made in the NICE Guidelines for Depression will be covered in more depth under Medication Management (see Section 3). It may be appropriate to have more frequent contact when psychosocial support is being offered or during liaison with secondary care and the arrangement of further support from other agencies.

First interview

The first session with the patient is described in detail and illustrated using case studies in Assessment (see Chapter 3.3). The basic structure looks like this:
- Introduction: role and function
- Patient-centred problem assessment, risk assessment, problem summary and negotiation of goals
- Symptom assessment (e.g. PHQ-9, CORE-OM, WSAS)
- If on antidepressants: medication effect and side-effect assessment
- Treatment plan agreed (e.g. medication management, psycho-education, behavioural activation, and other self-help approaches, scheduled contact)
- Feedback to GP

Second interview

The typical format of the second interview is:
- Confirmation of the problem summary
- Risk assessment (to self and others)
- Medication effects and side-effects – assessment
- Managing medication difficulties –

psycho-education and shared decision-making
- Implementation of agreed support programme
- Feedback to GP if treatment programme requires adjustment

Subsequent interviews

All further sessions follow a typical format:
- Review of symptoms (e.g. using PHQ-9, CORE-OM, WSAS)
- Risk review (to self and others)
- Medication effects and side-effects assessment
- Managing medication difficulties – psycho-education and shared decision-making
- Monitoring and delivering of a psychosocial support programme
- Feedback to GP at scheduled intervals and when treatment programme requires adjustment

Example CD-ROM 3 contains an audio clip of a telephone contact in which mental health worker Katie discusses with Sarah the side-effects Sarah has been experiencing with her medication. A transcript of the clip is given below.

Audio: Telephone skills

Sarah: Hello.

Mental health worker (Katie): Hello, is that Sarah Goodfellow?

Sarah: Yes.

Katie: Hi Sarah, it's Katie Walsh here, the mental health worker from Cochrane Park Health Centre. We arranged that I would call today.

Sarah: Yes, I was expecting you to ring.

Katie: Right, good. Now, we've got 10 minutes as usual. Last time we spoke you were experiencing some unpleasant side-effects from the antidepressants Dr Mehra prescribed you. Now, that was a week ago and I was wondering how things are now. Is it okay to focus on this today?

Sarah: That sounds fine. The dry mouth did get a bit worse but started getting better a few days ago. Sucking the sweets helped a bit too, and I haven't felt sick at all for the past two days.

Katie: That's really good news. Have you noticed any other effects of the antidepressants?

Sarah: I haven't had any more side-effects, but I think they might be starting to work a bit now.

Katie: What makes you say that?

Sarah: Well, I had my first good day for ages yesterday, and I've been feeling quite good today too.

Katie: I'm really pleased to hear that. It seems to fit with what we talked about last time – that many people experience side-effects in the first couple of weeks or so but these tend to subside and the person starts to notice the benefits after 3–4 weeks. Did you get the opportunity to read the leaflet?

Sarah: Yes, I did glance at it, and it explained the types of side-effects that I might experience; but I haven't had most of the problems on the list.

Katie: I'm glad you found time to read it and that it made sense. Have you got an appointment with Dr Mehra coming up soon to review how you're getting on with the medication?

Sarah: Yes, I'm due to see him on Tuesday.

Katie: Okay, well you'll have the opportunity then to talk about how you had some unpleasant side-effects at first, and how you are feeling by then. Is there anything else you would like to talk about today?

Sarah: No, not at the moment. I know we've got another telephone session booked next week to talk about the self-help booklet you gave me to read. I actually just started reading it today because I feel like I can concentrate a little bit better.

Katie: That's good to hear. Maybe you could try to read some more of it before we meet up next week, and then we can look at it together in more depth.

Sarah: Okay, I will.

Notice how they agree items to discuss and the order in which they will be addressed.

Time management

Most face-to-face and telephone contacts will take no longer than 30 minutes and some calls may be as short as 10 minutes. The time spent on each component in the interview will greatly depend on the specific clinical situation (e.g. if the patient has discontinued medication without medical advice, then the majority of the session will be spent on medication review).

Managing risk

If for any reason the mental health worker believes that there may be a concern over the safety of a patient (risk either to themselves or to others), this should be immediately communicated to the patient's GP. If the situation is deemed to be an emergency and the patient's GP is unavailable, the duty GP should be contacted. If there is any doubt whatsoever about the patient's safety, it is always good practice to contact the GP and to express concern. The clear message here is **do not take risks with risk.**

It is not the role of a mental health worker in primary care to design and deliver risk management plans for patients. This should be done by the GP and any specialist mental health worker involved in the patient's care. However, mental health workers in primary care must always reassess risk at each contact and, if in any doubt, they should contact the patient's responsible health professional (e.g. their GP or specialist mental health worker) without delay.

On no account should a primary care mental health worker take responsibility for managing a patient who is at significant risk of harming themselves or others. If a patient is actively suicidal, they should not be left alone until the support needed has been obtained. It is imperative that risk is assessed every time contact is made with the patient. Refer back to Chapter 3.3 (Assessment) for the key questions to ask when assessing risk.

Reducing frequency of contact

If the patient has received frequent contact and psychosocial support has been provided, then spacing out sessions prior to ending contact can help reduce the risk of relapse by promoting self-reliance. According to the recommendations of the *Enhanced Services Specification for Depression under the new GP contract* (2004), scheduled contact should be offered every two months for a period of twelve months, and then twice at six monthly intervals for patients treated at step 3; and every month for twelve months and then twice at six monthly intervals for patients treated at step 4. However, for all patients, it is often appropriate to arrange follow-up sessions a few weeks after active therapeutic contact has ended (e.g. at three and six months).

Offering follow-up contact can sometimes alleviate a patient's fears about their ability to maintain gains alone. The patient can be advised that they can call in if experiencing any difficulties between appointments.

In reality, just knowing the facility is available is often enough to help patients through any difficult patches.

During the follow-up phase, it is hoped that when a patient experiences a setback they are sufficiently equipped at this stage to deal with the problem alone. It is only when they are unable to resolve their problems alone that they call the mental health worker. The mental health worker can then help the patient to identify why they had not been successful in tackling the problem and agree with the patient, using shared decision-making, what they need to do differently if a similar problem arises in the future. Follow-up contact also maintains momentum to help the patient remain motivated to practise what has been learned during the therapeutic contact.

Relapse prevention

Relapse prevention represents an important final phase of any therapeutic intervention in preparing the patient for moving on. The aim is to help the patient maintain their achievements and reduce the likelihood of problems recurring. It is important that the patient is prepared to deal with a relapse prior to any discontinuation of contact with the mental health worker.

Right from the start, the patient is made

Useful questions to prevent relapse

'What have you learned during our contact?'
'What made you vulnerable to this problem?'
'What life stressors triggered your current difficulties?'
'What helped to maintain the problem?'
'What techniques have you learned during our contact to deal with your problems?'
'How can you build on what you have learned to continue self-help?'
'What situations might you come across that are 'high-risk' for a setback?'
'What strategies can you use to prepare for these 'high-risk' situations?'
'What will you do if a setback occurs?'
'What goals can you set for the coming month?'
'What goals can you set for the next three months?'

aware that the therapeutic intervention will not continue indefinitely and that they, in effect, are taking responsibility for learning how to tackle their problems alone without the help of the mental health worker in the future.

Setbacks

It is relatively unusual for a patient to sail through a therapeutic intervention without any setbacks and, therefore, they should be prepared for this from the outset. By letting the patient know that setbacks are expected, they are less likely to catastrophize if or when a setback does occur. The patient should know that setbacks are considered a helpful part of the therapeutic process, offering an ideal opportunity for them to tackle obstacles, preparing them to tackle any setbacks which may be encountered after contact has ended.

The Relapse Prevention Plan

Before the end of therapeutic contact, the mental health worker and the patient draw up a 'Relapse Prevention Plan', which emphasizes continued practice of skills learned and includes details on how to deal with setbacks.

The patient is encouraged to set short- and long-term goals to plan how to continue tackling any unaccomplished targets during the therapeutic contact and to continue work on any remaining difficulties.

The box (left) contains a list of helpful questions for the patient to answer when drawing up the plan. This can be done either together during a contact, or as an exercise which is then discussed in the following contact.

For each 'high-risk' situation that is identified, the mental health worker and the patient make a plan of how to handle it.

Early warning signs

Within the Relapse Prevention Plan, the patient also lists 'early warning signs' of relapse (e.g. emotional, physical, cognitive and behavioural symptoms such as an increase in negative automatic thoughts, reduced activity, disturbed sleep, lowered mood, etc.) that would alert them to possible relapse (see Box). The patient can then bring into play all the techniques that were learned during therapeu-

Example of an early warning signs list

Emotions	Feeling lower in mood (especially in the morning) Irritable with the kids
Physical	Waking up early Appetite reduced Feeling tired a lot of the time
Cognitive	Increase in negative thoughts Poor concentration Self-blame
Behaviours	Avoiding answering the telephone Not going out as much as usual Staying in bed

tic contact to tackle such problems (e.g. behavioural activation techniques, problem-solving, evaluating thoughts, etc.). The patient should be encouraged to act promptly at the first signs of relapse in symptoms.

Self-help sessions

The patient can be encouraged to make time to address, formally, by themselves, any arising difficulties, just as is done during therapeutic contact with the mental health worker. The patient can set an agenda, review what they have been doing, identify problem areas, use strategies to address these difficulties and set relevant tasks. They might find this idea a little strange at first, but they can practise self-help sessions when frequency of contact with the mental health worker is being reduced. The patient can then be encouraged to continue these sessions on a monthly basis initially, then reduce them to bi-monthly and then every six months. This reinforces the idea of self-help, as the patient is effectively carrying out regular self-booster sessions alone.

Section summary

- Case management involves providing telephone and face-to-face contact with patients following clear treatment protocols
- The five main components of good case management are: assessment; psycho-education; shared decision-making; feedback to the GP; coordination of follow-up care
- The GP should be contacted immediately if the mental health worker is concerned about risk of harm to self or others
- Primary care mental health workers do not deliver risk management plans. GPs should seek expert assistance from secondary mental health services
- A clear protocol for assessing risk is available in Chapter 3.3
- Relapse Prevention is an important final phase of therapeutic contact
- Setbacks offer opportunities for patients to practise coping strategies learned during

contact, and encourages them to continue with self-help after it has ended
- Offering follow-up or booster sessions can be helpful to the patient
- Each patient has an individualized Relapse Prevention Plan to guide them in dealing with setbacks
- Patients should be encouraged to set short- and long-term goals to work on after contact has ended
- Patients are encouraged to set time aside for formal self-help sessions

References

National Institute for Health and Clinical Excellence (2004a). *Depression: the management of depression in primary and secondary care.* London: National Institute for Health and Clinical Excellence. www.nice.org.uk.

National Institute for Mental Health in England North West Development Centre (2004). *Enhanced Services Specification for depression under the new GP contract.* Hyde, Cheshire: National Institute for Mental Health in England North West Development Centre.

Test yourself

 To check your progress, locate this section on CD-ROM 3 and work through the interactive questions at the end.

Section 3: Medication management

Introduction

Antidepressant medication is a first-line treatment for most people with depression, with or without other therapeutic interventions. Unfortunately, adherence to medication prescribed by GPs is often poor. Patients prescribed antidepressants can benefit from information and support to increase their likelihood of adherence. Telephone support for monitoring antidepressant treatment constitutes a major part of the work of the mental health worker in primary care, and is part of the case management role as described in the previous section. The most appropriate patients for this type of intervention are those depressed patients who have been newly prescribed antidepressants. However, the mental health worker may also be asked to provide medication management for all those patients on the GP's list who are currently on antidepressants.

There is a clear distinction to be drawn between the goal, which is adherence, and the process by which mental health workers engage with patients. Traditional compliance strategies are deeply engrained in medical practice.

Compliance implies passive agreement by the patient to the treatment regime, with the mental health worker merely monitoring compliance as directed by the expert prescriber, usually the GP. These customs and practices are being increasingly questioned, as evidence emerges that attempts to enforce compliance are unlikely to achieve the high level of patient adherence required for therapeutic benefit from antidepressant medication (Royal Society, 1997).

Collaborative working with patients based on the principles of concordance recognizes the importance of understanding the individual patient perspective on taking medicines. The Royal Society (1997) provides advice on interview strategies to improve adherence to treatment regimes. Concordance is also addressed in Chapter 1.3, Section 5 and Chapter 2.2, Section 1.

Aims of medication management

The aims of medication management are to:
- Monitor the patient's adherence, side-effects and response to medication
- Provide information to the GP regarding the above
- Provide education and support to improve the chances of adherence to medication and help prevent any unplanned discontinuation
- Provide appropriate follow-up care, including referral to secondary services if appropriate ('stepping-up'). See Section 1 for Stepped Care

Components of scheduled telephone contact

The normal length of time for a scheduled telephone call will vary, but usually lasts anything from 10 to 30 minutes. The content of each call will include:
- Assessment of patients' difficulties
- Checking how they are responding to treatment
- Checking if they are adhering to antidepressant treatment and any other intervention
- Education about their difficulties and treatment interventions
- Shared decision-making of treatment interventions
- Agreeing and organizing any follow-up care

All calls should be followed up by feedback to the GP. The focus of the telephone conversation will vary from patient to patient, depending on what is appropriate to discuss. For example, almost an entire telephone contact may be spent dealing with a patient's discontinuation of antidepressant medication and finding out why the person is having difficulties, and discussing the pros and cons of re-engaging in this treatment intervention.

However, another patient may be experiencing no difficulty with the antidepressant medication they are taking and, therefore, the focus is more on self-help strategies such as behavioural activation.

Mental health workers do not make recommendations and there is nothing that they should do to change the advice given by the GP, unless they note something dangerous (e.g. an increase in suicidal ideation). Their role is to help patients access and understand publicly available information about medication. For this purpose, you may find it helpful to access the pharmacy section on the website of Norfolk and Waveney Mental Health Partnership NHS Trust (at www.nmhct.nhs.uk/pharmacy) for useful information on antidepressants that can be downloaded and given to patients.

Frequency of contact

The first contact with the patient will usually take place within a few days of being prescribed antidepressants by the GP, and may be done face-to-face or by telephone. Patients commencing antidepressants who are considered to present a suicide risk (including all patients under the age of 30) should always be seen after one week of taking the medication. Ongoing scheduled contact will usually take place at 2, 4, 8, 12 and 16 weeks following the patient's commencement of antidepressant medication. This is the minimum recommendation for frequency of contact for medication management and, therefore, more frequent contact may be required. Further contact may also be needed to offer psychosocial support and coordination of care with secondary services.

Recommendations on advice given to patients taking antidepressants

The following recommendations are taken from the NICE Guidelines for Depression. Please access the full guidelines for the complete list of recommendations in Chapter 3.1, Section 1.

Commencing treatment

1 Antidepressant medication should be routinely offered before psychological interventions to patients with moderate depression.
2 Any concerns that the patient may have regarding addiction or that taking medication is a sign of weakness should be addressed.
3 Patients being prescribed antidepressants should be advised, from the outset, about possible side-effects and the risk of symptoms on discontinuation.
4 Any patients starting antidepressant medication should be informed that the positive effects will be delayed, about the time-course of treatment and the importance of taking the medication as prescribed. Appropriate written materials

offering information about medication should be made available to the patient.

Monitoring risk

1 Patients commencing antidepressant medication and who are considered to present a suicide risk (including all patients under the age of 30) should normally be seen after one week of taking the medication.
2 Patients considered to be a high suicide risk should be prescribed limited quantities of antidepressant medication.
3 For patients who remain a high risk of suicide, consideration should be given to providing additional support, such as more frequent face-to-face contacts from primary care staff.
4 Particularly in the early stages of selective-serotonin reuptake inhibitor (SSRI) antidepressant treatment, healthcare professionals should actively seek out signs of akathisia, suicidal ideation, and any increase in anxiety and agitation. Patients should also be advised of the risk of these symptoms in the early stages of treatment and to seek help promptly if they are at all distressing.
5 If a patient develops marked and/or prolonged akathisia whilst taking an antidepressant, the use of the medication should be reviewed by the GP.

Continuing treatment

1 Patients taking antidepressants who are not considered to be at an increased risk of suicide should normally be seen after two weeks. Thereafter, they should be seen on a regular basis (e.g. at intervals of 2–4 weeks in the first three months and greater intervals thereafter if there is a good response).
2 Treatment using antidepressants should continue for at least six months after remission of a depressive episode, as this greatly reduces the risk of relapse.
3 When a patient has taken antidepressants for six months after remission, a review with the GP should take place to determine the need for continued antidepressant

treatment. This review should include consideration of the number of previous episodes, presence of residual symptoms, and concurrent psychosocial difficulties.

First session

The format for Session 1 can be found in Chapter 3.3, Assessment. In addition to the standard format for this session, the mental health worker should pay particular attention to checking that the patient is taking the antidepressants as prescribed, and to asking the patient about the effects and side-effects of the medication.

Ongoing telephone session format

Each telephone contact will follow a set agenda, but the time spent on each item will vary from patient to patient depending on need. The usual session format is as follows:
- Ensure that you are talking to the right person and state name and role
- Negotiate the agenda with the patient and state estimated length of call
- Review symptoms (this may include the patient answering the questions from the PHQ-9 and the WSAS)
- Assess risk (see questions in Chapter 3.3 on assessment for how to ask patients about risk)
- Assessment of medication effects and side-effects
- Troubleshooting difficulties using psycho-education and shared decision-making
- Implementation and monitoring of any agreed interventions (e.g. behavioural activation, etc.)
- Revisit the problem summary to check that it still fits and amend as necessary (see problem summary in Chapter 3.3, Assessment)
- Ask for any final questions or concerns
- Negotiate next contact
- End call

The main points from every telephone contact should be recorded and followed up by feedback to the GP, if any adjustments need to be made to the treatment interventions.

Assessment of medication effects and side-effects

- Find out the fine details of the patient's medication use – behaviour
- Find out the specific nature of the patient's fears and worries – thoughts and feelings
- Find out what they have actually experienced with the medication – physical symptoms
- Find out the patient's views about the 'pros and cons' of taking medication - beliefs

Troubleshooting difficulties

Patients can discontinue or reduce their intake of medication for a number of reasons. Some of the most common reasons are that the patient:
- does not find it to be of any benefit (e.g. 'It's not helping', 'It doesn't do any good')
- believes that it is no longer needed ('I don't need it any more', 'I don't need as much as that')
- uncomfortable side-effects ('They made me feel sick', 'I'm worried I'll experience problems on a higher dose')
- has concern about the safety of taking the medication ('I don't think they are safe', 'I've read that they can be dangerous')
- worries about becoming addicted ('If I take too many I'll become hooked')
- sees medication as an inappropriate treatment for their difficulties ('Tablets are just a crutch' 'I feel like a failure for taking antidepressants')
- has concern over what others do or might think about taking medication ('My family are against me taking tablets', 'I'm worried my family will find out I'm on medication and disapprove')
- has concern that medication will only mask symptoms and stop the person from doing what they really need to do, which is deal with problems directly ('They'll make me a zombie')
- is forgetful ('Sometimes I forget to take it', 'I forgot to renew my prescription')

If the patient has stopped taking their medication or is only taking a sub-therapeutic dose, it is important to establish the reasons why. Questions around the possible reasons listed on the previous page will help ascertain the patient's reasons for stopping taking antidepressant medication as prescribed. Establishing the reason will also help the mental health worker in targeting the education they give the patient about their medication. If the reason is because of adverse side-effects, then exactly what side-effects have been experienced should be established and reported back to the GP.

The procedure in dealing with discontinuation or reduced intake is:

1 Assessment
2 Education
3 Shared decision-making

The patient does not find the medication to be of any benefit

When a patient reports that the medication is producing no benefits, it is important to ascertain what, if any, benefits they have experienced and any side-effects that may have been problematic.

The patient may have strongly-held beliefs about medication not being effective, so it is useful to discuss these with them to find out what their beliefs are.

It is also important to establish whether the patient has been taking the medication as prescribed and for how long. If the patient has been taking the medication in a haphazard way or stopped taking it after only a couple of weeks, it is unlikely that they will have derived any real benefit from it. Through assessment and discussing the pros and cons of taking medication, it may be that the patient will decide to re-try the medication at the proper dose for an adequate trial. However, if the patient has been taking the medication for more than four weeks and has derived no benefit, a review of the medication by the GP is indicated.

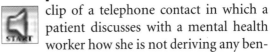

Example CD-ROM 3 includes an audio clip of a telephone contact in which a patient discusses with a mental health worker how she is not deriving any benefits from the medication that she is taking. A transcript of the clip is given below.

Audio: Medication management – The patient does not find medication to be of benefit

Mental health worker: Okay, so you've not been feeling too great since we last spoke. That isn't so good. How are things going with the medication Dr Bilham prescribed?

Patient: I stopped taking it a few days ago, actually.

Mental health worker: Oh, really? Was there any particular reason for that?

Patient: Well, it didn't seem to be doing me any good, so I thought 'Why bother?'

Mental health worker: Right. Did you experience any benefits at all from taking it?

Patient: No, not that I noticed, that's why I stopped them.

Mental health worker: What about side-effects?

Patient: Not really, a bit of dry mouth but nothing else.

Mental health worker: How long were you taking it for?

Patient: About two weeks.

Mental health worker: Right. Is it okay if I give you some information about how antidepressants work?

Patient: Yes, that's fine.

Mental health worker: Okay, I'll tell you a bit about how they work. Were you aware that it usually takes about 3–4 weeks for people to start noticing any improvement with antidepressants?

Patient: That's what Dr Bilham said when he prescribed it, and you said that too, the first time we spoke.

Mental health worker: Yes, that's right. It sounds like things aren't getting any better without it. From what you say, too, you only had mild side-effects. The good news is that side-effects are usually at their worst early on, and usually improve, with the benefits of the medication building up slowly over a period of a few weeks.

Patient: Okay, so do you think I should start it again?

Mental health worker: Well, you say you're not feeling any better, the side-effects you felt were mild, and you weren't taking it for long enough to derive any benefit. Do you have any other concerns that would put you off restarting it?

Patient: No, it was just that I felt it wasn't helping, but from what you've said, I didn't really give it a proper chance. I think I'll give it another go.

Mental health worker: Okay, well how's about starting to take it again today, and then take it daily for the next four weeks; then we can review again then how it's going?

Patient: Okay, that sounds fine.

Mental health worker: Good, well I'll make a note of this on your records so that Dr Bilham is aware of the situation, but I'd also like to call you next week just to see how you are getting on.

Patient: Okay then.

Mental health worker: Okay, I'll phone you at the same time next week.

The patient believes that medication is no longer needed

If a patient has discontinued or reduced their medication because they think it is no longer necessary, it is important to review the severity of depressive symptoms that the patient is experiencing. The patient may well be keen to discontinue medication because they are feeling better, and the patient's GP should be made aware of this.

It is important to note that there is strong evidence that there is an increased risk of relapse if medication is discontinued before at least six months of remission of depression, and this should be shared with the patient. If the patient's depression remains the same or has deteriorated, it is important to advise the patient about how antidepressants work and to discuss the pros and cons of taking medication.

The patient may then decide it would be a good idea to restart antidepressants on this evidence.

If the patient decides not to restart medication, the mental health worker should inform the GP. The patient should be encouraged to see the GP to discuss their concerns. If they are not keen to do this, then the mental health worker can advise the GP of the situation and ask the patient if they can be called back in the next couple of weeks to check how they are getting on. If symptoms persist, this offers a further opportunity to use shared decision-making to discuss the potential benefits of recommencing medication.

Example CD-ROM 3 includes an audio clip of a telephone contact in which a patient discusses with a mental health worker discontinuation of medication and what they agree between them to do next. A transcript of the clip is given below.

Audio: Medication management – Belief that medication is no longer needed

Mental health worker: So you're saying that you stopped taking the antidepressants a couple of days ago because you feel that they are no longer necessary.

Patient: Yes, that's right. I've been feeling pretty good for a few weeks now, so I thought it would be time to stop them. I don't need them any more.

Mental health worker: Do you think that the medication has helped you?

Patient: Well yes. As you know, I was really down, really depressed four months ago, but they did help me lift my mood and feel more able to deal with what life was throwing at me. But, as I say, I just feel loads better now and, well, I've done quite well really.

Mental health worker: Well, I'm delighted to hear that you are feeling so much better. That's great news. I'm just a little concerned that the antidepressants may still have a role to play in you getting better for a while longer. There's quite a bit of evidence to suggest that people taking antidepressants should keep taking them for even up to six months after they start to feel well. This has been shown to reduce the chance of relapse. As you say, you really were quite depressed and I think Dr Houlders had thought you might continue the medication for a while longer. Would you be prepared to recommence the medication?

Patient: I didn't know I would be increasing my chances of relapse. I don't know, I feel fine. As you know, I've never been keen on taking tablets, so I don't know, I'd like to give it a go without. An extra six months sounds like an awfully long time when I don't need them.

Mental health worker: I suppose it's like if you break a bone. It can take a while for the bones to knit together again, and when they have, you're still not able to put you're full weight on it for a while longer. It takes a bit longer before everything's fitted right back into place.

Patient: Yes, I see what you mean, but I'm a little bit disappointed about the idea of staying on antidepressants that long. I mean, I'm not really convinced I should restart them.

Mental health worker: Okay, well I'll make a note of that and let Dr Houlders know that you've decided to stop taking the medication. I think it might be a good idea to talk to him about it, though. Would you be prepared to come in to see him?

Patient: Yes, I'm due to see him Friday anyway, so I can talk to him about it then.

Mental health worker: Okay, great. Sounds like a good idea.

The patient is experiencing uncomfortable side-effects

Some possible side-effects of antidepressant medication include:

- Nausea
- Diarrhoea
- Headache
- Sleep disturbance
- Dry mouth
- Constipation
- Weight gain/increased appetite
- Weight loss/decreased appetite
- Blurred vision
- Dizziness
- Tremor
- Change in sexual function
- Tiredness
- Muscle tightness
- Sweating
- Difficulty urinating

The mental health worker asks patients if they have noticed anything unusual that might be caused by the medication they are taking. When a patient has been experiencing problems with side-effects, it is important to establish exactly what they are and whether they could actually be considered as potentially dangerous.

Symptoms that the mental health worker should be alert to include: an increase in suicidal ideation; signs of akathisia, manifested as pacing and a total inability to sit still. If forced to sit still, the person experiences extreme anxiety and agitation. In bad cases, the anxiety and agitation may get worse even while the person is moving, and they may experience an increase in anxiety and agitation. In these circumstances, the mental health worker should inform the GP immediately and ask the patient to come in to see the GP.

It is also important to discover whether the patient has discontinued the medication, and, if so, when. If they have discontinued the medication within the first three weeks of starting to take it and the side-effects were mild and not considered to be dangerous, it may be that the patient would benefit from information about antidepressants and how they work, which may lead them to start taking it again. The patient can be advised that the side-effects are likely to stop once they have been taking the medication for a while, or the patient may learn to tolerate them if the benefits end up outweighing the discomfort of mild side-effects.

Example CD-ROM 3 includes an audio clip of a telephone contact in which a patient discusses with a mental health worker the unpleasant side-effects that she has experienced and what they agree between them to do next. A transcript of the clip is given below.

Audio: Medication management – The patient is experiencing uncomfortable side-effects

Mental health worker: Okay, you've mentioned that you're thinking of stopping taking the medication that Dr Richards has prescribed you. What are your main reasons for feeling that stopping the medication is going to be necessary?

Patient: It's just the side-effects. I don't think I can take any more. I just don't think I'm getting enough benefits from them to outweigh the horrible side-effects.

Mental health worker: Right, well that isn't so good. What side-effects are you experiencing?

Patient: I've been having this sort of quivering in my legs and arms that I can't sit still, I find it hard to sit down and stay there for any length of time without needing to get up. It's just horrible.

Mental health worker: That does sound horrible. Have you taken a tablet today yet?

Patient: No, not yet.

Mental health worker: Okay, well what I would suggest is you do stop taking it right away. I'm going to discuss this with Dr Richards when I come off the phone. Is there any chance that you can come in for another appointment to see him in the next day or so?

Patient: I could come in anytime tomorrow.

Mental health worker: That would be really good. I tell you what, I'll organize an appointment and give you a ring back with the time.

Concern about the safety of taking antidepressant medication

Some patients may be concerned that there are some dangers associated with taking antidepressant medication. When this is the case, it is important to establish exactly what the patient fears about antidepressants. It is also important to distinguish between those symptoms that are actually experienced by the patient and those that they fear will happen but have not actually occurred. It should also be established where these fears have come from. For example, the patient may know someone, a friend, colleague or family member, who experienced a negative reaction to antidepressants or they may have read about some side-effects. If the patient has actually experienced some unpleasant side-effects, this should be addressed, as described under the previous topic, 'The patient is experiencing uncomfortable side-effects'.

Otherwise, education about medication and its effects should be given and pros and cons discussed, with a view to recommencing medication if the patient agrees that it is appropriate to do so.

Example CD-ROM 3 includes an audio clip of a telephone contact in which a patient tells the mental health worker her concerns about the safety of the medication she has been prescribed. A transcript of the clip is given below.

Audio: Medication management – Concerns about the safety of taking antidepressants

Mental health worker: You say that you haven't tried the medication that Dr Light prescribed for you. Is that because you have any specific concerns about it?

Patient: I'm a bit worried they might not be safe to take. I had a neighbour who was prescribed antidepressants, she had terrible side-effects. You know, she was worse off than before she even started them.

Mental health worker: Right, I can see why that would bother you and influence your decision about taking them. Side-effects aren't uncommon, to be honest, but most are usually only mild and improve with time. It sounds like the side-effects that your neighbour had were an unusual reaction, and thankfully that is rare. Is your neighbour okay now?

Patient: Oh yes, she's fine now. I mean, as soon as she stopped taking them, the side-effects just went away.

Mental health worker: That's good. Okay, well it sounds like she had an unpleasant experience. All the side-effects that we know about that can occur with taking antidepressants do go away though after stopping the medication. There's no evidence at all of people having delayed effects of antidepressants either. I suppose what we need to take into consideration is whether the potential benefits of the medication could outweigh any downsides. We don't know if you will experience any side-effects and, if so, how unpleasant they're going to be. So I guess that although you are obviously a bit worried about their safety, you're also keen to feel the benefits of them.

Patient: Yes, that's right. But, well, to be absolutely honest with you, I'm still not sure.

Mental health worker: Okay, well that's fine. I tell you what, I'll make a note of that on your records. What about if I arrange an appointment for you to see Dr Light so you can discuss it with him, and what alternatives there might be.

Patient: Alright, if you think so. You don't think he's going to be cross with me, do you?

Mental health worker: Oh no, not at all. I think it would be a good idea to see him to talk things through. What about if I call you later with an appointment, and arrange for us to talk again in a week's time maybe?

Patient: Yes, okay, that sounds fine.

Notice how the mental health worker addresses the patient's concerns.

Worries about becoming addicted

Some patients may be concerned that they will become dependent on antidepressants and worried that they will undergo terrible side-effects on withdrawal from the medication. It may be that the patient is confusing antidepressants with 'tranquillizers' and that, having seen or read about the effects of withdrawal, or known someone who has experienced difficulty discontinuing such medication, may have concerns about taking antidepressants. Again, education is called for here, with discussion of the pros and cons of taking medication, so the patient can make an informed decision about recommencing medication.

Example CD-ROM 3 includes an audio clip of a telephone contact in which a mental health worker addresses a patient's concerns about becoming addicted to antidepressant medication. A transcript of the clip is given below.

Audio: Medication management – Concerns about becoming addicted to antidepressants

Mental health worker: You mentioned you're taking your antidepressants on days when you feel particularly low, rather than every day as prescribed by Dr Moor. Is that right?

Patient: Yes, I've been really worried about getting addicted to them, so I reckon I can keep a bit better control this way.

Mental health worker: What's led you to believe that they're addictive?

Patient: I remember reading something a long time ago about tranquillizers being really addictive, and there were some awful stories on a documentary I saw about people having a lot of trouble coming off of them. I don't want to really go through that.

Mental health worker: No, of course, I can fully understand that. No-one would. Well, the good news is that the antidepressant that Dr Moor prescribed, and antidepressants across the board, are not the group of drugs classed as tranquillizers. You're quite right, though, people who have been taking tranquillizers for a while can have real difficulty when they come to stopping them. That's why they don't get prescribed very often these days, and when they do, it's only for short periods so that someone becoming dependent on them is quite unlikely. The type of medication that you've been prescribed comes from a completely different group of drugs, and research has shown that people don't get addicted to them. This means that you won't have any cravings for them like you might get for a cigarette, say, and you won't build up a tolerance and need more and more to obtain the same effect. This doesn't mean that depression doesn't sometimes come back after stopping taking the tablets, but equally, that's not a sign that you're addicted either, it just means that the medication still has a job to do, and at that point in time your depression still needs treatment. What do you think about what I've just said?

Patient: I feel a bit better about taking them now, but must admit that I haven't noticed any improvement since I started them. Maybe they just won't do any good anyway.

Mental health worker: Well, I think it's important to give them a chance before reaching that conclusion. They need a chance to build up in your system, that's why it's really important to take them daily as prescribed. You should start to notice some improvement in the next 3 to 4 weeks, but you're unlikely to notice anything much in the way of improvement before then. Is it worth giving them a fair crack of the whip? You did say earlier that you've been feeling pretty low at the moment; maybe they can help.

Patient: Okay, I'll give it a go and see how I get on with taking them properly.

Mental health worker: That sounds good. I'll make a note on your records for Dr Moor to that effect. At least that way, you'll know within the next month whether they are going to help or not. If you find that they are not helpful, then we'll look at some alternatives. How's about I phone you next week just to see how you're getting on with it all?

Patient: I'd appreciate that.

Mental health worker: Okay. Let's see when a good time might be.

Seeing medication as an inappropriate treatment for their difficulties

When a patient does not see antidepressant medication as being the appropriate treatment for their depression, it is important to ask what it 'means' to them to be prescribed antidepressants. The patient may perceive medication as being merely a kind of crutch or as meaning that they are a failure, for example. These kinds of thoughts can lend themselves well to thought evaluation (see Section 4e, Working with Thoughts). Identification and successful evaluation of these types of thoughts can help the patient feel able to make an informed decision as to whether they will resume medication. If they still feel that they do not wish to continue with antidepressant medication, the GP should be informed and the patient encouraged to see him or her to discuss it further.

Example CD-ROM 3 includes an audio clip of a telephone contact in which a mental health worker deals with a patient who sees taking antidepressants as a crutch and who is reluctant to recommence medication. A transcript of the clip is given below.

Audio: Medication management – Seeing medication as an inappropriate treatment

Patient: I've decided not to take the medication I've been prescribed. It's just a crutch and I don't think it'll help.

Mental health worker: Are there any potential benefits that you can see at all that you might get from medication for your depression?

Patient: I know that they are supposed to help with physical symptoms like tiredness and poor sleep, and that it can help lift my mood, but as I say, they're just a crutch, and

I don't like the idea of being reliant on them to make me feel okay.

Mental health worker: Okay, so from what you are saying, you can see that there are benefits that can be gained, both in terms of physical symptoms and your mood, but you are still not keen because you see them as a crutch and you really don't believe in them.

Patient: Yes, that's about it.

Mental health worker: You know, it's something like 15% of the population will experience depression at some point in their lives for various reasons. No matter what the reason, though, antidepressant medication is generally effective for most people. Antidepressants can help to alleviate some of the symptoms of depression like depressed mood, low energy, lack of interest in things, difficulty concentrating, and even feelings of guilt or worthlessness. They won't change the important life problems that you are facing, but what they can do is make you feel more able to deal with these problems more effectively, by helping you feel less overwhelmed. Now it really is up to you to decide what way you want to take this forward, but what may be worth considering is whether your personal beliefs about antidepressants being a crutch are getting in the way of going for a treatment that is potentially going to really help.

Patient: I hear what you're saying, but I'm not going to change my mind on this one.

Mental health worker: Okay. Would you be prepared to talk to Dr Gell in the next few days so that you can discuss it with him?

Patient: No, I really don't want to discuss it any further at the moment. I'll just see how I get on with this self-help stuff you're sending me out.

Mental health worker: Okay, I'll make a note for Dr Gell that you've decided not to take antidepressant medication and don't feel the need to discuss it with him at the moment. How's about if I check in with you next week and see how things are going with the self-help information that I'm sending you?

Patient: Yes, that would be fine.

Concern over what others say or might think about taking medication

Sometimes patients worry about what others might think or say about their taking medication. 'She said that I should just pull myself together and that I didn't need to be taking anything like that', 'He thinks that medication is never the answer', 'She would be ashamed of me if she knew I was taking tablets'. These are some examples of what patients might say. Here, it is crucial to differentiate between what has actually been said and what the patient perceives that someone else might be thinking. Again, these types of thoughts can lend themselves well to thought evaluation (see Section 4e, Working with Thoughts). If someone has actually said something that has influenced the patient's decision to stop taking medication, the mental health worker can offer education to ensure that the patient is making a decision informed by correct information.

Example CD-ROM 3 includes an audio clip of a telephone contact in which a patient is concerned about what her husband thinks about her taking medication. A transcript of the clip is given below.

Audio: Medication management – Concern over what others might think about them taking antidepressants

Mental health worker: You say you've stopped taking the medication that Dr Prosser has prescribed you, and that's because your husband was cross with you about taking antidepressants?

Patient: Yes, he said that I don't need to take anything and that I should try to get on without it; that they won't really help my problems and they'll still be there when I come off them.

Mental health worker: Well, it's not uncommon

for people to believe that antidepressants won't really help. Is there any chance that you and your husband could maybe come in in the next few days, so that we can discuss some information about the effects of antidepressants?

Patient: I can certainly have a word with him. I know he's on a late shift on Friday, so we could come and see you in the morning.

Mental health worker: Oh well, that would be really good. I could do 10 o'clock – how does that sound?

Patient: Yes, that would be fine.

Mental health worker: Okay, well let's meet up then, just the three of us on Friday, and then we can discuss in more depth what antidepressants can and can't do to help with depression. In the meantime, what I'm going to do is make a note on your records so that Dr Prosser is kept well informed.

Notice how the mental health worker arranges to see the husband and patient together to advise them about what medication will and will not do.

Concern that medication will only mask symptoms and stop the patient from facing their real problems

When this is the case, it is important to ask the patient about their specific concerns and where they come from. Is it from past experience or from what family and friends have said, or perhaps from something they have read? Some of the basic facts about antidepressants can be discussed with the patient, including information about what medication will and will not do. For example, antidepressants can help lift mood, increase energy levels, improve concentration, and reduce feelings of guilt and worthlessness. What they will not do is change a person's personality or change any of the life problems that need to be addressed. However, it may help the patient to feel less overwhelmed by problems and more able to deal with them.

Example CD-ROM 3 includes an audio clip of a telephone contact in which a patient is concerned that taking antidepressants will change his personality. A transcript of the clip is given below.

Audio: Medication management – Concern that medication will only mask symptoms

Patient: I'm frightened that the tablets will change my personality so that I'm just not myself anymore.

Mental health worker: It sounds like it would be worth talking through what medication can and can't do. What antidepressants will do is help alleviate some of the symptoms of depression, like depressed mood, low energy, lack of interest in things, difficulty concentrating, even feelings of guilt or worthlessness. What they won't do is change your personality or make you into a different person. Neither will they change the important life problems that you are facing, but what they can do is make you feel more able to deal with the problems effectively. They can help you feel less overwhelmed by problems, but they will not make you feel high.

Patient: Oh, I think maybe I've been worrying unnecessarily, from what you are saying.

Mental health worker: Perhaps I can send you a leaflet on medication which reiterates what I've said, as a kind of reminder. What do you think?

Patient: Yes, I think that would be helpful.

Mental health worker: Okay, I'll do that. In the meantime, how do you feel about taking the medication as it is prescribed rather than just now and again?

Patient: Okay, I'll give it a go.

Mental health worker: Okay, that's great. Let's talk through some of the side-effects you might experience and how best to handle them, and then perhaps we should arrange to talk again in a couple of weeks' time. I'll also make a note on your records to keep Dr Baguley up to date with how you are getting on.

Note the education that the mental health worker provides, and how a review of progress is planned when the patient decides to recommence medication following the information given.

Forgetfulness

Sometimes patients report that they forget to take their medication as prescribed, which results in them taking a reduced and sub-therapeutic dose. Mental health workers should try to ascertain if there are any concerns the patient holds that result in their forgetting (e.g. worries about addiction or side-effects). If it is purely a case of forgetfulness, the mental health worker and the patient can discuss strategies for remembering (e.g. keeping the tablets beside the coffee jar, so that the patient will be reminded to take their medication when they make their first cup of coffee in the morning, etc.). If the patient is forgetting to pick up prescriptions, it can perhaps be arranged that they are given a larger supply or strategies can be developed to help the patient remember (e.g. when they pay their bills at the end of each month, this can be a prompt to pick up their prescription).

Example CD-ROM 3 includes an audio clip of a telephone contact in which a patient describes how she finds it difficult to remember to take her medication as prescribed. A transcript of the clip is given below.

Audio: Medication management – The patient is forgetful in taking medication

Mental health worker: You say that you've been forgetting to take your tablets some days. Do you have any concerns about the medication that might be contributing to your forgetfulness?

Patient: No, it's just that since I've been depressed I am more forgetful, and I'm just not used to taking tablets, so I forget.

Mental health worker: Right. Well, some people find that when they are forgetful, that it's helpful to establish a routine and learn to associate it with something else. This might be an idea that could be helpful for you. Maybe we just need to give some thought to your daily routine to see whether there is anything you do every day, about the same time, that you could use as a prompt.

Patient: Right, well, the first thing I do every morning is come downstairs and make a drink. I could keep my tablets next to the teabags as a reminder to take one first thing.

Mental health worker: I think that's a really good idea. Okay, well, to really get the benefits of taking antidepressants, you really need to be taking them regularly and continuously. What I'll do is, I'll just make a note on your records to keep Dr Whitford up to date with what's happening. What about if we speak again in a couple of weeks time, and see how the teabags next to the tablets routine is working out?

Patient: Fine.

Notice how the mental health worker builds on what the patient has suggested to agree a routine to help prompt her to take the medication at the correct time, and organizes a review date.

Exercise

Ask a colleague to take on various roles of patients experiencing difficulties with their medication, while you take the role of the mental health worker.

- Work with the patient to resolve their difficulties.
- Ask your colleague for feedback after each role-play.
- If there are any scenarios that you find difficult or your colleague has given negative feedback on, role-play these again until you feel more proficient at handling these problems.

Psycho-education for depressed patients

Depending on the patient, topics for education will include:

- Facts about depression (see Chapter 3.1, Section 1)
- Effects of medication
- Time to experience beneficial effects of medication (up to four weeks)
- Side-effects of medication (see earlier in this section)
- Likely duration of side-effects

For information about medication, the mental health worker should consult a copy of the British National Formulary (BNF). You can visit the BNF website at www.bnf.org. Psycho-education is discussed in more depth in the next section.

Shared decision-making

Shared decision-making has already been covered in Case management (Section 2) and is summarized below:

- Review and summarize difficulties
- Present options
- Discuss arguments for and against each option (pros and cons)
- Help patient choose an option
- Plan how to implement option
- Make follow-up arrangements

Section summary

- The aim of medication management is to help monitor patients' adherence to medication, provide information to the GP, provide education and support to improve adherence, and provide follow-up care and onward referral as appropriate
- Components of telephone contact include: assessment, checking patients' response and adherence, education, shared decision-making and agreeing follow-up care
- A typical schedule of contacts includes: initial contact within a few days of the GP identifying the patient as depressed, with

follow-up contact at 2, 4, 8, 12 and 16 weeks after first contact (this is the minimum frequency of contact for medication management).

- Contacts may be more frequent, especially in patients with increased suicide risk, and patients under the age of 30 who should always be seen after the first week or within a few days of being prescribed anti-depressants
- A protocol should be followed for each contact with the patient

References

British Medical Association and Royal Pharmaceutical Society of Great Britain (2004). *British National Formulary.* London: British Medical Association and Royal Pharmaceutical Society of Great Britain. www.bnf.org.

National Institute for Health and Clinical Excellence (2004a). *Depression: the management of depression in primary and secondary care.* London: National Institute for Health and Clinical Excellence. www.nice.org.uk.

Royal Society of Great Britain (1997). *From compliance to concordance: achieving shared goals in taking medication.* London: The Royal Society.

Useful website

www.nmhct.nhs.uk/pharmacy. Norfolk and Waveney Mental Health Partnership NHS Trust offers useful information in their pharmacy section.

Test yourself

 To check your progress, locate this section on CD-ROM 3 and work through the interactive questions at the end.

Section 4: The self-help framework

Introduction

The self-help framework is all about supporting patients to handle their own problems and to exercise their own control to tackle difficulties and improve the outcome of situations. It involves helping patients to build on their own strengths, while recognizing weaknesses and working to improve them. The mental health worker supports the patient in working on their own thoughts, feelings, behaviours and skills development. Contact with the mental health worker is brief and the responsibility rests with the patient to work on their problems outside of the therapeutic contacts.

A self-help approach may be something that the patient has not encountered before, and they may require additional support and encouragement in using this method to tackle problems. On the other hand, people are often well informed about their particular problem (and, unfortunately, sometimes they are misinformed too). Information may have been obtained through the media, friends and family, local support groups, the internet or from an array of self-help books available from bookshops and libraries for all types of problems.

We must never underestimate a patient's inner resources and abilities to overcome their own problems with our support and guidance, rather than assume that the mental health worker's role is to provide 'treatment'. The mental health worker in primary care is not a therapist.

It helps if a patient feels enabled to deal with their problems. Feeling helpless decreases a patient's efforts and increases feelings of anxiety and depression. If a person believes that they are powerless when they aren't, this is clearly problematic; however, if a person assumes they have more control than they actually do, then they may blame themselves inappropriately for events that are not their fault. Patients who feel powerless to overcome their difficulties will require encouragement to show them that they have adequate personal resources to overcome their difficulties and that they can learn better coping skills to deal with problems.

Types of self-help

A person may join a support group (either through their own volition or signposted by the mental health worker) and get ideas and encouragement to manage their life better; they may read a book or other literature; access the internet; watch a talk show; talk to a friend or mental health worker – and use this as a way of helping themselves. By using self-help, the person is assuming full responsibility for change.

Self-help is not just about dealing with current problems but about developing life-long skills to possibly enable the person to prevent future problems or at least deal with them effectively when they arise.

Steps of self-help

The aim is to help patients to:
1 Analyse problems, break them down into meaningful parts, and make connections between symptoms to assist in greater understanding
2 Choose appropriate evidence-based self-help strategies to deal with the problems
3 Evaluate progress and modify how they are dealing with the problem accordingly

All the therapeutic approaches covered in this section are about helping the patient to help themselves, using a self-help framework. Sometimes patients can put these strategies into practice with minimal support; others may require guidance and encouragement outside the confines of what can be offered in the primary care setting, and may require referral to secondary services or signposting to other agencies.

Issues related to self-help are also addressed in Chapter 1.3, Section 4 and Chapter 2.2, Section 3.

The box on the next page illustrates the strategies that will be covered in this Chapter, and for which problems they are most appropriate.

Recommended reading

Department of Health (2003). *Self-Help Interventions for Mental Health Problems.* London: Department of Health.

Newcastle, North Tyneside and Northumberland Mental Health NHS Trust (2002). *Self-help guides for controlling anger, depression, depression and low mood, panic, shyness and social anxiety, sleep prob-*

Problem areas and their most appropriate strategies

Strategies	Problem areas
Psycho-education	All problems
Behavioural activation	Depression
Problem-solving	All problems
Graded exposure	All phobias, Panic Disorder
Working with thoughts	All problems
Controlled breathing	Panic Disorder, other disorders where the patient is experiencing panic attacks
Relaxation	Anger problems, Generalized Anxiety Disorder, sleep problems, stress
Sleep hygiene and improving the sleep environment	Insomnia
Lifestyle strategies	All problems

lems, stress, stress and anxiety. Morpeth: Northumberland, Tyne and Wear NHS Trust www.nnt.nhs.uk/mh.

World Health Organisation (2000). *WHO Guide to Mental Health in Primary Care.* London: The Royal Society of Medicine Press Ltd.

Useful websites

The websites in this list offer a variety of resources for patients and professionals. This list is not exhaustive but offers some of the most helpful websites currently available. You may know of some others.
www.bbc.co.uk/health/conditions: BBC health.
www.babcp.com: British Association for Behaviour-

al and Cognitive Psychotherapy.
www.depressionalliance.org: Depression Alliance.
www.mentalhealth.org.uk: Mental Health Foundation.
www.mentality.org.uk: Mentality.
www.mind.org.uk: MIND.
www.nimhe.org.uk: National Institute for Mental Health in England.
www.phobics-society.org.uk: National Phobics Society.
www.nhsdirect.nhs.uk: NHS Direct.
www.nopanic.org.uk: No Panic.
www.patient.co.uk: Patient UK.
www. primhe.org: Primary Care Mental Health Education.
www.whoguide mhpcuk.org: World Health Organisation.

Test yourself

 To check your progress, locate this section on CD-ROM 3 and work through the interactive questions at the end.

Section 4a: Psycho-education

Introduction

Psycho-educational approaches have been developed to increase patients' knowledge of, and insight into, their illness and its treatment. The aim is to improve a patient's ability to cope with their problems in a more effective way by increasing their understanding of their condition and of evidence-based approaches to overcome it. Although patients are generally the best managers of their own personal problems, they can often lack the information and support to manage them in the most effective way. Offering patients high-quality health information helps empower them to self-manage their mental health problems.

Content of psycho-education

- What is 'the disorder' (e.g. Generalized Anxiety Disorder)?
- What are the symptoms?
- Prevalence

- Prognosis
- What treatments are available and how effective are they?
- What can patients do to help themselves?
- The role of medication

The disorders

Mental health workers should have a good working knowledge of the disorders that a patient presents with. ICD-10 and DSM-IV-TR give the diagnostic criteria for the majority of disorders likely to be seen in the primary care setting. In addition, each of the sections in Common Mental Health Problems (see Chapter 3.1) give information on recognized disorders, as well as those problems commonly encountered in primary care but not recognized by ICD-10 or DSM-IV-TR.

The symptoms

In addition to the symptom lists and diagnostic criteria in ICD-10 and DSM-IV-TR, this book also provides lists of common emotional, physical, cognitive and behavioural symptoms for the disorders a mental health worker is likely to encounter in the primary care setting – both those recognized by ICD-10 and DSM-IV-TR and those not yet recognized (e.g. anger problems).

Prevalence

It can be helpful to tell the patient about how common their problem is in the general population, so that they know that they are not alone. The disorders that mental health workers are likely to encounter in the primary care setting are very common, hence the term 'common mental health problems', as opposed to more serious mental health problems which are less common and more likely to be treated in secondary care. Go back to the sections on the various disorders to check on prevalence.

Prognosis

Knowing the prognosis for individual disorders can help elicit hope in a patient. In general, patients with common mental health problems have a good prognosis. For more precise information on prognosis go back to Chapter 3.1.

What treatments are available and their efficacy

Patients should be offered a choice of treatments that are evidence-based. NICE Guidelines offer a comprehensive guide to what treatments should be available for a number of disorders, and a list of these can be accessed at www.nice.org.uk. Medication and CBT strategies are currently the preferred treatment approach for many common mental health problems.

How patients can help themselves

Helping patients to help themselves is a major role of mental health workers. They should be able to provide patients with support to use self-help strategies, signpost them to appropriate agencies and organizations, and facilitate referral to other services as appropriate. Self-help puts the onus on the patient to take responsibility to overcome their difficulties.

The role of medication

Many patients who are seen by a mental health worker in the primary care setting will be prescribed medication (predominantly antidepressants). As part of the role of the mental health worker is to provide medication management (see Section 3) for patients, they should be well versed in the uses, effects and side-effects of all the psychiatric medications usually prescribed in their work setting. Every mental health worker should also have ready access to an up-to-date copy of the British National Formulary.

What about causes?

Identifying causes has not been listed under the content of what is covered in psycho-education because, for many patients, it is not possible to determine the exact causes of their problems. Moreover, as there will be little that can be done about the causes, there is no point in spending valuable time surmising what they might be, especially as they may actually be incorrect. However, knowledge about the onset of the problem is extremely informative, and when triggers are elicited, it can be very useful to discuss these with the patient to prepare them for similar future occasions. Any patient who wishes to focus primarily on causal factors may be more likely to benefit from long-term psychotherapy, and referral to an appropriate professional may be what is called for in this instance.

Example CD-ROM 3 includes a video clip in which mental health worker Katie provides psycho-education to her patient Tim. A transcript of the clip is given below.

Video: Psycho-education

Mental health worker (Katie): Okay, I want to spend a little bit of time discussing stress: what the symptoms are, how common it is, and what treatments are available that might help.

Tim: Okay.

Katie: Okay. Now, stress is extremely common, in fact a recent survey in the UK suggested that over half a million people felt that they were experiencing work-related stress to the point where it was actually making them unwell.

Tim: That's a lot.

Katie: It is very common, so you are not alone. Now, for some people, the stress is short-lived: for example, if they are moving house or something like that; but for other people, where the situation is ongoing, the stress continues.

Tim: Like in my case.

Katie: Exactly. Now, when a person perceives that the demands placed on them are too high and exceed their capabilities, that's when we begin to suffer stress. Let me show you what I mean. If I draw you this graph … (draws bell graph) okay. Here we have performance level, and here we have the level of demand. Now, what

happen is, at the left-hand side, if there is very little demand, a person is unable to focus their energies on that task in hand, and there is little incentive for them to do so; but as demand increases, we reach what is known as the optimum level of performance where a person is able to focus their energies on the task in hand, but without suffering stress. However, as demand increases, a person's level of performance drops and this is the area where someone will begin to suffer stress.

Tim: Yes, that's exactly where I am. (points to right-hand side of graph)

Katie: I think that's right. Now, ongoing demands like this are not good because they can lead to all sorts of physical consequences, such as ulcers, irritable bowel syndrome, high blood pressure and, in some cases, even heart attacks.

Tim: Yes, that's what I was worried about when Dr Mehra said my blood pressure was up.

Katie: And it's not only the physical consequences; there are psychological consequences as well, and these include things like panic attacks and depression. But the good news is that there are a range of treatments available that have been shown to help, and these include things like taking relaxing activity, taking a practical approach to problem-solving, and looking at upsetting thoughts. I'll talk through each one of these in turn and explain what they mean, and also what treatments are available that might help in these cases.

See Figure 7 for the graph drawn by Katie.

Section summary

- Psycho-education aims to increase patients' knowledge of, and insight into, their illness and its treatment
- Psycho-education covers: disorders; symptoms; prevalence; prognosis; treatments; self-help; role of medication
- Mental health workers in primary care should have ready access to a copy of the British National Formulary

Exercise

Ask a colleague to role-play each of the patients we have met so far in this part of the programme.
- Practice providing psycho-education for each of the different problems using information from Chapter 3.1.
- Ask your colleague for feedback on how you have done with each of the role-plays.
- If possible, record these role-plays and play them back to yourself for self-reflection.

References

American Psychiatric Association (2000). *Diagnostic and Statistical Manual of Mental Disorders: DSM-IV-TR: Fourth Edition Text Revision.* Washington DC: American Psychiatric Association. www.psych.org.

British Medical Association and Royal Pharmaceutical Society of Great Britain (2004). British National Formulary. London: British Medical Association and Royal Pharmaceutical Society of Great Britain. www.bnf.org.

World Health Organisation (1994). ICD-10 International Statistical Classification of Diseases and Related Health Problems. World Health Organisation, Geneva. www.who.int.

Recommended reading

World Health Organisation (2000). *WHO Guide to Mental Health in Primary Care.* London: The Royal Society of Medicine Press Ltd.

Test yourself

 To check your progress, locate this section on CD-ROM 3 and work through the interactive questions at the end.

Section 4b: Behavioural Activation

Introduction

People are often less active when they are depressed. Loss of routine is common and patients also frequently reduce or even stop doing pleasurable activities. Patterns of behaviour in depressed patients can actually serve to exacerbate the depression and prevent the person from addressing problems in their lives which, if done, could ultimately have a positive effect on them. For example, a patient who stays in bed because they feel so depressed and does not feel able to face the day ends up keeping out of contact with people and activities that may actually help to improve their mood. In addition, this behaviour results in a decreased likelihood of the person experiencing situations that might bring a sense of pleasure or accomplishment.

It is not unusual for a depressed patient to stay in bed until late in the day, skip meals, and stop calling friends, which all serve to disrupt the patient's routine. The consequence is that the patient's negative mood is worsened. In addition, it is likely that the depressed person's concentration and attention span is impaired and motivation low. An effective way of treating depression is to re-establish routine and increase activity, including those activities that bring about a sense of achievement and pleasure.

Theory

In brief, Behavioural Activation is based on the idea that depressed (reduced) behaviours are partly functional in that they serve the function of reducing the impact of external negative factors.

There are persuasive arguments that the environmental factors trigger depression (e.g. life events, etc.) and, from a pragmatic view, it could be argued that depression can be treated by looking at external factors rather than 'inside the sufferer for explanations'. Patients themselves often talk about depression as a contextually experienced emotion; social explanations look at the interaction of the individual with their social environment for explanations of depression.

Rationale

Based on a negative feedback analogy, the rationale focuses on depressed behaviour as an avoidance strategy (e.g. sleeping, not doing anything, stopping previously enjoyed activities, stopping normal routines, socially isolating oneself). These avoidant behaviours ensure that sufferers reduce negative reinforcement from the environment. However, avoidance leads to a reduction of positive reinforcement as well, as it reduces normal activities and creates other problems, such as loss of work, reduced social interaction, etc. Further, because social and environmental routines maintain emotional stability, disturbed routines lead to increased depression.

Thus, regaining routine and confronting avoidance will lead to change. Treatment aims to re-establish routine and establish opportunities for positive reinforcement in behaviour change.

Why increasing activity levels in depression is helpful

Patients with depression will present with a variety of emotional, physical, cognitive and behavioural symptoms. As all symptoms influence each other, change in any one is likely to bring about change in the others. Focusing on behaviour, as one of the symptoms most amenable to change and likely to bring about significant and rapid improvement to the other symptoms is a reasonable approach. Increasing activity levels (i.e. focusing on a patient's behaviour) has been shown to have a positive effect on a depressed person's mood, physical symptoms and negative thoughts, as they actually begin to give themselves credit for their efforts. Even though an aim of this approach is to increase the patient's engagement in pleasurable activities as well as re-establishing routine, it is unlikely that they will experience any real enjoyment at all to begin with. The emphasis should be on re-establishing routine.

The mental health worker helps the patient to make attempts at engaging in activities despite feeling sadness and low levels of motivation.

By doing this, the patient is being encouraged to work from the 'outside-in', by changing their behaviour rather than waiting for a change in mood (i.e. 'inside-out'). It is not uncommon for a depressed patient to believe that they should wait until they feel a bit better before trying to re-establish their old routine. However, it has been shown that helping patients to become more active has a positive effect on mood and therefore behavioural activation should be a strategy used to help patients with depression.

It is important that patients are encouraged to increase their activity levels rather than passively wait to feel better. This intervention is particularly useful for patients who have difficulty motivating themselves and who have lost interest in doing things. In doing this, it is helpful to obtain a baseline of activity, and therefore patients can be asked to complete an 'Activity Schedule' for a few days to check exactly what they are doing. These Activity Schedules are simple diaries that break down each day of the week into hourly blocks of time, and they can be used in a number of different ways (i.e. monitoring activities, rating moods and planning activities).

A sample Activity Schedule in PDF format is included on CD-ROM 3 (activity schedule.pdf), and reproduced in the Appendix to this book.

Stages of Behavioural Activation

1   Establish a baseline by monitoring activity level
2   Scheduling Activities and grading of tasks
    a   Gradual introduction of low-intensity tasks (e.g. short walk)
    b   Gradual introduction of concentration tasks (e.g. reading)
    c   Focus on life problems (e.g. payment of unpaid bills)
3   Focus on external events (e.g. working, level of social contact, etc.)
4   Gradual withdrawal of diary

Note: At each stage, difficulties should be pre-empted to reduce the chance of failure. Like any other intervention, behavioural activation is set up as a no-lose exercise.

Stage 1: Establish a baseline by monitoring activity levels

The mental health worker is particularly interested in what the patient is doing or not doing each day. The patient is therefore asked to record behaviours on an hour-by-hour basis in an Activity Schedule. Firstly, the patient can be asked to record their activities for a week to establish baseline information.

The next step is to look at the relationship between activity and mood. The patient enters what they are doing on an hourly basis and rates each activity for sense of achievement (0–10) and level of pleasure (0–10). The higher the scores, the greater the sense of achievement and pleasure experienced. For example, eating a cream cake may give a sense of pleasure but not much in the way of achievement, while sorting through a pile of unopened mail may give a patient a sense of achievement and not pleasure. It can be helpful for patients to learn how to distinguish between the impact activities have on feelings of achievement and of pleasure.

Monitoring also helps identify activities that occur too often and those that do not occur often enough. For example, a patient may return with a diary that shows that they are spending much of their time in bed. By examining the diary together, the mental health worker can point out that the patient is spending a good deal of time in bed and ask the patient what impact they think this is having on their mood. If both parties agree that this behaviour may be contributing to the patient's depression, they can consider scheduling activities, which is the next step in behavioural activation.

The patient is asked to fill out the diary as close to the time they finish the activity as possible, to ensure that what has been done is not forgotten and to help maintain accuracy of ratings. However, it is not always possible for the patient to complete the diary at the time of the activity. If this is the case, patients can be asked to complete the diary at three-hourly intervals or at specified time-points throughout the day (e.g. lunchtime, teatime and bedtime). The patient is instructed to bear in mind their current mood state rather than comparing themselves to pre-depression functioning.

Introducing the Activity Schedule

While it makes perfect sense to the mental health worker that monitoring behaviours at baseline is an important task, it is not always clear to patients. A clear rationale should be presented for why recording activities is important. The mental health worker can tell the patient that they want to get an understanding of what the patient's life is like and, as it is impossible for them to follow the patient around all day, that a visual presentation in way of a diary detailing the patient's activities would be the next best thing. They can then go on to say that what the patient does on a day-to-day basis is a rich source of information and can be used to target the treatment approaches that are most likely to be of benefit to the patient. Once the patient understands that the activity schedule is an important tool to help understand their difficulties, and that it will help the mental health worker truly appreciate what they are experiencing, most patients agree to complete the diary.

Common difficulties

It is important to note that keeping a diary like this can be tedious, therefore it is understandable if the patient returns with a partially completed diary, or even only a few hours completed for an entire week. If this is the case, the patient can be encouraged to write something for a whole day, then two days, etc., until they feel more comfortable in keeping detailed records of their activities. The thing to remember is that any information is better than none.

A problem can also arise when patients do not view what they do as 'activities', or they see them as being too mundane to record. Diary sheets can be returned that report 'did nothing' or may just be left blank. In these instances, the mental health worker should encourage the patient to record even inactive activities such as 'lying in bed', or 'sitting looking out of the window', as this information is just as valuable and allows the introduction of the concept of rumination as an activity that has a consequence on mood. For example, the patient may be sitting staring at the wall, thinking about the loss of a job, or a relationship, etc., which results in distress and further rumination, and so on.

Reviewing Activity Schedules

It is crucial that the diary is carefully and thoroughly reviewed with the patient at each session, whether this be in a face-to-face session or through telephone contact. Reviewing the diary helps the mental health worker get a clear picture of what the patient is actually doing and not doing, and a patient may quickly give up the laborious task of completing such a diary if their hard work is given scant attention.

Monitoring activities can provide the mental health worker and patient with a great deal of useful information.

Why monitoring of activities can be useful:

- Provide data on the patient's current level of activity
- Demonstrate the relationship between mood and activity
- Identify activities that occur too frequently (e.g. staying in bed ruminating for long periods)
- Identify activities that do not occur frequently enough (e.g. eating proper meals)
- Establish what activities give highest and lowest achievement and pleasure ratings
- Highlight any excessively high standards held by the patient that are getting in the way of their ability to give themselves credit for completing tasks made more difficult because of the depression

---

Stage 2: Scheduling activities and grading of tasks

Scheduling activities

The next step is to increase activity to pre-depression levels by scheduling activities. The emphasis is always on attempting the planned activity and not on its successful completion.

Once the current level of activity has been established and those activities connected with positive and negative feelings are identified, the same schedule can be used to plan activities associated with positive moods for the coming week. The aim is to increase activity, re-establish routine and maximize levels of achievement and pleasure. Planning activities in advance can help alleviate patients' difficulties with indecision and procrastination. Some patients get stuck at this point because they have little motivation to do the things they are currently doing, let alone increase their activity levels. In these circumstances, the mental health worker can encourage the patient to use the 'outside-in' principle and to use the monitoring diary to guide the patient as to when they should plan activities. The patient writes a plan of activities for the coming week, which they then attempt to follow. It is important to bear in mind that patients with depression may see engaging in enjoyable pursuits as self-indulgent or selfish and feel guilty as a result.

The plan should be sufficiently flexible to allow for unforeseen circumstances (i.e. if it is raining heavily at the time the patient plans to go for a walk, they need to appreciate that there is no obligation to complete this task). Missed activities can be re–scheduled for another time. Planning tasks in this way increases the chances of them being carried out and increases the amount of time the patient spends involved in pleasurable activity.

The patient continues to rate activities for achievement and pleasure. Patients can also be asked to make a prediction on achievement and pleasure levels for agreed activities, then record the actual scores which can then be used for comparison.

Grading tasks

To maximize the chances of success in completing agreed activities, the mental health worker may work with the patient to break any activities down into small manageable steps. This can be done by specifying time limits, rather than by completion of the full task (e.g. 'spend 10 minutes cleaning out a drawer' as opposed to 'clean out a drawer') – which could end up becoming onerous and unmanageable. Alternatively, the level of difficulty of the activity can be graded (i.e. going for a 10-minute walk and building this up, prior to spending a day out with the ramblers).

Patients can sometimes set over-ambitious targets that increase their chances of failure, and this serves only to make them more depressed. Grading tasks increases the patient's chances of success. This strategy can also be useful when helping patients to enter anxiety-provoking situations. The aim is to gradually re-establish routine; therefore, by grading activities, the patient can progressively get back into doing the things they used to do prior to their depression, which will ultimately improve mood and restore regular everyday activity.

2a: Gradual introduction of low-intensity activities

When the patient has completed or partially completed a diary of monitoring activities for a few days, the mental health worker and the patient can use the information in the schedule to make some appropriate changes to what the patient does over the coming week. The patient may need to be helped to develop a more realistic view of their sense of achievement if they are comparing themselves unfavourably with pre-depression performance rather than taking into account how they are feeling now. For example, a person who regularly reads a book in a day might now find reading a single chapter takes considerable effort. Therefore, this achievement should be rated accordingly.

Patients can sometimes be reluctant to start activities until their mood improves. The mental health worker can explain that increasing activity can often improve one's mood. This hypothesis can then be tested, by comparing more active days with less active days.

Activities at this stage can vary hugely, depending on the patient's current level of activity. The aim is to help patients re-establish their old routine. An early task may be for the patient to go to bed to sleep each night rather than to sleep in an armchair, or it may be that a patient agrees to get out of bed earlier in the day (e.g. to get up at 10am each day rather than at noon), cook a simple meal, telephone a friend, or go for a 10-minute walk, etc.

2b: Gradual introduction of concentration tasks

Concentration difficulties are common in depression. Many patients will have stopped reading, or have difficulty concentrating on films all the way through, or watching television programmes that they previously enjoyed. Levels of concentration can gradually be increased with practice. The task may be to watch the main items on the news, read a few pages of a book, or one article from a newspaper. Each of these tasks can be progressively increased as the patient's concentration improves.

2c: Focus on life problems

Patients with depression may have stopped addressing important practicalities that need to be dealt with (e.g. paying bills, opening mail, etc.). Tasks can be negotiated so that the patient starts opening a certain number of letters a day and paying bills, etc. These tasks are particularly important for patients who may be experiencing financial difficulties and, as a result of their inattention to dealing with bills, may be incurring more debt.

Recap

These three examples of graded activity should be introduced within the first four contacts with patients who are depressed. By doing this, action is being taken early in helping the patient re-establish their routine. In this way, the pattern of inactivity which is serving to exacerbate the patient's depression is addressed early, thereby breaking the vicious circle of low mood and inactivity.

Stage 3: Focus on external events

When people are depressed, they may take time off work and reduce social contact. It is essential that these activities are re-established. When the patient is more active, a gradual return to work can be negotiated. Good social support is crucial; therefore, re-establishing links with friends should be introduced at this stage.

The patient may have withdrawn from seeing friends and family, and a gradual reintroduction of social contact of this kind is an important step in the patient's recovery.

Stage 4: Gradual withdrawal of the diary

Although an Activity Schedule provides a wealth of information, it is not practical, nor is it necessary, for the patient to keep a diary such as this in the long term. At which point the diary is withdrawn is really up to the patient. Having kept the diary fully, the patient may reduce entries to important events only, then gradually stop completion altogether and just make notes of important events to tell the mental health worker during their contacts.

Activity Schedules provide an excellent opportunity for the mental health worker to gain access to some of the patient's thoughts about the planned activities, especially as some thoughts may get in the way of the patient successfully completing the task.

Example CD-ROM 3 includes an audio clip in which Sarah and her mental health worker, Katie, plan activities for the coming week. A transcript of the clip follows.

Audio: Behavioural Activation

Mental health worker (Katie): It's been really helpful talking through your activities in the diary. Well done for having completed it over the last week. I know that it was quite an effort for you, but it is really helpful in showing exactly what you are doing on an hour-by-hour basis each day.

Sarah: Yes, it was a bit of an effort, but I do think it really highlights that I'm not doing very much at all.

Katie: That's helpful, though. Using this diary as a baseline, we know what we need to build on. We can come back in a few weeks and compare your level of activity, and see how it has changed from the diary of this past week. Now, you already know that people with depression tend to be less active than those who are not, and one of the early steps in overcoming depression is to try to re-establish routine, and get more active.

Sarah: Yes, I remember we talked about this last week.

Katie: Yes, we talked about it when I asked you to fill in this diary. Now that we've got the baseline, I think we are ready to look at how we can get you more active and re-establish some routine.

Sarah: Yes, but part of my routine was working, and I'm not doing that now.

Katie: Well, that's true, but even so, I'm sure there are ways of getting you more active with a view to looking for work at a later stage.

Sarah: I suppose you're right. I'm staying in bed a lot, so I couldn't look for another job at the moment until I sort that out and feel a bit better in myself.

Katie: Exactly, so perhaps your sleep routine is a good place to start. All the activities we look at are also aiming to help you start feeling better in yourself, too. Do you have a copy of the blank diary?

Sarah: Yes. I've got it here. Should I write things down as we go along?

Katie: I think that would be a good idea, so you have it as a prompt. Right, let's look at your sleep pattern. There's quite a few entries here where you are lying in bed late in the morning but not actually sleeping, and there are a couple of times when you've gone back to bed in the afternoon.

Sarah: Yes, I spend too much time there, I know.

Katie: Well, I wonder whether you could perhaps start getting up a bit earlier in the day, maybe shortly after you wake up, and then we can look at what you can do with that time?

Sarah: Yes, I don't suppose there's any point in getting up and heading straight for the sofa.

Katie: No, that's right. Now, I remember you saying that you used to take a lot of pride in your flat, and that Karen has taken over all of the housework these days. Could that be a good place to start?

Sarah: Yes, I would like to do a bit more about the place. It's not fair on Karen to do everything. I used to do all the ironing for both of us, because I actually enjoyed it, would you believe? But I haven't done any for ages. There's quite a pile actually, but I haven't been able to face it.

Katie: That sounds like a really good place to start, though I can see how a big pile of ironing would feel overwhelming to tackle. Is there any way of breaking this down into smaller steps? Some people find that doing a task for a certain length of time, say 20 or 30 minutes, is more manageable than doing the whole thing in one go. Could this be something that could work here?

Sarah: I think I might be able to do that.

Katie: Okay, that's great. How long do you think you could manage without it feeling too much?

Sarah: Probably about half an hour. Maybe I could do that in the morning? It would give me something to do rather than stay in bed.

Katie: That sounds like a good idea. Now, how often do you think you could do that?

Sarah: What about three times over the next week?

Katie: That would be great. Okay, so far, we have that you'll get up shortly after waking up, can we say within an hour of waking up?

Sarah: Yes, that sounds okay.

Katie: And to do half an hour's ironing three times over the next week. Do you think this is doable?

Sarah: Yes, I'll give it a go.

Katie: That's what it's all about, giving it a go, and if it doesn't work out, and you find that half an hour is too long, then shorten it; doing a little is always better than doing nothing. Is there anything you think you might be able to do on the days you're getting up a bit earlier, but not doing ironing?

Sarah: I used to go out running, but I haven't done anything for ages. I just don't have the energy, but maybe I could go for a short walk to get a bit of fresh air?

Katie: That sounds like a good idea. A bit of fresh air would be good. We also know that exercise is really good as a mood lifter, so going for a walk would be a good start. What about if we plan for you to have a short walk each day that you are not ironing – depending on the weather of course?

Sarah: Yes, I think that sounds fine.

Katie: Now, how long do you think these walks should take?

Sarah: Would 15 minutes be okay?

Katie: That sounds fine.

Exercise

Print off a copy of the Activity Schedule PDF on CD-ROM 3 and keep a diary for a week. Try to assign each activity to one of the following areas: your daily routine; a concentration activity; a general life activity; or whether it is something physical that you are doing.

- Once you have completed your entries, look to see what proportion of your life is spent in each of the activity areas.
- If a colleague is doing the same exercise, compare your activities to identify similar and different activity areas.

Section summary

- People with depression are often less active and frequently lose their normal routine
- An effective way of treating depression is

- to increase activity levels and re-establish routine
- An Activity Schedule can be used to monitor activities, rate moods and plan activities
- The patient rates each activity for sense of achievement and sense of pleasure
- The Activity Schedule can be used to monitor other moods, such as anxiety or anger
- Scheduling activities involves planning with the patient what they will do on a daily basis over the coming week (for a part of each day)
- Grading tasks enables the mental health worker to help the patient break down tasks into smaller, manageable steps
- The emphasis is always on attempting the task, not on its successful completion

Recommended reading

Jacobson, N., Martell, C.R. and Dimidjian, S. (2001). Behavioural activation treatment for depression: Returning to contextual roots. *Clinical Psychology: Science and Practice* 8 (3) 255–270.

Hollon, S.D. (2001). Behavioural activation treatment for depression: a commentary. *Clinical Psychology: Science and Practice*, 8 (3) 271–274.

Martell, C.R., Addis, M.E. and Jacobson, N.S. (2001). *Depression in Context: Strategies for Guided Action*. New York: Norton.

Test yourself

 To check your progress, locate this section on CD-ROM 3 and work through the interactive questions at the end.

Section 4c: Problem solving

Introduction

A problem-solving approach can be used as a straightforward and effective technique for dealing with life problems. It is an extremely useful technique for tackling the practical aspects of a problem. When someone feels overwhelmed by life problems, it is often difficult for them to see a way of addressing these difficulties satisfactorily. It can often feel impossible even to know where to start. Using a problem-solving approach enables a person to take a step back from their problems and consider what solutions exist. A step-by-step approach is used, and one problem is dealt with at a time.

The stages of problem solving

Stage 1: Identify the problem

This first step in problem solving is to identify the problem as clearly and precisely as possible. This can be straightforward, but sometimes it can be difficult to pinpoint exactly what the problem is. If the patient has difficulty identifying the precise problem, they can be encouraged to talk to someone they trust to help identify it exactly. The exact problem is then written down. Each problem is broken down into its constituent parts to aid problem solving. For example, a problem with disturbed sleep may be broken down into: intrusive thoughts on going to bed; and waking during the night with difficulty getting back to sleep.

Stage 2: Write down as many solutions as possible

Patients are encouraged to list all the ideas they come up with, no matter how silly or ridiculous they may seem. This may help in fostering a more flexible approach to dealing with problems. Patients may also find it helpful to consider what ideas other people they know would suggest. The more ideas the person generates, the more likely it is that an acceptable solution will be found.

Stage 3: Consider the pros and cons of each possible solution

The patient then works through the list of possible solutions and assesses the main advantages and disadvantages of each one.

Stage 4: Select the best or most promising solution

The next step is to choose the solution that can be carried out most easily with present resources (e.g. time, money, etc.) and is most likely to result in a positive outcome.

Stage 5: Plan how to carry out the chosen solution

This step involves listing the resources needed, the main problems that need to be overcome and the steps needing to be undertaken. Difficult steps can be practised and notes made of what information is needed. The steps should be specific and realistic. It should be clear what steps are going to be taken and when they will be carried out.

Stage 6: Put the plan into action

The person puts the plan into action, following the steps identified at Stage 5.

Stage 7: Review what happens

The chosen solution may work perfectly, or it may not. If it doesn't, the person is encouraged to go back to their list of solutions and try something else. Many solutions are helpful, but do not provide the complete answer. Whether the person's solution has worked completely, partially or not at all, they should be encouraged to praise themselves for their efforts. Plans may need to be revised, but the person is encouraged to continue with the problem-solving process until they have resolved their problem or achieved their goal.

An example of a problem-solving action plan is reproduced in the Appendix to this book.

Example CD-ROM 3 includes a video clip in which Julie and her mental health worker, Samantha, use a problem-solving approach for the issues around Julie's Mum's illness and the awareness that her Mum may not always be able to cope alone. A transcript of the clip is given below.

Video: Problem solving

Mental health worker (Samantha): Now, Julie, one of the things that we talked about was to see whether using a problem-solving approach would be any good for your types of problems. So we were going to try that out today, and you were going to bring a problem with you for us to work on. Have you managed to think of a problem?

Julie: Yes, I think I'd like to look at the problem around my Mum's illness.

Samantha: Okay; she's not been too well recently, has she?

Julie: No, no. I'm really worried about what might happen when she can't look after herself.

Samantha: Right, is that the aspect of the problem you would like to look at?

Julie: Yes.

Samantha: Okay. Well, I've actually got a 'Problem Solving form', and I think we should use this, so I'd like you to write it if that's okay. I've got something for you to lean on, and I've got a pen here, so could you just write that in the 'Identify the problem', here at the top?

Julie: Okay. (writes it down)

Samantha: So what have you put there?

Julie: Mum becoming unwell and unable to look after herself.

Samantha: Okay, good. Right, what we do next is to try and come up with as many solutions as we can. Can you think of any solutions for this problem?

Julie: Well, the first thing that's obvious to me is that perhaps she could come and live with us in our house.

Samantha: Okay, good. Can you write that under the first one there?

Julie: (writes it down)

Samantha: Any others that you can think of?

Julie: (thinks for a moment) I vaguely remember that David's Dad had prostate cancer and we saw him in a hospice, and that seemed to be quite nice.

Samantha: Okay, can you put that down under number 2?

Julie: (writes it down)

Samantha: Great. Any others you can think of?

Julie: No, I'm a bit stuck now.

Samantha: Okay. Well let's just think about this for a moment. Do you know of anyone else who has been in a similar situation? It doesn't need to be that their parents have been terminally ill, say, but maybe someone that has had a poorly parent or relative?

Julie: I think the neighbour has been unwell, and I know that he's had some people come to his home and help him wash and dress, and I think the nurse has been in a few times.

Samantha: Alright, okay. Well what about putting that one down too?

Julie: Okay. (writes it down)

Samantha: Right, any others you can think of?

Julie: No, I can't think of anything else about being at home really, no.

Samantha: Right, okay. What about, have you got any other relatives, any brothers or sisters?

Julie: Yes, I've got one sister.

Samantha: Is that another possibility, your Mum going to stay with your sister?

Julie: But it's not one that I'd like because it's a long way, but my sister would look after her. Maybe it is an option, I don't know.

Samantha: Okay. Well should we put it down as a possibility anyway? And then we can look at the pros and cons of each of them later.

Julie: Okay. (writes it down)

Samantha: Great. Okay, can you think of any others, then?

Julie: No, I can't think of any more, no.

Samantha: How many have we got there so far?

Julie: Four.

Samantha: Four, so that's not bad. We could work with them, I'm sure. Okay, well, the next step is to go through all the different solutions and look at the pros and cons of each. So we'll look at the first one.

Julie: Right, okay; that's her coming to live with us.

Samantha: That's living with you. So what would be the pros of that, do you think?

Julie: Well, I guess I could keep an eye on her a bit more, and we'd be quite close.

Samantha: Okay, put that down.

Julie: So I can get help if she needs it, because I can see what's required really. (writes it down)

Samantha: Yes, I can see that, that's good. What about any other advantages of that one then?

Julie: I guess she'd still be near her friends and things. (writes it down)

Samantha: Good. What about on the downside, what about the cons of that one?

Julie: I think one obvious one is that my husband, David and her, they don't get on that well, so that could be a bit difficult really. (writes it down)

Samantha: No, I can see that. Okay, so that's a disadvantage of that one. Any others?

Julie: I guess there's a space problem. I know that Colin's leaving soon because he's getting married, but obviously I wouldn't be able to have her there until he's gone really. That would be difficult. (writes it down)

Samantha: Okay, anything else?

Julie: I can't think of anything.

Samantha: Okay, good. (fade out and fade in later)

Samantha: Okay, so what we've done is we've identified the problem, we've come up with four solutions, and now looked at the pros and cons of them. We're ready to move on to the next step, and that's actually on the next sheet. We'll need these visible for us to look at. So, what we need to do is decide which solution is probably going to be the best one to go with at the moment out of the ones we have been weighing up the pros and cons.

Julie: Well, I think the best one would be to look at investigating helping her to stay at home by the looks of it, because I think she keeps her own world a bit more that way. That's the one I think would be best for her.

Samantha: Yes, okay. So that's solution number 3, then. So, write that in, and that's 'to stay at home'. Let's look at how we would need to plan how to carry this out, and this is getting the help for your Mum at home.

Julie: I guess I need to find out how long it's going to take to get some help and also whether that's what Mum wants.

Samantha: Right, okay. So there's two issues really that need to be addressed there.

Exercise

From the PDF on CD-ROM 3, print out the problem-solving form, or make a copy of the version in the Appendix to this book.

- Use the problem-solving approach to address Sarah's problem of not having a job.

Julie: Yes, that's right. So, I guess I could talk to her GP, Dr Richards, because she could talk to my Mum.

Samantha: So that's the first step; but how do you feel about talking to your Mum's GP though?

Julie: I don't mind, because she's my GP as well, so that will be alright. So I can talk to her about it when I see her next myself.

Samantha: Okay. Let's look at what we've done here, then. You identified the problem with your Mum's deteriorating physical health, you've come up with four credible solutions, and then we've looked at the pros and cons of each of them; then you've come up with the best one, which is getting care for your Mum at home. Then what we've done is looked at the steps towards the plan of what you are going to do next. The next step is to follow through with the plan, and then we need to review how that's gone. Now, in problem solving it's not always that the first solution is the best one, so sometimes, when you review it, you come back to the drawing board and go with another solution, but we can try this one out, go ahead with the plan and then come back and review it. How does that sound?

Julie: That sounds like it's a good idea.

Samantha: Have you found this exercise a useful thing to do?

Julie: Yes, I have. I've learnt a lot. I could use this perhaps on other things.

Samantha: Right, well that would be good, because I've got some blank problem solving forms that I can give you to take away today, and then maybe what you could do between now and next time is to see

whether you can use it for any other problems that arise?

Julie: Okay, that's fine.

Section summary

- A problem solving approach is helpful for life problems
- Problem solving is a step-by-step approach dealing with one problem at a time
- Problem solving comprises seven stages

Recommended reading

Williams, C.J. (2001). 'Practical Problem Solving', Chapter 2.1 in *Overcoming Depression: A Five Areas Approach*. London: Arnold.

Test yourself

 To check your progress, locate this section on CD-ROM 3 and work through the interactive questions at the end.

Section 4d: Graded exposure

Introduction

Graded exposure has been proven to be a particularly useful technique for treating phobias, especially Specific Phobias (e.g. heights, dogs, spiders, etc.), and for Agoraphobia and Social Phobia, in conjunction with cognitive approaches.

The first step in using this approach is for the patient to compose a hierarchy of fearful situations from the least anxiety-provoking to the most-feared situation. The patient is then encouraged to start with the target associated with the least anxiety and practise this step until the anxiety subsides before moving to the next step. It is vital that the patient experiences some degree of anxiety, otherwise they will learn little from the experience. Practice should be prolonged (usually one hour is recommended) and repeated regularly (typically daily practice). The patient carries on working through the hierarchy until they are able to face the most fear-evoking step, thereby conquering the phobia.

Many factors can affect the amount of anxiety experienced by the patient (e.g. time of day, number of people around, being unaccompanied, etc.). When composing the exposure hierarchy, moderating factors such as these should always be considered.

To elicit this information, useful questions to ask the patient are 'What would make this situation easier for you?' and 'What would make this situation more difficult for you?'. Then the situations can be placed accordingly on the hierarchy.

Example: a patient with a phobia of dogs

A 17-year-old male with a phobia of dogs is referred to a primary care mental health worker. The patient is unable to remember the onset of his difficulties, but he has been troubled with the phobia since childhood and is particularly frightened of large dogs. He is planning to move away to university in the near future, and because of this increased independence he is keen to tackle his fears. The box (right) shows an example of a graded exposure hierarchy for dog phobia.

Exercise

Suppose you have been asked to see a patient with a severe heights phobia. She has trouble crossing bridges, either on foot or in a car, and is unable to go higher than the second floor of a building without feeling anxious.

• Write down what you think an exposure hierarchy might look like for this patient.

Note: In a real situation you would not construct this hierarchy alone. This would be done collaboratively with the patient.

Common difficulties

Some problems can arise when using graded

Dog phobia, a graded exposure hierarchy example

1 Look at pictures of large dogs.
2 Watch a video of large dogs.
3 Sit in room with small dog on lead several feet away.
4 Sit in room with small dog on lead close enough to touch.
5 Sit in room with small dog unleashed.
6 Sit in room and stroke small dog while it is on a lead.
7 Sit in room and stroke small dog while it is unleashed.
8 Sit in room with large dog on lead several feet away.
9 Sit in room with large dog on lead close enough to touch.
10 Sit in room with large dog unleashed.
11 Sit in room and stroke large dog while on a lead.
12 Sit in room and stroke large dog while it is unleashed.
13 Take large dog for a walk.

(If the patient's anxiety subsides quickly, they may be able to work through several steps on the hierarchy within the space of one session)

---

exposure. Firstly, some tasks are difficult to grade (e.g. an aeroplane journey, or signing one's name in front of others). Secondly, some patients have a number of what appear to be unrelated fears (e.g. standing in queues, using lifts, sitting at the back of a bus, etc.). This means that a number of hierarchies may need to be devised. However, if a recurring theme emerges (e.g. feeling trapped) then one hierarchy can still be used. Finally, sometimes tasks are naturally very brief (e.g. passing a dog in a garden, signing one's name, etc.). In this instance the task should be repeated more regularly.

A simple diary can be used to record tasks and the level of anxiety experienced by the 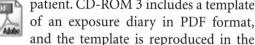 patient. CD-ROM 3 includes a template of an exposure diary in PDF format, and the template is reproduced in the

Appendix to this book for you to copy and use with patients.

Note: It is important to remember that, to be most effective, whenever possible exposure should be graded (using a hierarchy), prolonged (at least one hour) and repeated (daily practice).

How does exposure work?

Exposure works on the principles of habituation (a waning of a response such as anxiety). The graph in Figure 11 shows what happens when someone escapes from a situation. This is illustrated by the red line. Note that anxiety goes down but only brings about short-term relief as, the next time the patient enters the feared situation, they will feel just as anxious as last time. The black line shows what happens when the patient stays in the situation. Note that anxiety peaks, but levels off after a while and starts to decrease. The blue line shows what happens with repeated exposure (i.e. the patient's anxiety peaks lower and the anxiety comes down quicker until they experience minimal anxiety). This graph is extremely useful when demonstrated to patients in session, when the mental health worker can emphasize that exposure is graded, prolonged and repeated for best results.

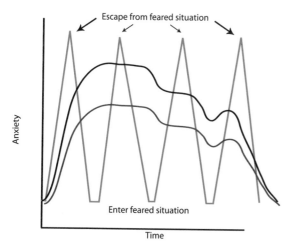

Figure 11: A habituation graph

Example 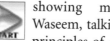 CD-ROM 3 includes a video clip showing mental health worker, Waseem, talking to Lorraine about the principles of exposure practice, having just demonstrated the habituation graph to her. A transcript of the clip is given below.

Video: Graded exposure

Mental health worker (Waseem): Now that you've seen how anxiety works from the graph, what would you think is the best way of tackling your phobia?

Lorraine: Well, I can see on this graph that I need to stop avoiding driving because, if I don't, my anxiety will get worse. If I start driving again, it will actually get easier, just as it has with me in the passenger seat.

Waseem: Yes, that's absolutely right. We call it 'exposure', in fact. We need to slowly get you driving again. We'll break it down into three stages for you. First of all you need to do it in very slow steps. There's not much point in throwing you straight at it, you'll get too scared and won't do it. Secondly, you have to be able to do it for a length of time, so it needs to be reasonably prolonged, because, of course, when you get into the car you're going to feel a little bit scared, and if you don't stay there long enough to know that nothing will happen, then you'll never get over the problem. So we tend to say around about an hour works. Thirdly, if you are going to do it for an hour, it's pointless doing it for an hour then never doing it again, so we have to repeat it, and usually we say repeat it on a daily basis, and that makes things easier. So, just to try to summarize that for you – because there is quite a lot there: it's called 'exposure'; you need to do it on a graded basis; you need to do it for a length of time, maybe about an hour at a time; and you need to repeat it, probably on a daily basis. How does that sound to you?

Lorraine: Well, I can certainly give the time to it, but it does sound a little scary though.

Waseem: Yes, I'm sure it does, and there's no doubt that you probably will feel more anxious when you first start doing it; but what we'll make sure is that we do it in steps, so you're not running before you can walk, if you like. So we'll do it in little chunks, so that you are in total control of it. We'll make sure you are perfectly happy with the first stage before we go on to the second stage, and so on.

Lorraine: Okay, that sounds okay.

Waseem: I'm going to give you this 'Exposure Diary', which I'd like you to fill in as you're doing this.

Lorraine: Okay.

Waseem: Okay, let's spend a bit of time developing a list of steps, so we can decide on the first steps to getting you back to driving again.

Exercise

Ask a colleague to role-play the patient introduced in the previous exercise who has presented for treatment for her height phobia (she has trouble crossing bridges, either on foot or in a car, and is unable to go higher than the second floor of a building without feeling anxious), while you take the role of the mental health worker.

- Describe to the patient the role of habituation, using a graph similar to that shown in Figure 11, and then discuss the principles of exposure.
- Ask your colleague to give feedback when you have finished the role-play.

Section summary

- Graded exposure is a useful technique for tackling phobic anxiety
- A hierarchy is developed to provide the steps of exposure
- Exposure is based on the principles of habituation
- To be most effective exposure should be graded, prolonged and repeated

Recommended reading

Marks, I.M. (2001). Chapter 12, 'Self-Help for Your Fears and Anxiety', in *Living With Fear* (second edition). London: McGraw-Hill.

Norman, I. and Ryrie, I. (2004). Chapter 15, 'The person with an anxiety disorder', and Chapter 24, 'Behavioural Techniques', in *Art and Science of Mental Health Nursing: A Textbook of Principles*. Maidenhead: Open University Press.

Test yourself

 To check your progress, locate this section on CD-ROM 3 and work through the interactive questions at the end.

Section 4e: Working with thoughts

Introduction

Automatic thoughts describe the thoughts and images that come into our minds automatically throughout the day. These tend to be brief and rapid, unlike the constant stream of conscious thoughts that may be running through our minds, such as 'I wonder what I should do this evening. Maybe I should go to the cinema or call Pamela to see if she wants to go out for a meal', and so on. Automatic thoughts tend to just pop into our minds. In depressed patients, these automatic thoughts are often negative in content, harsh, usually highly convincing and laden with negative emotion (e.g. 'I am so stupid for not knowing the answer to the question my boss asked me', or an image of oneself fainting in a supermarket and no-one coming to help). We are often more aware of the emotion that has occurred as a result of the thought than of the thought itself.

Identifying negative automatic thoughts

Evaluating negative and upsetting thoughts can be a useful skill to teach patients. The aim is to help the patient develop a more realistic view of situations. Becoming aware of negative automatic thoughts and their effect on emotion is the first step in this process. Some thoughts and images seem to be hotwired to the emotion and are therefore often referred to as 'hot thoughts'. Figure 12 shows an example of a thought diary in four columns, and CD-ROM 3 includes a template of the diary in PDF format. The template can also be found in the Appendix.

When hot thoughts are correctly identified, the associated mood should make sense (e.g. being in the post office and having the thought, 'It's terribly crowded in here', does not correspond with a high anxiety state, whereas the hot thought, 'I'm going to collapse', does).

We all have thousands of thoughts going through our minds every day; some will be dysfunctional, some won't. Some events will be upsetting to almost anyone (e.g. rejection, failure, death of a loved one). However, people with anxiety and depression often misinterpret neutral or even positive events and see them as having a negative or threatening connotation (e.g. 'David said I did a good piece of work today. He obviously thought I made a mess of things yesterday.'). It is useful to remember that patients with depression are more likely to blame themselves for negative events, whereas they have a tendency to attribute positive events to others, and to minimize achievements while maximizing perceived failures.

How to help patients elicit their negative automatic thoughts

Negative automatic thoughts may come in the form of words (e.g. 'I am pathetic') or images (e.g. seeing oneself homeless and destitute). Therefore, the mental health worker does not ask patients what they were thinking during a given situation,

but rather 'What went through your mind?' This is a key question to ask when using this approach. When a mental health worker spots a change in a patient's emotion, it is helpful to ask 'What's going through your mind right now?'

If the hot thought is not identified using this question, the implication for the thought needs to be clarified (e.g. in the case of the thought 'Ian is often bad tempered when he comes in from work', the implication may be 'It's all my fault, I'm a hopeless wife; so he dreads coming home because he doesn't love me anymore.'). To elicit the implication of the thought, questions such as 'What did you make of that?' and 'What did that mean to you?' can be particularly useful. The patient is thus trained to check what's going through their mind when they notice increased feelings of sadness, or anxiety, or anger.

Remember: The hot thought should always explain the emotion that is evoked.

Next, it is important to ask the patient to rate their belief in the thought (0–100%) and to rate the level of emotion (0–100%) that is associated with the thought.

Identifying your own negative automatic thoughts

To help patients identify their negative automatic thoughts, it is useful to learn how to identify your own negative automatic thoughts effectively first.

What to do when a negative thought is reported in question form

You may find that patients can sometimes report their automatic thoughts in the form of a question, making evaluation very difficult (e.g. 'Do they think I'm stupid?'). As it is difficult to rate your belief in a question, it is important to help the patient to express the negative thoughts in statement form by getting to the distressing and implied subtext (e.g. 'They think

Date	Situation	Emotions Rate intensity 0–100%	Thoughts Rate belief 0–100%
15.06	In the post office standing in a long queue	Anxious 85%	It's terribly crowded in here 80% I can't cope 80% I'm going to collapse 90%

Figure 12: Four-column thought diary

Exercise

A template for the four-column thought diary is included on CD-ROM 3, and is reproduced in the Appendix to this book. Think of a time recently when you felt a strong emotion in reaction to something. Then, using a copy of the template, write the situation in the corresponding column and the emotion you experienced in the 'emotion' box. Rate from 0–100% how strongly you felt that emotion.

- Now ask yourself '*What was going through my mind?*' Write your automatic thought or image in the 'thought' column. Now rate from 0–100% how strongly you believed that thought or image.
- If the thought or image you have recorded is not the 'hot thought', ask yourself '*What did I make of that?*' or '*What did that mean to me?*'.
- Does the thought make sense when you consider the emotion you felt and how strongly you felt it?
- Make some more copies of the four-column thought diary and keep a record of your automatic thoughts over the next week.

I'm stupid'). The patient can then rate how much they believe this thought.

Teaching patients to catch their hot thoughts using the four-column diary

Helping patients become aware of negative automatic thoughts is an important self-help activity. The mental health worker models using the thought diary in session to access the patient's thoughts, then the patient is encouraged to try this at home.

Use copies of the four-column thought diary to help patients record their automatic thoughts. Continue to catch your own auto-

matic thoughts. The more confident you become at identifying your own thoughts, the better you will become at helping patients to access theirs.

Example CD-ROM 3 includes a video clip in which mental health worker Katie introduces Andrew to the four-column thought diary, and negotiates with him the task of catching more thoughts in between their contacts. A transcript of the clip follows.

Video: Working with thoughts: eliciting a hot thought

Mental health worker (Katie): I'd like to show you the diary that I mentioned recently that we can use to help you examine your thoughts. Now, the first step is to learn how to catch these thoughts, and then at a later stage we can come onto how you examine them. Would that be alright?

Andrew: Yes, that's fine.

Katie: Okay, here's the diary. Now, I think you're better to write in it than me. The best way for me to show you how this operates is to use a real example, so, can you think of a situation in which you felt socially anxious recently?

Andrew: What about when my friend dropped me in it at the party?

Katie: Yes, I think that's a great example. So, let's put that in. First put the date in.

Andrew: It was the first.

Katie: Okay.

Andrew: (writes it down)

Katie: Okay. Now, here, we need a brief description of what happened.

Andrew: How about 'I'm at party and my friend introduces me to a woman and I panic'?

Katie: Good, I think that's nice and succinct, and that covers all the main points. Let's put that in.

Andrew: (writes it down)

Katie: Right, can you remember what emotion you felt at the time?

Andrew: Anxiety.

Katie: Okay, let's put that in here.

Andrew: (writes it down)

Katie: And how intense was that anxiety if we use the scale of 0–100, where 0 is not a problem and 100 is really, really anxious. Where would you say you were on that?

Andrew: 90.

Katie: Okay, let's write that in here.

Andrew: (writes it down)

Katie: Now, thinking back, can you remember what went through your mind at the time?

Andrew: Yes, I felt like I was making a fool of myself, and I thought that she would think I was pathetic.

Katie: Okay, well that sounds like two separate thoughts. So let's put both of those in here.

Andrew: (writes it down)

Katie: Okay, was there anything else that went through your mind?

Andrew: Well, I could just picture myself standing there with a bright red face and sweating like a pig.

Katie: Okay, well, do you want to put that in here then?

Andrew: (writes it down)

Katie: Okay, now, the next step is to fill in here how much you think you believed each of these thoughts and the image. So, can you do that?

Andrew: That would be 90, 100 and 100.

Katie: Okay, so you've given it 90, 100 and 100. Well done. Next week we'll look at how you evaluate these thoughts. So would you be able to use a diary like this over the coming week and practise that, and then next week we can look at how we evaluate them?

Andrew: Yes, yes, I could.

Evaluating negative automatic thoughts

Once patients are adept at using the four-column diary for identifying hot thoughts, it is time to move on to learning how to evaluate them. The aim is to help the patient to evaluate their thoughts unaided. However, this can be a difficult task for some patients and, therefore, the evaluating of thoughts together on a few occasions can really help put patients on the right track.

A negative interpretation of an event is only one of a number of different interpretations that can be made, and the patient may find that another interpretation may actually be more realistic. However, it is important to note that sometimes a negative interpretation is not necessarily unrealistic (e.g. 'I have few friends'). In these circumstances, the mental health worker can work with the patient to make changes to the problem situation by using a problem solving approach (see Section 4c) or help the patient develop more effective coping strategies (e.g. joining a fitness club).

Once a hot thought has been elicited, the patient rates their belief in the thought, identifies the associated emotion, and rates its intensity. If the distorted thought is believed strongly and is causing distress, the patient can be taught how to evaluate the thought. The mental health worker may collect more information first about physiological symptoms, what the patient did in reaction to the thought, and other thoughts occurring in the same situation.

At this point the full nine-column diary can now be introduced (CD-ROM 3 includes a template of the nine-column diary in PDF format). The template is also included in the Appendix.

Examining thoughts

One of the key techniques for helping patients evaluate their hot thoughts is looking at the evi-

---

Exercise

Consider the following statements, and in each case decide whether it is based on fact or interpretation.

- 'I have pains in my chest'
- 'Aidan thinks I'm pathetic'
- 'Everyone can see I'm anxious'
- 'Something always goes wrong'
- 'Nick was crying when I told him'
- 'There were five people in the queue ahead of me'
- 'I've never succeeded in anything'

dence for and against the thoughts. The evidence should be fact-based rather than based on other thoughts or interpretations. For example, 'Jackie did not return my call' is factual evidence, whereas 'Jackie did not return my call because she thinks I'm not important' is not factual evidence unless Jackie has actually said 'I think you are not important'. Evidence against the automatic thought is usually the hardest for people to identify, especially when they are experiencing a distressing emotion associated with the negative automatic thought.

Using evidence to evaluate hot thoughts

Once the hot thought and associated emotions have been rated, the patient is asked to provide evidence to support the thought (e.g. 'What's the evidence that you have for this thought?', or 'What makes you come to that conclusion?'). The mental health worker must be careful to accept only factual evidence and not other thoughts or interpretations. This evidence is written in the nine-column diary's *Evidence for the hot thought* column.

When as much evidence to support the hot thought as possible has been established, the next step is to elicit evidence that does not support the hot thought (e.g. 'Is there any evidence that does not support this thought?'). This evidence is written in the *Evidence against the hot thought* column. This may prove to be a more difficult task, as the information may not be easily accessed by the patient who is currently experiencing a strong emotion.

Useful questions

We know that depressed people are more likely to blame themselves for negative events, while positive events tend to be attributed to others. Depressed people use a different set of standards to judge themselves as compared to others. For that reason, a useful question to ask a patient when evaluating their negative automatic thoughts is 'What would you tell a friend if they were in the same situation?'.

The box (below) contains some more useful questions to use when helping patients evaluate negative automatic thoughts. However, it is important to note that not all questions will be appropriate on every occasion. This list is also included on CD-ROM 3 in PDF format. You can also give the list to your patients to help them when they are evaluating their thoughts on their own.

It is important to take as much time as is needed to establish evidence for and against hot thoughts. The evaluation of thoughts is likely to be unsuccessful if the patient does not believe that all the evidence supporting the thought has been considered. Equally, if there is little – or only weak – evidence that does not support the hot thought, the patient will find the evaluation unconvincing.

Once all the information for and against the hot thought has been collected, this information is used to arrive at a more balanced alternative, which is written in the nine-column diary's *Alternative or balanced thought* column.

Questions to use when evaluating negative thoughts

1 What evidence do you have that supports this thought?
2 What evidence is there that does not support this thought?
3 Is there another way of looking at this situation?
4 What is the worst thing that could happen if this thought is true?
5 If the thought is true, will it still matter in five years time?
6 How would someone else think about this?
7 What would you tell a friend if they were in the same situation?
8 If you were not depressed, would you believe this thought?
9 Are you applying unrealistic standards to yourself?

Establishing whether the evaluation of a thought was effective

It is very important to establish whether the evaluation of a thought has been successful. This is done by asking the patient to re-rate their belief in the original hot thought and the intensity of the associated emotion. This information is written in the nine column diary's '*Re-rate belief in hot thought and intensity of emotion*' column. By doing this, the mental health worker and the patient can easily assess how successful the thought evaluation has been. If the patient is not asked to re-rate the hot thought and emotion, the mental health worker may make the mistake of believing the evaluation of the thought has been a success when in fact it has made no difference to how the patient thinks and feels.

Why evaluation of thoughts is not always effective

Sometimes no shift in belief in the hot thought is attained. Here are some reasons why this might be the case.

- The evaluated thought was not the hot thought but a more peripheral thought
- The evidence supporting the hot thought has not all been elicited
- The evidence against the hot thought is not convincing to the patient
- The hot thought is actually a deeper held belief (e.g. 'I am a bad person') that is being articulated as a thought and, therefore, it is more difficult to shift and may need more formal CBT work from a qualified therapist

Often the evaluation of a negative automatic thought leads naturally to an action, and that is what the final column '*What to do next*' in the diary is used for. For example, a patient may have evaluated a negative automatic thought related to how they think their partner will not understand, or care, about their difficulties.

Through evaluation of the negative automatic thought, it becomes clear that the patient's partner is actually generally very sup-

portive of the patient and is likely to be supportive on this occasion too. The action in this case may be for the patient to spend some time talking to the partner to tell them how they feel, thereby testing out their initial prediction that the partner will not understand or care about their difficulties.

(The preceding text has been adapted from the Praxis CBT Distance Learning Programme, with permission.)

Example CD-ROM 3 includes a video clip in which Deborah evaluates a thought with her mental health worker, Waseem. A transcript of the clip follows.

Video: Working with thoughts: Evaluating a hot thought

Mental health worker (Waseem): Deborah, I see how you've filled out the first four columns of the thought diary. We'll have a look at a few of these things and try and evaluate these thoughts.

Deborah: Okay.

Waseem: Now, it looks like you were doing some exposure training in the supermarket last Tuesday, which is good. But unfortunately you felt very anxious and you thought you were going to faint.

Deborah: I felt terrible. I was so lightheaded and felt really, really dizzy.

Waseem: It must have been very scary for you if you've put down that you thought you were going to faint – 90%, that's quite a lot.

Deborah: Yes.

Waseem: Okay, well let's try and make sense of these, then, shall we? What evidence do you think that you had, to think that you were going to faint?

Deborah: Well, because I felt really light-headed and my heart was beating very fast and I felt hot I think as well, yes, really hot.

Waseem: Okay, let's write that down in the column there.

Deborah: Okay. Dizzy, lightheaded. (writes it down)

Waseem: Right. Anything else? Any other reason

that made you think that you were going to faint?

Deborah: I had palpitations.

Waseem: You had palpitations, okay.

Deborah: (writes it down)

Waseem: Can you think of anything else to make you think that you were going to faint?

Deborah: No.

Waseem: No, that summarizes it. Alright, well let's see what we can put in the next column. What evidence do you think you've got against the thought that you would faint?

Deborah: Well, I suppose I never have actually fainted.

Waseem: Good point. I think we could write that down.

Deborah: (writes it down)

Waseem: You've got no history of fainting in the supermarket. There's something else: remember we spoke about what happens to your blood pressure when you're anxious and what happens when you faint, and how they are not really compatible – because it goes up when you're anxious and down when you faint? So I think that would be worth writing down.

Deborah: That would be the evidence that my blood pressure was raised. (writes it down)

Waseem: Because when you're anxious it's raised, and to faint it would need to be lowered. Can we think of anything else, any other reasons against the thought that you might faint? We've got two there.

Deborah: No, I think that's it.

Waseem: Okay, well we'll leave it at that just now. So if you consider the evidence *for* the thought you were going to faint and the evidence *against* the thought that you were going to faint. If we balance these up, now, do you think you can put in the next column perhaps an alternative thought to your original thought?

Deborah: Well, instead of thinking I am going to faint, I could think that I'm not very likely to faint because my blood pressure is higher and it needs to be low for me to faint.

Waseem: Okay, shall we write it down in the next column?

Deborah: Okay. I'm not likely to faint ... (writes it down)

Waseem: Despite the fact you felt that way, perhaps?

Deborah: Despite the way I feel, my blood pressure is not low ...

Waseem: Right, that's a more balanced view now, isn't it, on the thought that you had? Right, now that we've had the reasons for and against your thought, you know you said that you thought 90% that you were going to faint. Would you like to re-rate it?

Deborah: I suppose it would actually be quite a lot lower when I think about it, and when I think about this thought here. Probably around 50%.

Waseem: Good, let's put that in that column.

Deborah: (writes it down)

Waseem: Good – which is quite a shift isn't it? It's lowered down quite a lot despite the fact that you felt anxious and you clearly thought you were going to faint. It has dropped quite a lot. The question is, how do we get it even lower than that?

Deborah: I suppose what I was saying earlier, that I actually left the supermarket when I was rating it about 90%, that I guess if I could just stay a bit longer in the supermarket I might be able to think this thought, have this thought in my mind, and maybe that would lower it to much more like 50%.

Waseem: If you stay in the supermarket it will start to reduce. It might feel a bit scary, you might feel a little bit nervous, but keep these thoughts in mind so you can evaluate this thought and this figure will start to slowly go down. Maybe we should write that in the last column: 'try and stay there a little bit longer'.

Deborah: To stay in the supermarket longer. (writes it down)

Notice how this process led to it being apparent what are the next steps Deborah has to take to overcome her agoraphobic difficulties.

Evaluating angry thoughts

Often people who get angry do not notice what is going through their minds at the time, but it is vital that, if the person is going to control their anger, they must learn to recognize their thoughts and to evaluate them.

People who have a propensity to getting angry tend to experience thoughts with similar themes again and again; e.g.:

- 'He's trying to make a fool of me'
- 'She's being so selfish'
- 'This is unfair'
- 'They should not be doing this'

Patients with anger problems tend to take things personally and often jump to conclusions about what others' intentions are. They often have high expectations of others, and when these are not fulfilled they feel angry. They expect their standards of behaviour to be followed by others (e.g. 'This driver should be more careful.').

Evaluating thoughts related to panic

In Panic Disorder, considering the evidence for and against a misinterpretation is used in the same way that it is used with other types of negative automatic thoughts.

Useful questions to use when evaluating catastrophic misinterpretations include the following. In the example questions, fear of fainting is used. However, this can be replaced with any other catastrophe (e.g. losing one's mind, hav-

ing a heart attack, suffocating, etc.).

- How many panic attacks have you experienced?
- How many times have you fainted?
- So you've had lots of panic attacks but you've never actually fainted. What do you make of that?
- Do you know what causes someone to faint?

These types of question are used to guide the patient to discover that their interpretation may actually be inaccurate, and to lead on to what the patient can do next to directly test the misinterpretation (e.g. stay in a situation long enough for the symptoms to pass).

Evaluating thoughts related to Social Phobia

The aim here is to help the person evaluate their negative interpretations so they learn to accept that, even if they make mistakes because of anxiety, people will not judge them adversely as a person, and are far more likely to think that something must have been troubling them on the day.

The need for practice

Once the mental health worker has demonstrated how to use the four- and nine-column diaries at least once, the patient can be given some blank copies of the diaries and asked to record negative thoughts and to attempt to evaluate the hot thoughts, by themselves, between contacts. It is emphasized that this is a new skill and that they may not find it an easy task, but with practice it will get easier. They are asked to give it a try and are reassured that any problems that arise will be discussed at the next contact.

Section summary

- Automatic thoughts can come in the form of thoughts or images hence the question *'What's going through your mind?'* rather than *'What were you thinking?'*
- Clarify the implication of a thought using questions like *'What did you make of that?'*

and '*What does that mean to you?*'

- The thought most connected to emotion is often referred to as the 'hot thought'
- Thoughts reported as questions need to be

Exercise

Having elicited some of your own negative automatic thoughts, now use the nine-column diary to evaluate your thoughts (print one from the PDF on CD-ROM 3, or make a copy of the example in the Appendix). Ensure you have identified a hot thought, and rated your belief in the thought and the intensity of the emotion. Then look for evidence for and against your hot thought (columns 5 and 6). Remember that only factual evidence should be used. Now ask some of the other questions described in this section to evaluate the thought, then, using all your evidence, come up with a more balanced thought (column 7). Next, re-rate your belief in the original thought and intensity of the associated emotion (column 8). Finally, consider whether some action now needs to be taken (column 9). Continue to practise identifying and evaluating your thoughts over the next two to three weeks. You will find that it gets easier to do with practice.

---

turned into statements thereby eliciting the implied subtext

- The associated emotion should always be elicited
- Thoughts and emotions should always be rated in terms of belief and intensity from 0 to 100
- Learning to become aware of one's own thoughts is an important step in helping others to identify theirs
- The hot thought and associated emotion are rated before and after the thought has been evaluated
- Examining evidence for and against a hot thought is a key technique in evaluating thoughts
- Evidence used should always be fact-based

- Evaluating thoughts is a skill which will require practice for you and the patient to become proficient

Reference

Newcastle, North Tyneside and Northumberland Mental Health NHS Trust (2003). *Praxis CBT Distance Learning Package.* Morpeth: Northumberland, Tyne and Wear NHS Trust. www.praxiscbt.com.

Recommended reading

Beck, J.S. (1995). *Cognitive Therapy. Basics and Beyond.* New York: Guilford Press.
Greenberger, D. and Padesky, C.A. (1995). *Mind Over Mood, A Cognitive Therapy Treatment Manual for Clients.* London: Guilford Press.

Test yourself

 To check your progress, locate this section on CD-ROM 3 and work through the interactive questions at the end.

Section 4f: Controlled breathing

Introduction

When someone is anxious or panicky, they will breathe more quickly to increase the amount of oxygen in their system and provide more energy. The person's heart will beat faster to carry blood to the main muscle groups and brain, and they will start to sweat to stop the body from overheating. This is a biological reaction to prepare the body for fight or flight. It is the effects of these symptoms, and of over-breathing in particular, which results in the person trying to take in more oxygen and consequently breathing out too much carbon dioxide. This can increase some of the physical symptoms of panic, including lightheadedness and dizziness.

Note: this does not increase the risk of fainting. For someone to faint, they must first experience a sharp drop in blood pressure. During a panic attack blood pressure rises. Therefore the two states are incompatible.

Evidence-based approaches for the treatment of panic attacks have changed radically over recent years. The use of strategies to control panic symptoms is now considered outmoded. When using a formal CBT approach, it is now seen as inappropriate to teach controlled breathing and relaxation exercises, as these can merely serve to add to the patient's repertoire of safety behaviours, which help to maintain the problem.

However, as an interim treatment for patients in primary care, it is acceptable to teach patients relaxation (see Section 4g) and controlled breathing techniques.

Principles of controlled breathing

If a patient can learn to control their breathing during a panic attack, symptoms may be reduced. The patient practises how to breathe calmly and slowly. This may not be as easy as it first appears. An effect of over-breathing is that the person feels that they need more air, and so, naturally, it is extremely difficult to do something that makes the person feel as though they are getting even less air. Practice should firstly take place when the patient is not panicking, for a minimum of three minutes. The patient should be advised that this technique works best when the symptoms of panic have just started, rather than waiting until they are in the midst of a full-blown panic attack.

Stages of controlled breathing

These instructions are reproduced from a self-help stress booklet from Newcastle, North Tyneside and Northumberland Mental Health Trust, available online at www.nnt.nhs.uk/mh and selfhelppsychology@nmht.nhs.uk.

The patient should be instructed as follows:
1 Fill your lungs with air. Imagine you are filling a bottle, so it fills from the bottom up. Your stomach should push out too.
2 Do not breathe in a shallow way, from the chest, or too deeply.
3 Keep your breathing slow and calm.
4 Breathe in through your mouth and out through your nose.
5 Try breathing in slowly, saying to yourself 'one elephant, two elephant, three elephant, four'.
6 Then let the breath out slowly to six: 'one elephant, two elephant ... six elephant'.
7 Keep doing this until you feel calm.
8 Sometimes looking at the second hand of a watch can help to slow breathing down.

Remember: even if you don't manage to control your breathing, nothing bad will happen.

It is important to reinforce this final point to ensure that the patient does not believe they are learning this technique because their symptoms are actually dangerous. They are not, and it is important that this fact is reinforced. This technique is used to demonstrate to the patient that they can exercise a degree of control over their symptoms.

The most important strategies to use to tackle panic attacks are to guide patients to discover that panic attacks are not dangerous. The best way to do this is to help patients evaluate their anxious thoughts (see *Working with Thoughts* in Section 4e) and to encourage them to face avoided situations using exposure techniques (see Section 4d).

Example CD-ROM 3 includes a video clip in which mental health worker Waseem teaches Alison how to do controlled breathing.

Video: Controlled breathing

Mental health worker (Waseem): Okay, I said today that we would look at some of the problems that you are having during your panics, and today we will pay attention to the difficulties you have with breathing. You know you said that sometimes you find it difficult, and your breathing gets very fast when you're having your attacks. So what I'm going to teach you today is how to breathe slower and calmer.

Alison: Okay.

Waseem: It will help reduce some of the dis-comfort you feel. When you're breathing in, the tendency is to breathe very short breaths and gasp a little bit. What I'd like you to do is breathe really slowly and calmly. Watch me first. We'll breathe like we are filling a bottle, so we are breathing from the bottom upwards, and you'll notice that, as well as my chest, my stomach will go out. Okay? Breathing in really slowly through the mouth, then out through the nose. Just try that ... Let's try it again.

Alison: (breathes slowly)

Waseem: Nice and calm, slowly in through the mouth and out through the nose. Okay, this time as you breathe in, I'm going to count. One elephant, two elephant, three elephant, four elephant. Now out through the nose. Good. If you keep this going nice and slow-ly, it will help you feel much calmer.

Alison: Okay. Why elephants?

Waseem: Only because 'one elephant' is more or less one second, so it helps you time it so it helps you regulate the speed at which you are breathing.

Alison: Okay.

Waseem: You might find that if you looked at the second hand of a watch, that might help you as well. The main thing is to do it nice and slowly and calmly, and also to repeat it. So if you repeat it regularly, probably better to do it when you are not feeling panicky, so you can get used to doing it.

Alison: Right.

Waseem: And if you repeat it regularly, say up to three minutes a day, then that will help you a lot.

Alison: Okay, I'll give it a go.

Waseem: Good. Okay. And one last thing: whether or not you use these techniques to control some of the symptoms that you're having during the panic attack, nothing bad will happen.

Alison: Okay.

Waseem: I'm teaching you these techniques so that you can reduce some of the discomfort that you have during the panic attacks.

Notice how Waseem reinforces that nothing bad will happen regardless of whether Alison manages to control her breathing during a panic attack or not.

Section summary

- Over-breathing is a symptom of the fight or flight response
- Over-breathing does not increase the like-lihood of fainting
- Controlled breathing can help give a patient control of over-breathing
- It is important to reinforce to patients that nothing dangerous would happen if they continued to over-breathe

Reference

Northumberland, Tyne and Wear NHS Trust (2002). *Self-help guide for Stress.* Morpeth: Northumberland, Tyne and Wear NHS Trust. www.nnt.nhs.uk/mh.

Test yourself

 To check your progress, locate this sec-tion on CD-ROM 3 and work through the interactive questions at the end.

Section 4g: Relaxation

Introduction

Relaxation techniques are not indicated as an intervention of choice for many mental health problems, and can actually be unhelpful for some (e.g. Panic Disorder or phobic disorders when undertaking exposure practice). However, relaxation can be very useful in help-ing patients with anger problems, stress prob-lems, Generalized Anxiety Disorder and sleep difficulties, and anyone who has difficulty unwinding. Being able to relax is a useful skill for all of us to have, but many people do this in less formal ways.

Patients can be taught relaxation techniques, learn to notice the first signs of physical tension, and then put these techniques into practice, thereby nipping physical tension in the bud. Some people find it easier to relax using less formal strategies, such as listening to a favourite piece of music, reading, watching television, exercising, etc., which is equally as acceptable.

Most forms of relaxation are based on variations of progressive muscle relaxation, which was first developed by Jacobson in 1938. If it is appropriate to teach a patient how to relax, here is a typical relaxation routine based on a sequence of exercises described by Ost (1987).

Relaxation Exercise 1

The mental health worker explains to the patient that they will be asked to tense (for about 10 seconds) and then relax various muscle groups. These are demonstrated to the patient before starting. The muscle groups are:

1 Lower arms: Tightening the fists and pulling them up towards the body
2 Upper arms: Tensing the arms by the side of the body
3 Lower legs: Extending the legs and pointing the feet up
4 Upper legs: Pushing the legs together
5 Stomach: Pulling it in towards the spine
6 Upper chest and back: Inhaling and holding for a count of 10
7 Shoulders: Pulling them up towards the ears
8 Back of the neck: Tilting the head back
9 Lips: Pursing the lips but without clenching the teeth
10 Eyes: Tightly closing the eyes
11 Eyebrows: Frowning and so pushing them together
12 Upper forehead: Raising the eyebrows

The patient can do the exercise while sitting in a chair. An audio tape can be used to assist with this, and the patient should be encouraged to practise the relaxation exercise at home.

It should be emphasized that relaxation is like any new skill: it needs to be practised for the person to become accomplished at doing it. Some people do not like this formal type of

relaxation, and can find that it actually makes them more tense; therefore it may not be useful for everyone. Once the patient is able to relax using the tape then they should be encouraged to proceed without it.

The problem with relaxation in this form is that it is not easily transferred to stressful situations (e.g. if a person gets agitated or anxious in a supermarket queue, it is impossible to just find a chair and sit down to relax). Therefore, this is just the first stage of the relaxation training programme and there are a number of further exercises to help the patient learn to relax more quickly.

Relaxation Exercise 2

Once the patient is adept at Exercise 1, they progress to the next stage, which involves larger muscle groups:

1 Whole arms: Slightly extend the arms with elbows bent and fists tightened
2 Whole legs: Extended with toes pointing upwards
3 Stomach: Pulling it in towards the spine
4 Upper chest and back: Inhaling and holding for a count of 10
5 Shoulders: Pulling them up towards the ears
6 Back of the neck: Tilting the head back
7 Face: Scrunching up the eyes and lips
8 Forehead and scalp: Raising the eyebrows

The patient is encouraged to practise this exercise without the use of a tape.

Relaxation Exercise 3

Once the patient is adept at Exercise 2, they are ready to progress to the next stage:

1 Whole arms: As before
2 Upper chest and back: As before
3 Shoulders and neck: Lifting the shoulders and tilting the head back
4 Face: As before

This exercise can be practised in a number of situations, including walking around, driving, sitting at a desk, etc.

Relaxation Exercise 4

In this version of the relaxation exercise, the patient does not tense muscles, but focuses on the various muscle groups to try to notice if there is any tension present, then relaxes the muscles without tensing first. Again the patient practises this in real-life situations.

Relaxation Exercise 5

The patient must be completely competent at exercise 4 (release-only relaxation) before moving onto this stage. When the patient is relaxed, they are instructed to take one to three deep breaths and to think of the word 'relax' with each exhalation, while scanning their body for any tension, which – if found – is released. Once the patient is able to do this, they are encouraged to practise without it being preceded by the release-only relaxation and only with the word 'relax'. By doing this, the word 'relax' becomes a signal to the patient to relax. The patient is then encouraged to practise this type of relaxation several times throughout the day in various settings. It can be helpful to discuss cues that the patient can use to remind themselves to relax (e.g. whenever the phone rings, sitting at traffic lights, making a drink, etc.).

Relaxation Exercise 6

The patient is encouraged to apply what they have learned to situations where it is most needed (e.g. anger-provoking situations, or when the patient is tense and anxious). The patient

Exercise

Make an audiotape of yourself giving relaxation instructions for Relaxation Exercise 1. Give a copy to your supervisor to try. If your supervisor feels that it is of sufficient quality and at the right pace for relaxation, you can give copies of this tape to your patients when appropriate.

should now be well aware of the early signs of anger, anxiety or stress, and be prepared to apply the relaxation techniques well before the symptoms are very intense.

Example CD-ROM 3 includes an audio clip in which mental health worker Samantha discusses relaxation with Ben. A transcript of the clip follows.

Audio: Relaxation

Mental health worker (Samantha): Okay, Ben, the next thing we've got down for discussing today is how you've been getting on with the second relaxation exercise that we tried out when we met up a couple of weeks ago in session. How did you get on with it?

Ben: Yes, okay, thanks. I found it a bit more difficult than the first exercise, but I soon got used to it, and I'm getting on fine now.

Samantha: Okay, that's good. Are you able to achieve a state of relaxation when you're doing the exercise?

Ben: Yes, I would say I've been doing it successfully for about five days or so now.

Samantha: Well, that's good. Do you think it's a good time to move onto the third stage in the relaxation process?

Ben: Yes, I'd like to.

Samantha: Okay, great. Well, basically, in this one you're going to use larger muscle groups, so instead of the eight muscle groups that you've been used to working on so far, we're going to reduce it to four.

Ben: Okay, I'll give it a go.

Samantha: Right. Let me just run through the muscle groups then. They are your whole arms, just like you were doing them before; your upper chest and back, just as you were doing that before too; then your shoulders and neck, by lifting your shoulders and tilting your head back; and your face, just as you were doing that before too.

Ben: Okay, I've written those down. I'll give it a go. If it's anything like last time, it'll probably seem a bit weird at first, but I'll soon get used to it.

Samantha: Okay, well it does seem that you're

taking to this really well, which is great. Can I just get you to read those four back to me, though, Ben, because I know I rattled through them pretty quickly there.

Ben: Yes, okay. My whole arms; my upper chest and back; my shoulders and neck by lifting my shoulders and tilting my head back; and my face.

Samantha: Great, yes. Do you think you'll get a chance to try that out over the next week, then we can maybe talk again?

Section summary

- Relaxation can be useful for patients with anger problems, stress problems, Generalized Anxiety Disorder and sleep difficulties
- Patients learn to notice the first signs of physical tension and put these techniques into practice, thereby nipping them in the bud
- Deep muscle relaxation is just the first stage of the relaxation training programme, followed by a number of exercises to help the patient learn to relax more quickly

References

Jacobson, E. (1938). *Progressive relaxation*. Chicago: University of Chicago Press.

Ost, L.G. (1987). Applied relaxation: description of a coping technique and review of controlled studies. *Behaviour Research and Therapy* 25, 397–410.

Test yourself

 To check your progress, locate this section on CD-ROM 3 and work through the interactive questions at the end.

Section 4h: Sleep hygiene and improving the sleep environment

Introduction

Encouraging patients to learn good sleep hygiene and to optimize their sleep environment can have a dramatic effect on their sleep difficulties. Here are some of the most helpful changes a person can make in working on their problems sleeping.

Helping a patient with sleep problems

1: Sleep hygiene

Establish a regular wake-up time

Learning to wake up at the same time each morning is an important first step in establishing a regular sleep cycle. This helps to set all of a person's body rhythms. Patients are advised that they should establish a getting-up time and should not vary this by more than an hour, even at weekends or days off. A person who gets up at 11am on a Sunday morning, as opposed to 7am on weekdays, is likely to have difficulty getting to sleep that night, and a cycle of tiredness and poor sleep may continue for a few days before the rhythm is re-established.

Go to bed only when sleepy

Many people with sleep problems make the mistake of going to bed when they are not sleepy.

When someone has had a difficult time sleeping the night before, they often go to bed early in the hope of catching up. Going to bed when sleepy results in quicker sleep onset, while going to bed when wide awake can often lead to ruminating and physical alertness. If the person fixes the time they get up in the morning and can become more flexible about the time of going to bed, then their body will begin to tell them how much sleep is needed.

Avoid napping

Napping during the day can disrupt the body's sleep rhythm, resulting in difficulty sleeping at night. It is therefore important to encourage patients to avoid sleeping during the day. Often mid-afternoon or early evening is a danger time for catnapping, so patients can be encouraged to engage in activities that are non-conducive to dropping off to sleep (e.g. physical exercise).

Caffeine

Patients should be encouraged to avoid consuming caffeine within six hours of going to bed. Coffee, tea, cola drinks, hot chocolate, etc., contain caffeine, which is a strong and long-lasting stimulant that interferes with one's ability to sleep.

Alcohol

Despite alcohol being a depressant, which can actually aid relaxation and sleep if timed correctly, it can lead to disrupted and non-restorative sleep. Therefore, it is important to encourage patients to avoid consuming alcohol within two hours of going to bed.

Smoking

Smokers should be advised to reduce their intake prior to bedtime as, like caffeine, nicotine is a powerful stimulant.

Physical exercise

Exercise can assist in improving a person's sleep, but not if it is done too close to bedtime. Patients should be encouraged to exercise regularly but to avoid strenuous exercise after 6pm if possible.

Supper

If someone goes to bed hungry, this can lead to difficulty in getting to sleep. If this is the case, a light snack, such as crackers, milk or a slice of toast, consumed shortly before bedtime, is appropriate. Chocolate or other sugary foods should be avoided. Any snacking in the middle of the night should be discouraged, as this can lead to habitual waking at that time each night feeling hungry. Any bedtime drinks should not contain caffeine; milky, malty drinks are best and have been found to be beneficial to sleep (e.g. Horlicks).

Medication

Some medicines and other drugs can affect sleep because they contain stimulants such as caffeine. Ask patients what medication they are taking and check with their GP or the pharmacist if they may contain any substances non-conducive to sleep. For example, some medication used in the treatment of asthma and migraine headaches contain stimulants; paracetamol contains caffeine.

Dealing with worry

Some patients may find that they ruminate over their problems when they get to bed. If this is a problem, patients can be encouraged to get out of bed and write down the problems that are troubling them. They can then use a problem-solving technique (see Section 4c) to tackle the difficulties earlier in the day.

Establish a bedtime routine

A bedtime routine helps us prepare for sleep and is an opportunity to unwind from the stresses of the day. Energetic activities are discouraged at this time, and, instead, the patient should be encouraged to engage in quiet and relaxing pursuits such as a warm bath, reading, or watching television. A predictable bedtime routine can help the onset of sleep and can include activities like brushing teeth, setting the alarm, applying creams, closing the curtains, etc. Good sleepers tend to have a set bedtime routine, so it is a good idea to encourage poor sleepers to develop these kinds of routines too.

2: Improving the sleep environment

Patients should be encouraged to make the bed and bedroom as conducive to sleep as possible (e.g. minimal noise, comfortable temperature, and a suitably dark room).

Associating the bed with sleep

Many poor sleepers do not associate their beds with sleep, but instead associate it with other activities such as reading, watching television, worrying, tossing and turning, etc. It is crucial that all activities other than sleep (sexual intercourse being the only exception) take place elsewhere. Patients should be encouraged to remove their televisions from the bedroom and to read elsewhere. The bedroom should be reserved for sleep, and all other activities should take place in another room.

What to do when sleep onset does not occur

The patient should be instructed to get up after about 10–15 minutes of going to bed if they have not fallen asleep. Most people can estimate when 10–15 minutes has elapsed and it is important that the patient is not encouraged to become a clock-watcher. The aim is to avoid the patient starting to get tense and anxious about lack of sleep. The person is encouraged to leave the bedroom and to go into another room and engage in a quiet activity (e.g. sitting listening to relaxing music) and only return to the bedroom when they are sleepy.

This step is repeated as often as necessary throughout the night for any ongoing initial insomnia, or if the patient wakes in the middle of the night and has difficulty getting back to sleep.

Example CD-ROM 3 includes a video clip in which mental health worker Samantha discusses with her patient Roger what to do if sleep onset does not occur immediately. A transcript of the clip follows.

Video: Sleep hygiene and improving the sleep environment

Mental health worker (Samantha): Okay, Roger, we've looked at some strategies to help with your poor sleep, and one of the things is to reduce your tea intake, especially in the evenings, because that seems to be interfering with your sleep. But now, what I'd like to do is to look at what actually happens when you get to bed. Now one of the things that has come up in your diary is that you seem to spend a long time in bed, but not much of that time sleeping; in fact I think it was just the other night it took 1½ hours to get to sleep.

Roger: Yes, that was a particularly bad night, but most nights it's usually an hour or so.

Samantha: Okay, let's see if we can do something about that. Now, we've talked about re-associating the bed and bedroom with sleep onset rather than lying there watching TV, worrying, eating, drinking, that kind of thing, and you've already agreed to take out the TV, and to stop eating and drinking in bed.

Roger: Yes.

Samantha: Okay, well part of that re-associating the bed and the bedroom with sleep is not to lie there for long periods without sleeping, but instead to get up.

Roger: Right. Well that should be okay, because quite often I get up anyway to make a drink.

Samantha: Okay, well, that's really good that you don't mind getting up, but what I'm proposing is just slightly different. What I'd like you to do is get up after about 10–15 minutes, say, if you don't fall asleep or even if you just lose that feeling of sleepiness; and then to get up and go into another room. But this time I don't want you to make any caffeinated drinks, like a cup of tea or anything like that, and preferably not a drink at all, but just to sit and do something relaxing like listening to a piece of music, nothing strenuous at all, and nothing too interesting – so say watching a TV programme that's pretty dull and uninteresting, not a thriller or a comedy or anything like that. Just something that you could leave after 2 minutes or 20 minutes, say, without any difficulty. How does that sound?

Roger: That sounds fine. As I said with the sleep hygiene stuff, I'd give anything a go. It's not as if I've got anything to lose.

Samantha: No, okay. Well, what I think we should do now is recap what we've covered so far and what you plan to do between now and the next session, and also to check and see whether you've enough diaries or not for next time.

In summary

All these strategies should help the patient get a better night's sleep. A sleep diary template is included on CD-ROM 3 in PDF format, and the template is reproduced in the Appendix to this book. Print out the PDF or copy the Appendix template and use it with patients to enable them to record their sleep pattern, both as a baseline and, when using the sleep techniques, to review progress and evaluate the effectiveness of the intervention.

A sleep diary such as this can be kept by the patient over a 1–2-week period, as a baseline. Doing this can produce lots of useful information about the sleep problem and help to identify important factors that even the patient is unaware of and that may be interfering with their sleep. In particular, estimates of the time spent awake during the night and the number of times a patient wakes up each night can provide a useful baseline that any interventions can be measured against.

Section summary

- The main techniques for helping patients with sleep problems are sleep hygiene and improving the sleep environment
- To improve sleep, patients should only go to bed when they are sleepy
- Patients with sleep problems should be encouraged to reduce their intake of stimulants (e.g. coffee)
- Patients with sleep problems should be encouraged to exercise early in the day
- If the patient does not fall asleep within 10–15 minutes, they should get up and go into another room

Recommended reading

Bearpark, H. (1994). *Overcoming insomnia.* Rushcutters Bay, Sydney: Gore and Osment Publications.

Bootzin, R.R. and Perlis, M.L. (1992). Non-pharmacological treatments of insomnia. *Journal of Clinical Psychiatry*, 53 (Suppl.) 37–41.

Lacks, P. (1987). *Behavioural treatment for persistent insomnia.* Oxford: Pergamon Press.

Lacks, P. and Morin, C.M. (1992). Recent advances in the assessment and treatment of insomnia. *Journal of Consulting and Clinical Psychology*, 60, 586–594.

Reite, M.L., Ruddy, J.R. and Nagel, K.E. (1990). *Concise Guide to the Evaluation and Management of Sleep Disorders.* Washington: American Psychiatric Press.

Test yourself

 To check your progress, locate this section on CD-ROM 3 and work through the interactive questions at the end.

Section 4i: Lifestyle strategies

Introduction

Aspects of a person's lifestyle can have a direct impact on their physical and mental health. In this section, key lifestyle strategies focused on healthy eating, physical activity, controlled drinking and smoking cessation are all discussed.

Healthy eating

Healthy eating habits are relevant to everyone. There is growing evidence that diet is an important factor in mental health, in particular, intake of Omega-3, folic acid and selenium, but this is something that is often ignored by mental health professionals. Balanced eating helps us feel energetic and reduces our risk of some illnesses. Eating healthily on its own will not prevent illness; however, healthy eating can help reduce our risk of some diseases. It is not easy to change our eating habits and, therefore, if working with a patient to improve their diet, this should be done in a gradual way. What is important is the preparation of well-balanced meals, making healthy food choices, and maintaining a healthy weight.

It is important to emphasize that eating a healthy diet does not mean stopping eating favourite foods altogether, but is about making healthier food choices and eating in moderation.

Some of the important components of a healthy diet are covered in more depth in this section and include: consuming a variety of foods; establishing regular meal times; and avoiding overeating.

Consuming a variety of foods

It is important that we eat a variety of different foods to ensure that we get all the essential nutrients we need. These include: carbohydrates, fats, proteins, vitamins and minerals. Some people take food supplements that include vitamins, but these are not as good as eating a well balanced diet which includes a variety of different food groups.

- *Carbohydrates* give us vital energy and should therefore make up the majority of our food intake each day. There are two types of carbohydrates, simple and complex. So-called simple carbohydrates refer to sugars which are found in fruit and some dairy produce. Complex carbohydrates can be found in pasta, rice, bread, grains, potatoes and other vegetables. Some carbohydrates are less good for us (sometimes called refined carbohydrates) and are usually high in sugar, (e.g. honey, cakes, syrup, processed foods). These tend to cause undesirable peaks and troughs in blood sugar levels and tend to offer little in the way of nutritional value.

- *Fats* fall into two main types, saturated and unsaturated (which includes polyunsaturated and monounsaturated fats). Fats help give us energy and are essential for helping us grow, gain strength and repair damaged tissue. However, excessive consumption of fats leads to them being stored in our bodies, resulting in weight gain and an increased risk of heart disease.

- *Proteins* provide us with energy and are required by our bodies to help maintain our immune system, help fight infection and repair tissues that have been damaged. Protein is contained in meat, fish, poultry, eggs and other dairy products. Some protein can also be found in nuts and seeds, as well as in some vegetables. Vegetable proteins are high in fibre and low in fat and contain no cholesterol.

- *Vitamins and minerals* help us to build strong bones and muscles. If we eat a good variety of foods, we are more likely to get the right amount of vitamins and minerals to ensure our bodies function properly. In the main, there is no need to take supplements of vitamins and minerals. However, some people, at certain times of their lives, may require additional vitamins or minerals. This should be recommended and supervised by the patient's GP, as too much of some vitamins or minerals can actually be detrimental to one's health.

A balanced diet

The Food Standards Agency recommend that a healthy daily diet should comprise the following:

- 30% fruit and vegetables
- 30% bread, potatoes, rice or pasta
- 15% milk and dairy products
- 15% meat and fish
- 10% fat and sugary foods

Fruit and vegetables

People who eat a lot of fruit and vegetables have been found to have a lower risk of disease, including some cancers and heart disease. It is therefore recommended that people eat at least five portions of fruit and vegetables every day, regardless of whether those vegetables are tinned, frozen, fresh, dried or cooked.

Bread, potatoes, rice and pasta

These foods contain the starchy carbohydrates that are the body's main source of energy, and are all very filling. Unrefined carbohydrates are a better choice than refined ones. Refined carbohydrates are those that have been manufactured in some way (e.g. white bread, pasta and noodles made from white flour). Unrefined carbohydrates contain whole grains and are higher in fibre and stop us feeling hungry for longer (e.g. wholegrain rice and bread, wholewheat pasta).

Protein

As well as meat and fish, this food group contains poultry, beans, nuts, soya products and vegetable protein foods. These foods are high in protein. As mentioned earlier, protein is essential in our diets as it helps maintain our immune system, fight infection and repair tissues that have been damaged. Vegetarians and vegans need to be extra careful to ensure that there is enough protein in their diets. Main sources of protein for vegetarians come from eggs, nuts, beans, seeds, pulses and soya. As vegans do not eat dairy products or eggs, they can obtain the required proteins by combining foods such as nuts, seeds, pulses and soya.

Milk and dairy products

As well as milk, also included within this food group are cheese, yoghurt and fromage frais. It is important to note that butter, margarine and cream do not fall into this group but stay in the Fatty and Sugary group of foods. The foods in this group are particularly rich in calcium, which is a mineral that strengthens bones and teeth. It helps us grow and gives strength to our bones. People who have not consumed enough calcium in their diets until the age of around 35 will have an increased risk of developing osteoporosis (a form of brittle bone disease). Vegans must look for alternatives to milk and dairy products to ensure adequate intake of calcium. This can be obtained from soya milk, dark green leafy vegetables such as spinach, broccoli and watercress, almonds, sesame seeds, and dried foods such as dates and figs.

Fat and sugar

This is the food group that we should consume only small amounts of, as it contains the least nutrients. As mentioned earlier, fats fall into two groups: saturated and unsaturated fats. Saturated fat is found in lard, butter, whole milk, hard margarine and those products that have any of these as ingredients (e.g. cakes, pies, pastries, biscuits, chocolate). It is best to keep consumption of saturated fat low, as it is linked with obesity and increased risk of heart disease. Unsaturated fat is much healthier than saturated fat and is found in vegetable, sunflower, soya, sesame and olive oils; soft margarine and oily fish (e.g. sardines, pilchards and mackerel).

Sugary foods tend to taste lovely and it can feel like a real treat having food from this group. However, it is best to keep them as treats, rather than a regular feature in one's daily diet, as they are often also high in fat and can cause tooth decay. Sugary foods include items like cakes, chocolate, pastries, etc.

How to cut down on fatty and sugary foods

- Make fresh and dried fruits available for snacks, instead of crisps and chocolate
- Buy only lean cuts of meat, and trim off any fat
- Reduce the amount of food that is fried, and instead use methods such as grilling, poaching, steaming and baking
- Switch to semi-skimmed or skimmed milk instead of whole
- Swap lard, butter and hard margarine for vegetable oil and low-fat spreads

---

The Department of Health recommends that fat intake should be no more than around 76g per day for the average woman and 100g per day for the average man.

Many of us enjoy sugary foods and it is unrealistic to expect people to cut them out of their diets altogether; the answer is to eat them sparingly as the odd treat.

Achieving and maintaining a healthy weight

Being a healthy weight is extremely important for all of us as it can have a direct impact on our health. This does not mean that we have to be skinny. Images portrayed in the media are often misleading and, in reality, being too thin can lead to health problems in itself. A person's healthy weight will be determined by a number of factors, including: age; genetics; activity level; how much of the person's weight is fat; and any physical problems that affect weight. If a person needs to change their weight, there are two main factors in doing so: eating habits and level of activity.

Eating habits

There are a number of common problems associated with eating habits that interfere with achieving and maintaining a healthy weight. Here are some of them:

Snacking

This is a common problem. It can be relatively easy to mindlessly munch one's way through a packet of biscuits, sweets or crisps while watching television or reading. The secret is to plan ahead, to make available more healthy snacks such as fresh fruit and raw vegetables, and to limit the amount of junk food available. Another useful technique is to eat only when there is no other stimulation (such as television), so an awareness is raised of exactly how much food is being consumed. A designated eating area can help here (e.g. at the dining table).

Comfort eating

Many people find themselves eating because of negative emotional states (e.g. boredom, unhappiness, loneliness, etc.). Like snacking, it is easy to lose track of how much has been eaten at these times. Again, availability of healthy foods is helpful (e.g. fruit, raw vegetables). However, there are times when healthy foods just don't hit the spot, and the person may have a craving for junk food that no amount of fresh fruit and vegetables will satisfy. It can be helpful at these times to keep a diary of eating and moods. By doing this, the person can begin to anticipate these situations and do something else instead (e.g. go for a walk, phone a friend, do a jigsaw puzzle, etc.). Some activity that is non-conducive to eating is the best kind of distraction technique.

A dislike for healthy foods

Eating healthily does not mean cutting out all foods that a person likes, but reducing the intake of non-healthy foods and increasing healthier options. This might mean cooking food in a different way (e.g. grilling as opposed to frying, increasing the amount of green vegetables and reducing the number of potatoes, etc.). It is unrealistic to go for a complete change in diet, which may only result in the person being unable to stick to the new regime and possibly giving up. If a person is partial to lots of chocolate, it is unreasonable to expect them to give it up altogether. However, limiting the amount of chocolate consumed to one bar instead of four would seem reasonable, and that one bar could be looked forward to as a real treat.

Making too much food and not wanting it to go to waste

This can be a particular problem for those people who live alone. It can sometimes be the case that the person ends up eating two meals. The recommendation, if this is the case, is for the person to measure out exactly the right proportion of ingredients for the meal. If there is any food left over, rather than have it sitting on the table and available for plate top-ups, it can be stored away and left for the next day or put in the freezer for another time.

Nutrition specific to mental health

Many mental health professionals know little about nutrition, and it is rarely used as a therapeutic approach to mental health problems. However, the public in general have been found to be increasingly interested in the role of nutrition in physical and mental health. Many people with mental health problems may already have experimented with dietary changes and may have found benefit in doing so. Some may have reduced sugar and saturated fat consumption and increased their intake of oily fish. *Nutrition and Mental Health*, published by the Northern Centre for Mental Health (2004), recommends that there be a stronger focus on applying the available evidence base around nutrition to mental health problems.

Omega-3

It has been found that people with depression tend to have low levels of Omega-3 fatty acid in the blood. It has been shown that the lower the blood level of Omega-3, the more severe the depression. Therefore, patients with depression should be recommended to increase their intake of Omega-3, either with food supplements or increasing their intake of oily fish. It has been found that relatively small amounts of Omega-3 fatty acids in the diet (as little as two fish meals a week) can help protect us against depression.

Folic acid

There is increasing evidence that a deficiency in folic acid is associated with depression. Encouraging patients to eat the recommended five pieces of fruit and vegetables a day and breakfast cereals fortified with folic acid helps to increase levels of folic acid in the blood. People who are unable or do not want to follow these recommendations are likely to benefit from folic acid supplements.

Selenium

Selenium is a mineral which helps enhance our immune system. There is evidence that low levels of selenium are linked to depression, anxiety and anger problems. The best source of selenium is Brazil nuts, and only one or two a day provides adequate selenium to meet full daily intake requirements. Selenium can also be found in meat, poultry and fish.

Caffeine

Drinks containing caffeine (e.g. coffee, tea, cola, etc.) should be consumed sparingly, as caffeine can increase the physical symptoms of anxiety, especially in those people who are prone to anxiety and panic attacks.

Physical activity

Regular physical activity is a vital part of a healthy lifestyle. Some people have never been very active and others may have given up physical activity because of depression, work overload or other problems.

Long periods of inactivity lead to weakness, tiredness, high blood pressure, weight gain and depression. The best cure for inactivity is exercise, which has been shown to help lift our moods and make us feel better about ourselves, as well as making us fitter and reducing our blood pressure, increasing energy levels, improving our levels of strength and stamina and helping us reduce weight and increase our self-confidence. Sometimes people think that exercise necessitates hours of painful hard slog at the gym, when it does not have to be that way. Even short periods of gentle exercise can improve fitness levels and a person's mood.

Becoming more physically active

One way of encouraging patients to become more physically active is to encourage them to set aside some time for a formal exercise programme which might include activities such as walking, jogging, swimming, aerobic exercise classes, exercise video tapes, or tennis, etc. However, little things like getting off the bus a stop early, gardening, dancing to a song on the radio, taking the stairs instead of the lift, leaving the car at home when the journey is relatively short, or parking further away from the final destination and walking instead, all help and should be actively encouraged. The important thing to get across to patients who need to become more physically active is that exercise does not need to be something that is dreaded; it can and should be fun.

When someone is depressed, increasing activity is a crucial step in recovery and can bring about rapid improvements in mood. It is important to ensure that the person is encouraged not to be overambitious – little is better than nothing, and even a small amount of physical activity can bring about significant improvement in feelings of well-being and better mood. Encouraging patients who haven't exercised at all for years to start a highly active exercise regime is likely to result in failure, which in turn will be discouraging for the person, who may give up before even really getting started. Therefore it is important to start slowly and increase gradually.

Barriers to exercise

Although most of us want to be fit and we know that it makes us feel healthier, it can be difficult to get started, and we can make excuses for not doing it. Some common barriers and possible remedies include the following:

Lack of time

Sometimes people say that they do not have the time for physical activity (e.g. overworked Tim with his busy job and high stress levels may find it difficult to see how he could possibly make time in his day for exercise). In reality, we all have the same amount of time, it is just that we choose to spend it differently or demands make it difficult to make time for ourselves. Really, we should all make some time for physical activity; it does not have to be a lot. As little as five minutes a day is a start, and is definitely better than no exercise at all.

Tiredness

Feeling down or depressed can lead to feelings of listlessness and lack of energy. This can also happen when a person is just out of shape. Regular exercise actually helps reduce tiredness, leads to increased energy levels and improves sleep.

Finding exercise boring

Exercise can be boring if the person forces themselves to do a physical activity that they do not enjoy (an hour at the gym does not appeal to some people). The important thing to emphasize is to make it as much fun as possible, by doing it with other people for instance, or playing favourite songs on a personal stereo while exercising. Variety in the types of exercises the person does is also important to stop boredom setting in.

Fear of failure

Some people avoid starting anything new in case they do not do it successfully. If this is the case, it is important for the person to learn to be proud of what they have done, rather than to focus on what they have not been able to do. Negative thoughts about failure lend themselves very well to thought evaluation (see *Working with Thoughts* in Section 4e).

Controlled drinking

The odd drink now and again does no harm, but, for some people, social drinking can lead to much heavier consumption which can increase the person's risk of developing serious health problems. Government-recommended 'sensible drinking' guidelines were developed on the basis of careful consideration of the harmful, and some beneficial, effects of drinking at different levels.

The 'sensible drinking' message was first referred to in the government's 1992 'Health of the Nation' White paper.

This recommended that men should con-sume no more than 21, and women no more than 14, units per week. However, consumption at these unit levels has been recommended by the Health Education Authority since 1987 (when the term 'units' was first coined), prior to which the message had been expressed in terms of 'standard drinks'.

In 1995, in recognition of the dangers of excessive drinking in a single session, the sensible drinking message was changed to focus on daily guidelines. It suggests:

- A maximum intake of 2–3 units per day for women and 3–4 for men, with two alcohol-free days after heavy drinking; continued alcohol consumption at the upper level is not advised
- Intake of up to two units a day can have a moderate protective effect against heart disease for men over 40 and post-menopausal women
- Some groups, such as pregnant women and those engaging in potentially dangerous activities (such as operating heavy machinery), should drink less, or nothing at all

(This text has been taken from the Alcohol Harm Reduction Strategy for England. Prime Minister's Strategy Unit: Cabinet Office 2004-11-16, and is acknowledged as Crown Copyright. www. strategy.gov.uk.)

Asking about alcohol problems: the CAGE questionnaire

1. Have you ever felt you ought to **C**ut down on your drinking?
2. Have people **A**nnoyed you by criticising your drinking?
3. Have you every felt bad or **G**uilty about your drinking?
4. Have you ever had a drink first thing in the morning to steady your nerves or get rid of a hangover (**E**ye-opener)?

Two or more 'Yes' responses yield a positive screen test for alcohol.

Note: one unit of alcohol is roughly the equivalent of half a pint of beer or cider, a pub measure of spirits (e.g. gin, vodka, rum, whisky), and a small glass of wine (125ml).

Someone who has problems with alcohol is likely to have:
- A strong desire to drink alcohol
- Difficulty controlling how much they drink
- An increased tolerance to alcohol
- Signs of withdrawal when without alcohol

The box contains the CAGE questionnaire, which can be used with patients when assessing alcohol problems.

If a patient has problems with excessive alcohol intake and has difficulty controlling their drinking when given common-sense information and encouragement, it may be appropriate to refer them to specialist services or signpost them to a specialist agency where people have specialist skills in helping with these types of problems.

Smoking

Stopping smoking is an obvious positive step towards a healthier lifestyle. Smoking cessation groups can offer a great help in supporting people who wish to stop smoking. Smoking increases a person's risk of developing cancer, heart disease and other serious illnesses. Stopping smoking is not easy and takes a great deal of willpower for the person to succeed. As the nicotine in tobacco is addictive, people will experience withdrawal symptoms on stopping smoking. This can result in the person feeling depressed, angry and irritable. People can also feel restless, anxious, find it difficult to concentrate and can have difficulty getting to sleep.

There are a number of products available to help smokers give up the habit. One option is nicotine replacement therapy (NRT), which continues to provide the body with nicotine but without the harmful chemicals contained in cigarettes. NRT is available in the form of patches, gum, inhalers and even a nasal spray. The NHS also provides help through smoking cessation clinics. Any patient who wants to stop smoking can be referred to one of these clinics for the appropriate help and support, and signposted to other appropriate agencies as needed. Help for stopping smoking is likely to include attending meetings and access to telephone support.

In summary

It cannot be underestimated how important lifestyle factors are to mental health. However, it is not realistic to expect patients to make all the changes necessary, immediately, to lead a healthy lifestyle by stopping smoking, exercising for 20 minutes a day, and eating a healthy diet. It is important to support gradual change and to break down these activities into small, manageable steps. An early step might be to switch from full-fat to semi-skimmed milk and to grill the main meal of the day instead of using a frying pan. A second step might be to start eating at least one piece of fruit a day and introducing light exercise.

Using a gradual, stepped approach is far more likely to bring about sustainable improvements than making radical changes in one fell swoop, which are unsustainable and likely to result in failure and despondency. It can be highly motivating and self-reinforcing if people can see what is being achieved; therefore, encouraging patients to keep a diary will help keep motivation going, show the patient how well they are doing and increasing their ability to deal with setbacks if they occur.

The mental health worker should emphasize the benefits the patient may gain from increasing their intake of Omega-3, folic acid and selenium, and decreasing their caffeine intake.

Section summary

- A healthy diet should comprise: 30% fruit and vegetables; 30% bread, potatoes, rice or pasta; 15% milk and dairy products; 15% meat and fish; 10% fat and sugary foods
- Patients with mental health problems may benefit from raising their levels of Omega-3,

folic acid and selenium, and reducing their caffeine intake

- Increasing activity can improve mood
- Alcohol recommendations are a maximum intake of 2–3 units per day for women and 3–4 for men, with two alcohol-free days after heavy drinking
- Intake of up to two units of alcohol a day can have a moderate protective effect against heart disease for men over 40 and post-menopausal women
- Smoking cessation clinics can offer help for patients wanting to stop smoking
- Patient's requiring help to increase the healthiness of their lifestyle should be encouraged to make changes using small, manageable steps

References

Department of Health (1992). *Health of the Nation White Paper*. London: HMSO.

Food Standards Agency. www.food.gov.uk.

Holford, P. (2005). *Optimum Nutrition for the Mind*. London: Piatkus.

Peet, M. (2004). *Nutrition and mental health*. Durham: Northern Centre for Mental Health.

Test yourself

 To check your progress, locate this section on CD-ROM 3 and work through the interactive questions at the end.

Chapter 3.5
Patient pathways

Aim

To provide an overview of pathways and outcomes for patients with common mental health problems managed in primary care.

Learning outcomes

By the end of this Chapter, the reader will be able to:

- Appreciate the overall management of a range of patients with common mental health problems
- Critically evaluate potential patient pathways in primary care
- Understand the role of clinical decision-making in managing the care of patients with common mental health problems in primary care

Introduction

Chapter 3.5 will follow the progress of all the patients featured in the programme. (You might find it useful to revisit the video and audio clips or their transcripts.) Particular attention is given to the clinical interventions and guided self-help received from their mental health workers. Although these are all hypothetical patients, each illustrates fairly typical presentations for those encountered in the primary care setting.

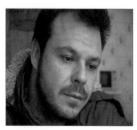

Nigel (Depression)

Session 1

Assessment: Nigel, 45, presented as moderately depressed, and, although his GP, Dr Rushforth, was keen for him to start anti-

depressant medication, Nigel was reluctant to go down this route. He did not present as a significant suicide risk.

Problem statement: Difficulty engaging in normal routine due to low mood since breakdown of marriage, resulting in being off work and social withdrawal.

Goals:
- To re-establish old routine to enable me to return to full-time work.
- To see friends twice a week for sport and other leisure activities.

Nigel was asked to complete a PHQ-9 and CORE-OM. His PHQ-9 score was 14 and his CORE-OM scores were: Subjective well-being 7; Problems 22; Functioning 19; Risk 1. From this assessment session, Nigel was asked to keep a monitoring diary of his activity levels for one week. A copy of Nigel's diary is available in PDF format on CD-ROM 3.

Sessions 2–4

Sessions 2 and 3 were conducted face-to-face, while the fourth session was conducted by telephone. All were held weekly. It was clear that Nigel's activity levels were limited and he was therefore encouraged to increase them gradually. For example, he was encouraged to get dressed within twenty minutes of waking up, gradually start dealing with unopened mail, and go for more walks, which had previously been part of his usual routine. He had been neglecting his garden which had previously been a source of great pleasure for him, so he began to gradually spend more and more time tending to the garden. This activity was time-limited to 10 minutes initially, and gradually increased. He also arranged to see his children over the weekend and went out for lunch with them, which brought about a sense of pleasure as he enjoyed spending time with them.

His mental health worker, Waseem, discussed Nigel's diet with Dr Rushforth and recommended that Nigel start taking Omega-3 and increasing his selenium and folic acid levels. Dr Rushforth agreed this was a good idea. Consequently, Waseem discussed Nigel's diet with him and, as he had a liking for oily fish but was not currently eating any and had a reduced intake of fruit and fresh vegetables, he agreed to increase his intake of these food products. He also liked nuts and agreed to eat two Brazil nuts a day to increase his selenium levels.

Sessions 5–7

By session 5, Nigel was beginning to notice some minor improvement in his mood with his change in diet and behavioural activation. At session 6 Nigel completed the measures again. His scores had improved. His PHQ-9 was now 11 and his CORE-OM scores were: Subjective well-being 5; Problems 17; Functioning 15; Risk 0. These three sessions were conducted over the telephone on a weekly basis.

Sessions 8–12

Nigel met with Waseem for session 8, when they discussed examining his negative automatic thoughts, particularly in relation to him seeing himself as weak and pathetic for suffering from depression.

Waseem kept in contact with Nigel via telephone over the next four sessions to monitor progress with behavioural activation and the introduction of working with his thoughts. By session 10, Nigel had made a gradual return to work and the frequency of appointments was reduced to fortnightly. At session 12, measures were completed again. His PHQ-9 score was now 7 and his CORE-OM scores were: Subjective well-being 3; Problems 9; Functioning 9; Risk 0. Nigel was now back at work full time and coping well. (See the PDF of Nigel's diary.)

Sessions 13–15

These sessions were all conducted over the telephone and spaced out by four weeks between each contact. At session 15 the measures were completed one last time. His PHQ-9 score was now 2 and his CORE-OM scores were: Subjective well-being 1; Problems 4; Functioning 5; Risk 0. Relapse prevention was also discussed at this stage, and Nigel completed an 'Early Warning Signs' sheet.

Nigel's Early Warning Signs	
Emotions	Feeling lower in mood (especially in the morning) Feeling irritated with self
Physical	Difficulty getting off to sleep Waking up early Appetite reduced Feeling tired a lot of the time
Cognitive	Increase in negative thoughts Poor concentration
Behaviours	Avoiding going out socially Letting the house get untidy Staying in bed longer than usual Not dealing with mail

Telephone session eight weeks later

A telephone call was made to Nigel and he reported that he continued to feel well. He acknowledged that the eight-week gap in the telephone calls was helpful, in that, although he was continuing to do well, he appreciated being able to talk through with Waseem how he was getting on. They negotiated that Waseem would continue to call him on a two-monthly basis for a further five occasions, and review what further help Nigel needed at that time.

Five more calls on a two-monthly basis

Nigel remained in remission from his depression. By the last of the five calls, Nigel had joined an internet dating agency, and, despite experiencing some initial anxiety about this, had found it a positive experience. He had been on three dates and, although he had not met anyone he felt he wanted to develop a long-term relationship with, he was continuing to enjoy it. Waseem and Nigel agreed to a telephone session in six months time, with a final session anticipated in a further six months.

Calls at 6 and 12 months

Nigel remained in good spirits and was continuing to work full-time. By the final telephone session, he was dating a woman he had met through the internet dating agency, and he reported that they were both enjoying being in a relationship. During this period he had met with Dr Rushforth to review progress. It was at this stage that Nigel and Waseem agreed that no further contact was required. Table 2 summarizes the amount of contact time Waseem spent with Nigel.

Table 2: Summary of Waseem's time spent in contact with Nigel.

Type of session	Number spent	Time	Total time
Face-to-face	1 x 40min, 3 x 20min	1hr 40min	
			4hr 50min
Telephone	19 x 10min	3hr 10min	

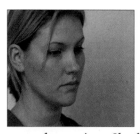

Sarah (Depression)

Session 1

Assessment: Sarah, 24, presented with a moderate depression. She had just started to take antidepressant medication, prescribed by her GP, Dr Mehra. Sarah was seen for assessment by her mental health worker, Katie, within a few days of having seen Dr Mehra. She was seen to be an ideal candidate for medication management and behavioural activation.

Problem statement: Lack of motivation and low energy levels due to low mood following redundancy, leading to loss of routine, no interest in finding another job, and withdrawal from an active social life.

Goals:
- To actively look for full-time employment.
- To see friends out socially at least twice a week.

Sarah was asked to complete the PHQ-9 and CORE-OM. Her PHQ-9 scores were 18 and her CORE-OM scores were: Subjective well-being 11; Problems or symptoms 29; Functioning 21; Risk 2. From this assessment session, Sarah was asked to keep a monitoring diary of her activity levels for one week. Sarah's partially completed diary, which she discussed with Katie at session 3, is included in PDF format on CD-ROM 3.

Session 2

This session was conducted by telephone one week after assessment, in keeping with recommended scheduled contact for medication management. Sarah was experiencing some side-effects of her medication (namely dry mouth and nausea), but felt these were tolerable and continued to take the medication. She agreed to read the antidepressant leaflet and complete the monitoring diary for the next session. She was also seen by her GP, Dr Mehra, for review, in keeping with NICE Guidelines for patients prescribed antidepressants who are considered to be a risk (e.g. all patients under the age of 30).

Session 3

This session was also conducted by telephone one week later. Fortunately, the side-effects of nausea and dry mouth had dissipated, and Sarah was beginning to notice a slight improvement in her mood at this stage. Sarah had completed the activity schedule used to monitor her activities for the week, which she discussed over the phone with Katie. The diary revealed that she lacked structure to her day and had limited levels of activity. Katie was keen to help Sarah re-establish some routine, and encouraged her to become more active. Sarah agreed to get up shortly after waking each day, do half an hour of ironing three days a week, and go for 15-minute walks on the days she was not doing the ironing.

Session 4

This session was conducted two weeks later by telephone. Sarah was starting to notice some more improvement in her mood and was beginning to be more active. She had no more problems with adverse effects of the medication. This session was used to look at how Sarah could build on her current level of activity, using behavioural activation strategies. Sarah and Katie agreed to talk again in two weeks time. Meanwhile Sarah was to continue to take the antidepressant medication and work on becoming more active.

Sessions 5–8

These sessions were all conducted by telephone and spaced at fortnightly intervals. By session 5, Sarah had been taking antidepressants for eight weeks and was noticeably brighter in mood. She was continuing to build on her confidence by going out again with her flatmate Karen, and was now feeling more able to fill her day with greater amounts of activity. The measures completed at assessment were repeated. Her PHQ-9 score was now 12 and her CORE-OM scores were: Subjective well-being 7; Problems 19; Functioning 14; Risk 0. Katie reported back to the GP about each contact she had with Sarah, using shared primary care records. At session 7, Sarah was also seen by Dr Mehra for a 12-week review of progress. It was also at session 7 that Sarah was being encouraged to look through the local newspaper to check the jobs section for employment that might suit her skills.

However, she was still somewhat concerned about her ability to return to full-time work. She was signposted to a local job club, which she attended and found to be of help in looking for opportunities and in completing application forms for jobs. At session 8, Sarah reported that she had applied for a part-time voluntary job in a local charity shop as a stepping-stone towards looking for paid, full-time work. Sarah's mood was clearly much improved at this stage. Sarah and Katie talked about what questions she might be asked in an interview and discussed ways of answering them. Sarah was continuing to find the help she was receiving from the local job club very useful.

Session 9

This telephone session was held four weeks later. Sarah was successful in her application for the voluntary work and was enjoying interacting with customers. She felt that her mood was brighter because she now had a reason to get up in the morning, giving structure to her day. She informed Katie that she had applied for two salaried jobs with help from the job club, and both interviews were to be held the following week.

Session 10

This was a telephone session held two weeks later. Sarah had been disappointed at not being successful in getting the first job she applied for and had spent an anxious few days waiting to hear how she had got on with the second one.

However, she was delighted to tell Katie that she had been successful in getting the second job, and was to start the following Monday. Despite the fact that Sarah had been working part-time in a voluntary capacity without difficulty, she was a little anxious about starting full-time paid employment. She had already used the thought diaries to address her concerns and had concluded that they were only natural under the circumstances.

Sessions 11–12

These sessions were both conducted by telephone on a four-weekly basis. At session 11, Sarah had started her new job and was beginning to settle in and enjoy it. The work was very similar to her previous job and she was pleased that her work colleagues were friendly towards her. At session 12, Sarah was coping well with work and enjoying a social life through her new job, as well as that already established with her flatmate Karen and other friends. Sarah completed the PHQ-9 and CORE-OM over the phone with Katie. Her PHQ-9 score was now 4 and her CORE-OM scores were: Subjective wellbeing 2; Problems 8; Functioning 6; Risk 0. It was agreed that Sarah was coping well and contact with Katie could be reduced to every two months for the next year and then reviewed again. Sarah had no objection to continuing medication for six months after remission. Katie sent Sarah information on relapse prevention and asked her to complete an 'Early Warning Signs' sheet for discussion next time they spoke.

Calls on a two-monthly basis for 12 months

Sarah's symptoms of depression remained in remission and she continued to enjoy work. She had completed her 'Early Warning Signs' sheet, which she talked through with Katie, as well as a plan of what she would do if she experienced any of these early warning signs. During this time she was reviewed by Dr Mehra, who was pleased with Sarah's progress. At the twelve-month stage, Sarah and Katie agreed to review progress after 6 and 12

Sarah's Early Warning Signs	
Emotions	Feeling lower in mood Feeling tearful
Physical	Waking up early Appetite reduced Feeling tired a lot of the time
Cognitive	Increase in negative thoughts Poor concentration
Behaviours	Avoiding going out socially Staying in bed longer Stopping exercising Not doing the housework

months by telephone.

Calls at 6 months and 12 months

Sarah continued to remain well and gradually reduced and discontinued her medication during this time. She remained well at final contact. Table 3 summarizes the amount of contact time Katie spent with Sarah.

Table 3: Summary of Katie's time spent in contact with Sarah.

Type of session	Number spent	Time	Total time
Face-to-face	1 x 40min	40min	4hr 40min
Telephone	10 x 15min, 9 x 10min	4hr	

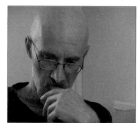

Julian (Depression)

Session 1

Assessment: Julian, 46, presented as being severely depressed and actively suicidal. His mental health worker, Waseem, was extremely concerned about his safety and stayed with Julian until he was seen by his GP (Dr Attenborough). Julian was admitted straight away to the local psychiatric hospital, where he underwent an assessment by the psychiatrist. He agreed to stay voluntarily and after a 4-week hospital stay was discharged home and into the care of the community mental health team (CMHT). He had no further contact with Waseem. Table 4 summarizes the amount of contact time Waseem spent with Julian.

Table 4: Summary of Waseem's time spent in contact with Julian.

Type of session	Number spent	Time	Total time
Face-to-face	1 x 30min	30min	30min
Telephone	0	0	

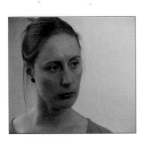

Alison (Panic Disorder)

Session 1

Assessment: Alison, 31, was experiencing frequent and disabling panic attacks that were occurring up to three times a week. She found that she was becoming preoccupied with concerns about when the next panic attack would occur. During a panic attack she would experience palpitations, tingling, shortness of breath and chest pain, which she would interpret as being a sign that she was experiencing a heart attack.

Problem statement: Panic attacks occurring unpredictably, leading me to be pre-occupied about when I may have one again; scanning my body for symptoms that may suggest I'm about to have a heart attack; resulting in escape from situations when the symptoms come on and avoidance of situations where they have previously occurred.

Goals:

- To go shopping twice a week with minimal anxiety to places where a panic attack has occurred previously.
- To use strategies to reduce anxiety and to remain wherever I am until symptoms pass.

Alison was asked to keep a diary of her panic attacks over the following week, using the four-column thought diary. The diary recording Alison's panic attacks for the week is included in PDF format on CD-ROM 3. She was also given literature to read about Panic Disorder and asked to complete the CORE-OM and WSAS for the next session.

Session 2

This was a face-to-face session held one week later. Alison had completed the two measures as agreed. Her CORE-OM scores were: Subjective well-being 5; Problems 21; Functioning 8; Risk 0. Her WSAS scores were: Work 2; Home management 5; Social leisure activities 6; Private leisure activities 2; Relationships 0; Total = 15.

Alison talked through the two panic attacks she had experienced over the week. Her mental health worker, Waseem, offered psycho-education about Panic Disorder and then introduced her to the nine-column thought diary (also available in PDF format on CD-ROM 3). They used the panic attack that she had experienced in the department store as an example, as this was the most severe of the two. Waseem helped Alison look at the evidence for and against the interpretations of her symptoms being a sign that she was having a heart attack.

Despite the overwhelming evidence that Alison was not about to suffer a heart attack, she remained somewhat sceptical. Evaluating a thought like this only once is unlikely to shift the belief in it completely, and may need to be repeated many times. Alison agreed to keep a copy of the balanced thought written on a card (this is sometimes referred to as a flashcard), so that she could easily remind herself that her symptoms were not dangerous when they came on.

Session 3

This session was conducted face-to-face one week later. Since the last session, Alison had used the flashcard during a panic attack to remind herself that her symptoms were not dangerous. Although this had helped to some degree, she had still felt the need to leave the situation. Waseem introduced the controlled breathing technique, which Alison was asked to practise over the following fortnight.

Sessions 4–6

Sessions 4 and 5 were conducted by telephone on a weekly basis. Alison continued to use her flashcard and practised the breathing technique with increasing success. By session 6, which was a face-to-face contact, she was now encouraged to stay in situations rather than escape, to give her symptoms an opportunity to pass without avoidant behaviour. Alison was initially reluctant to do this and Waseem spent time discussing the habituation graph again, which Alison agreed made sense.

Session 7

This session was conducted by telephone two weeks later. Alison reported staying in a supermarket where she experienced panic symptoms and, although she felt immense discomfort for around 20 minutes, the symptoms gradually passed. This gave her confidence to try this in other situations in which she experienced panic symptoms, and she agreed to go back to a supermarket she had been avoiding following a severe panic attack, prior to seeing Waseem.

Session 8

Again this session was conducted by telephone, three weeks later. Alison reported that she had visited the supermarket that she had been avoiding, and had managed to stay there despite experiencing some degree of anxiety and panic. She reported feeling much better and that panic symptoms were hugely reduced, resulting in her feeling that there was nowhere that she would avoid for fear of developing panic symptoms. Her belief that she had something wrong with her heart had reduced to 0% when she was calm and 10% when she was panicking. Waseem and Alison discussed relapse prevention and agreed to talk in four weeks' time to review progress, with a view to discontinuing contact if all was still going well.

Session 9

Alison reported in this telephone session, four weeks later, that she was continuing to make progress and now found that she was able to enter situations that had previously been difficult, without using the breathing technique or carrying the flashcard as a reminder. She had not had a panic attack for over six weeks. She repeated the two measures she had completed at assessment. Her CORE-OM scores were:

Subjective well-being 2; Problems 6; Functioning 2; Risk 0. Her WSAS scores were: Work 0, Home management 1; Social leisure activities 1; Private leisure activities 0, Relationships 0; Total = 2. No further contact was arranged. Table 5 summarizes the amount of contact time Waseem spent with Alison.

Table 5: Summary of Waseem's time spent in contact with Alison.

Type of session	Number spent	Time	Total time
Face-to-face	1 x 40min, 3 x 30min	2hr 10min	
			3hr 15min
Telephone	3 x 15min, 2 x 10min	1hr 5min	

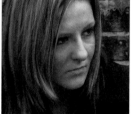

Lorraine (Specific Phobia)

Session 1

Assessment: Lorraine, 22, presented with a driving phobia, which developed after a road traffic accident. Post Traumatic Stress Disorder had been ruled out by her GP. Her problem was highly specific to driving.

Problem statement: Avoidance of driving due to symptoms of anxiety and fear of being involved in another accident, leading to lack of independence and reliance on my Mum to drive me places.

Goal:
* To drive alone, with minimal anxiety, in busy traffic, including using roundabouts and other junctions where stopping and starting are necessary, on a daily basis.

Lorraine was asked to complete the CORE-OM and WSAS for the next session, and given information to read about anxiety. She was also asked to consider the steps that would need to be taken to reach her goals, with a view to working together to devise a hierarchy at their next session.

Session 2

Lorraine had completed the two measures. Her CORE-OM scores were: Subjective well-being 5; Problems 21; Functioning 8; Risk 0. Her WSAS scores were: Work 4; Home management 0; Social leisure 6; Private leisure 0; Relationships 0; Total = 10. Lorraine and her mental health worker, Waseem, devised a hierarchy to tackle her driving phobia.

Lorraine's Driving Hierarchy

1 Sit accompanied, in driver's seat of car, with engine off.
2 Sit alone, in driver's seat of car, with engine off.
3 Sit accompanied, in driver's seat of stationary car, with engine on.
4 Sit alone, in driver's seat of stationary car, with engine on.
5 Having been driven to an industrial estate by someone, drive round at a quiet time, accompanied.
6 Having been driven to an industrial estate by someone, drive round at a quiet time, alone.
7 Drive accompanied, round quiet streets at times when there is little traffic, including roundabouts and junctions in journey.
8 Drive alone, round quiet streets at times when there is little traffic, including roundabouts and junctions in journey.
9 Drive accompanied, round busy areas, including roundabouts and junctions in journey.
10 Drive alone, round busy areas, including roundabouts and junctions in journey.

Sessions 3–5

These sessions were conducted by telephone on a weekly basis. Lorraine steadily worked through her hierarchy with the help of her Mum, who accompanied her for steps 1, 3, 5, 6, 7 and 9. She experienced some anxiety at each step, but each seemed manageable when it was

reached, and her anxiety soon dissipated as she engaged in prolonged, repeated and graded exposure. She used an Exposure Practice Diary (included in PDF format on CD-ROM 3) to record the steps she took and the anxiety she experienced, which illustrated the improvement she reported.

Session 6

By session 6, held two weeks later, Lorraine was able to drive to the appointment alone. At this, Lorraine's final session, relapse prevention was discussed, and Waseem arranged to telephone her in eight weeks' time to check progress with a view to that being their last contact if all was well. Lorraine also completed the measures again at this stage. She scored 0 on all the subscales of the CORE-OM and WSAS.

Follow-up telephone call eight weeks later

Lorraine continued to do well and was now driving alone with no difficulty whatsoever. They agreed that no further contact was needed. Table 6 summarizes the amount of contact time Waseem spent with Lorraine.

Table 6: Summary of Waseem's time spent in contact with Lorraine.

Type of session	Number spent	Time	Total time
Face-to-face	3 x 30min	1hr 30min	2hr 10min
Telephone	4 x 10min	40 min	

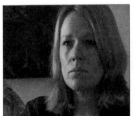

Deborah (Agoraphobia)

Session 1

Assessment: Deborah, 42, presented with a disabling Agoraphobia, which started during recuperation from a physical illness for which she had been hospitalized and that required a period of recovery at home. By the time she was physically able to go out, she found that she had lost her confidence and was fearful of fainting, despite the fact that this had never actually happened to her.

She was highly dependent on her husband, Paul, to do the shopping and other activities that required leaving the house. When Deborah came to see the mental health worker, Waseem, she was keen to regain her independence and to work on her difficulties, but she just wasn't sure how to start.

Problem statement: Avoidance of leaving home alone due to symptoms of anxiety and fear of fainting, leading to becoming increasingly housebound and dependent on Paul.

Goals:

- To go shopping with minimal anxiety, alone, at busy times at least once a week.
- To use public transport with minimal anxiety, alone, at busy times at least once a week.

She was asked to complete the CORE-OM and WSAS for the next appointment and given information to read about Agoraphobia.

Session 2

Deborah had completed the two measures two weeks later. Her CORE-OM scores were: Subjective well-being 4; Problems 12; Functioning 8; Risk 0. Her WSAS scores were: Work 7; Home management 6; Social leisure activities 6; Private leisure activities 6; Relationships 0; Total = 25. Waseem spent time educating Deborah about the nature of anxiety and the role of graded exposure, which he demonstrated using a habituation graph. Time was spent developing two hierarchies to help Deborah break down tasks into small manageable steps towards her two goals. She agreed to tackle the first step on the public transport hierarchy during the following week on several occasions.

Sessions 3 to 6

These sessions were all conducted face-to-face on a weekly basis. Over these four sessions, Deborah was introduced, firstly, to the four-column thought diary, then to the nine-column thought diary, to help tackle her fears of fainting. As Deborah had learned at the assessment session that fainting was not a symptom of anxiety, there had already been a slight change in how strongly she believed she would faint. However, when in an anxiety-provoking situation, she found it difficult to believe that this would not happen and this would lead to an escalation in her anxiety. A combination of evaluating this thought with Waseem and graded exposure, which encouraged her to stay in progressively difficult situations, was helping to shift this belief.

Deborah's Hierarchy for Tackling Public Transport

1. Stand at bus stop with Paul, and allow buses to go past until anxiety no higher than 20 on the 0–100 scale.
2. Stand at bus stop unaccompanied, and allow buses to go past until anxiety no higher than 20 on the 0–100 scale.
3. Get on bus and go on circular route at a quiet time (approximately 1 hour 10 minutes), sitting on the outside seat at the front of the bus with Paul sitting beside me
4. Ditto with Paul sitting in seat behind me.
5. Ditto with Paul sitting several seats behind me.
6. Ditto with Paul being present for half of the journey then getting off bus and getting back on when bus passes back on other side, twenty minutes later.
7. Ditto with Paul present for the first two stops only, and getting on for the final two stops.
8. Ditto with Paul seeing me off on bus and meeting me when I get off.
9. Do entire journey, including leaving and returning home, alone.
10. Ditto but at a busier time.
11. Ditto but at an extremely busy time.

By session 5, Deborah had progressed well with the public transport hierarchy and had sufficiently renewed confidence to begin working through the supermarket hierarchy. It was at this stage that it became clear that Paul was starting to have some difficulty in coping with Deborah's new-found independence, despite her need for him to support her through most of her hierarchies. At session 6, Waseem suggested that Paul join the carers' group held at the surgery, which he agreed to think about.

Sessions 7–10

At session 7 (a face-to-face session), Deborah was asked to complete the measures again. Her scores had improved. Her CORE-OM scores were: Subjective well-being 2; Problems 9; Functioning 5; Risk 0. Her WSAS scores were; Work 5; Home management 3; Social leisure 3; Private leisure 2; Relationships 0; Total = 13. Over the next three sessions, held fortnightly and conducted by telephone, Deborah continued to make good progress. By this time, Paul was now attending the carers' group, which he found helpful in offering him support. By session 10, Deborah was able to travel by bus unaccompanied at reasonably busy times, but she had not yet tackled rush hour. She was also able to separate from Paul in the supermarket for periods of up to 10 minutes when she would be unable to see what aisle he was in.

Sessions 11–13

These sessions were conducted by telephone on a fortnightly basis. Deborah continued to make good progress, and by session 13 was travelling by bus at busy times alone and was able to go to the supermarket unaccompanied at quiet times. It was acknowledged that there was still work to do, but Deborah was managing well with Paul's support. It was agreed that they would meet in four weeks' time to review progress, discuss relapse prevention and repeat the CORE-OM and WSAS measures again.

Session 14

In this face-to-face session four weeks later, Deborah reported that she was continuing to make progress and the previous day she had gone to the supermarket on the bus at a busy time and shopped alone with minimal difficulty. Relapse prevention was discussed and measures repeated, which mirrored the improvement that Deborah had reported. Her CORE-OM scores were: Subjective well-being 1; Problems 6; Functioning 3; Risk 0. Her WSAS scores were: Work 3; Home management 2; Social leisure 1; Private leisure 1; Relationships 0; Total = 7. It was agreed that no further contact was required. Table 7 summarizes the amount of contact time Waseem spent with Deborah.

Table 7: Summary of Waseem's time spent in contact with Deborah.

Type of session	Number spent	Time	Total time
Face-to-face	1 x 40min, 7 x 30min	4hr 10min	5hr 10min
Telephone	6 x 10min	1hr	

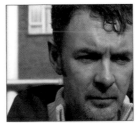

Andrew (Social Phobia)

Session 1

Assessment: Andrew, 34, presented with disabling social anxiety. He feared negative evaluation by others and, as a result, had difficulty interacting with people, particularly strangers. He also found eating in front of others particularly difficult. He would sometimes use alcohol to calm his nerves before going out socially in the evening, but he did not have an alcohol problem per se, as he was not alcohol dependent.

Problem statement: Difficulty facing social situations due to anxiety and fear of negative evaluation by others, leading to drinking alcohol before going out and avoidance of eating in front of others.

Goals:

- To go out socially with friends twice a week and speak to at least one stranger on each occasion, consuming a maximum of two alcoholic drinks over the course of the evening.
- To eat in the staff canteen in the company of others at least twice a week.

Andrew was given literature to read about social anxiety and asked to complete the CORE-OM and WSAS for the following session.

Session 2

Andrew had completed the measures as agreed by the time he was seen for his second session one week later. His CORE-OM scores were: Social well-being 8; Problems 25; Functioning 29; Risk 1. His WSAS scores were: Work 7; Home management 3; Social leisure 8; Private leisure 0; Relationships 6; Total = 24. Andrew's mental health worker, Katie, spent time explaining to him how his negative thoughts about what others thought of him were leading to anxiety, and how this was affecting the way his body reacted in these situations.

The role of safety behaviours, escape and avoidance, and how they only served to reinforce his fears, were also discussed. He was introduced to the four-column thought diary, which he was asked to complete over the coming week. He was also asked to complete two hierarchies of progressively difficult situations to help him work towards his ultimate goals.

Sessions 3–5

These sessions were all held face-to-face on a weekly basis. Andrew returned to Session 3 with two hierarchies for tackling his Social Phobia. He agreed to tackle the first step on the 'Eating in front of others' hierarchy). He felt that working towards talking to a stranger was more difficult and, therefore, it was agreed that this hierarchy would be left until a little later.

Andrew's Hierarchy for Eating In Front of Others

1. Eat a packet of crisps in pub in presence of friends
2. Eat a portion of chips in pub with friends
3. Eat a portion of chips in canteen in presence of one other
4. Eat a sandwich and crisps in canteen in presence of one other
5. Ditto in the presence of three others
6. Eat a meal in restaurant in company of immediate family
7. Eat a meal in restaurant in company of extended family
8. Eat a meal in restaurant with a minimum of two friends
9. Eat a meal in canteen in the presence of at least three others

---

Session 6

At this face-to-face session held a week later, it was clear that Andrew was making limited progress and remained severely debilitated by his Social Phobia. This was reflected in the repetition of the measures completed at assessment. His CORE-OM scores were: Subjective well-being 9; Problems 25; Functioning 31; Risk 1. His WSAS scores remained unchanged. Having discussed his case with his GP, Dr Rushforth, it was proposed to Andrew that he may require more formal therapy from a CBT specialist. Andrew agreed to this referral which was made on his behalf.

Table 8 summarizes the amount of contact time Katie spent with Andrew.

CBT treatment

Andrew was assessed by a CBT nurse therapist who felt that Andrew's Social Phobia was moderate to severe, and he was offered formal treatment. Andrew ultimately responded very well to CBT and, following 16 sessions with his therapist, he was discharged, having improved markedly. At discharge, he had achieved both end goals and was functioning well in social situations, although not symptom free.

Table 8: Summary of Katie's time spent in contact with Andrew.

Type of session	Number spent	Time	Total time
Face-to-face	2 x 40min, 4 x 30min	3hr 20min	3hrs 20min
Telephone	0		0

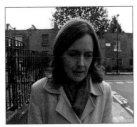

Julie (Generalized Anxiety Disorder)

Session 1

Assessment: Julie, 47, presented with excessive worrying about a variety of issues in her life, including her husband's potential redundancy, her mother's illness, her son's upcoming marriage, her daughter's well-being as she had recently moved away to university, the family dog, and ultimately worrying about the worrying itself.

Problem statement: Difficulty dealing with life problems due to excessive worrying, leading me to feel stressed and anxious, and concerned about my own mental well-being.

Goals:
- To use a problem-solving approach to tackle practical problems that occur in my life.
- To spend a maximum of 10 minutes worrying each day.

Julie was given reading material on anxiety and asked to complete the WSAS and the CORE-OM.

Session 2

Julie had completed the measures as agreed at the previous session, a week earlier. Her CORE-OM scores were: Subjective well-being 12;

Problems 28; Functioning 14; Risk 0. Her WSAS scores were: Work 4; Home management 6; Social Leisure 4; Private leisure 4; Relationships 5; Total = 23. Julie's mental health worker, Samantha, offered information about the nature of anxiety and worry and introduced Julie to a problem-solving approach to help tackle practical problems directly rather than spend time worrying needlessly. They also agreed a 'worry time' of half an hour each day at 6pm, when Julie was allowed to worry about whatever she liked. However, any worries that popped into her mind at any other time of day were to be written down on a piece of paper and kept for the 'worry time'.

Sessions 3–6

These sessions were held weekly and conducted face-to-face. Julie reported that she had found the scheduled worry time had helped, in that it freed up her mind during the day to get on with her life, and when it actually came to the agreed 'worry time', it was difficult for her to focus on her worries. She found the problem-solving approach difficult to engage in at first, and each session was used to tackle a problem together, to help her gain confidence in using the approach.

Sessions 7–9

These sessions were held fortnightly over the telephone. Julie reported that she had now reduced her worry time to the 10-minute goal and was beginning to use the problem-solving approach unaided. By session 9 she was clearly much improved and her ability to address concerns rather than worrying endlessly was also much improved. It was agreed that no further input was needed at present, but that Samantha would call her in four weeks' time to check on progress. A repetition of the measures showed improvement, which was in keeping with Julie's own reports. Her CORE-OM scores were: Subjective well-being 6; Problems 10; Functioning 6; Risk 0. Her WSAS scores were: Work 2; Home management 4; Social leisure 3; Private leisure 3; Relationships 3; Total = 15.

Follow-up call 4 weeks later

Julie remained improved. Her son's wedding had taken place the previous week and she had enjoyed it. She did notice an increase in worry the week before the wedding, but since then she had reverted to how she had been over more recent weeks and continued to make further improvement. Having discussed relapse prevention and jointly devised an 'Early Warning Signs' sheet, Julie and Samantha agreed to have no further contact at that time. Table 9 summarizes the amount of contact time Samantha spent with Julie.

Prior to the session, Samantha had posted Julie the measures to complete, which she had returned. Her scores for the CORE-OM were: Subjective well-being 3; Problems 7; Functioning 4; Risk 0. Her WSAS scores were: Work 0, Home management 3; Social leisure 2; Private leisure 3; Relationships 2; Total = 10.

Table 9: Summary of Samantha's time spent in contact with Julie.

Type of session	Number spent	Time	Total time
Face-to-face	1 x 40min, 5 x 30min	3hr 10min	4hr
Telephone	2 x 15min, 2 x 10min	50min	

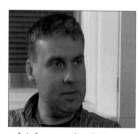

Tim (Stress)
Session 1

Assessment: Tim, 46, presented with high stress levels following redundancies at work which resulted in a marked increase in his workload. Dr Mehra had told Tim at a recent consultation that his blood pressure was raised. Tim had always thrived on stress but, more recently, he was finding it difficult to keep a balance with work and home life.

Problem statement: High levels of occupational stress leading to feeling under continual intense pressure, deterioration in the way I look after myself, problems in my relationship with my partner John and risk to physical health with high blood pressure.

Goals:
- To leave work on time at least three times a week.
- Go to the gym for an hour five times a week.
- Go out socially with John and/or friends twice a week.

Tim was given information to read on stress and asked to complete the CORE-OM and WSAS for the next session.

Session 2

One week later, Tim had completed the two measures as agreed. His CORE-OM scores were: Subjective well-being 11; Problems 19; Functioning 14; Risk 0. His WSAS scores were: Work 4; Home management 4; Social leisure 4; Private leisure 4; Relationships 2; Total = 18. Tim's mental health worker, Katie, spent time talking to him about the nature of stress and working with him to identify the main triggers. Katie also highlighted lifestyle factors that may be contributing to his stress, such as his diet, increased smoking and caffeine intake. Tim agreed that his health was at risk and, despite his fear of losing his job if he did not continue to work as intensively as he currently was, he could clearly see that his productivity was vastly reduced and that ultimately he had to put his health first. Tim agreed that he would arrange a meeting with his boss, Martin, and advise him that, although he was willing to put the work in to save the company, he could not continue working indefinitely at this pace. Tim was understandably anxious about doing this, but agreed that it was a necessary step. He had also been surfing the internet to find out further information about stress and had stumbled across a site about expert patients. He asked Katie if he could see the expert patient for his area. Katie agreed to organize a meeting for him.

Session 3–6

Sessions three and four were held face-to-face and sessions five and six were conducted by telephone. They were held on a fortnightly basis. At session 3, Tim reported that he had spoken to his boss about his inability to continue working at his current pace. His boss was very reasonable about it and confided that he was going through similar difficulties, and felt that he could not continue at this pace for much longer either. They agreed that both would work late together two nights a week, the rest of the week they would finish at 5.30pm, and they would review whether they were still getting as much done in two weeks time. When they reviewed how the two weeks had gone, they agreed that they had been able to focus more easily and concentrate on the tasks in hand when they had allowed themselves proper breaks. From this, they agreed to have lunch for half an hour away from their desks at least three times a week.

Tim had also vastly reduced his caffeine intake and was eating more healthily. However, his smoking remained high. Katie signposted Tim to a smoking cessation clinic, but he did not feel able to address this issue at this time and agreed to think about it in a few months as he was ultimately keen to stop smoking, and he knew that his partner John would support him in doing so.

In addition, Tim had seen the expert patient, who had encouraged him to try increasing his Omega-3, folic acid and selenium levels by changing his diet. In these four sessions, Tim was encouraged to learn how to use relaxation strategies to tackle times of stress and to begin accessing and evaluating any negative thoughts he was experiencing.

Session 7–8

Both of these fortnightly sessions were held over the telephone. Tim was feeling much better and was now spending less time at work and more time doing the things that he enjoyed, including going to the gym, and spending quality time with his friends and his partner, John.

His job seemed slightly less precarious, but he had been head hunted by another company. He was now considering the offer, although he had a great deal of loyalty towards his current employer. He had an appointment scheduled with his GP, Dr Mehra, between sessions 7 and 8. His blood pressure was taken during that consultation and it was found to be within the normal range.

At session 8, it was agreed that no further input from Katie was required at this time. A follow-up call in eight weeks time was agreed after they had discussed relapse prevention and early warning signs. Tim completed the same measures that he had been given at assessment.

His CORE-OM scores were: Subjective well-being 2; Problems 4; Functioning 5; Risk 0. His WSAS scores were: Work 2; Home management 0; Social leisure 1; Private leisure 1; Relationships 0; Total = 4.

Follow-up call 6 weeks later

Tim remained well and had recently started a new job with better prospects. Despite the new job and his eagerness to impress his new boss, he was continuing to maintain a good balance between work, home and social life. It was at this stage that Tim informed Katie that he had arranged to attend the smoking cessation clinic the following week.

Table 10 summarizes the amount of contact time Katie spent with Tim.

Table 10: Summary of Katie's time spent in contact with Tim.

Type of session	Number spent	Time	Total time
Face-to-face	4 x 30min,	2hr	3hr
Telephone	2 x 15min, 3 x 10min	1hr	

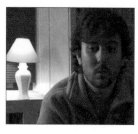

Roger (Insomnia)

Session 1

Assessment: Roger, 39, presented with a seven-year history of insomnia. This had particularly bothered him over the past seven months following a change of job. He had been a shift worker up until this point, but was now working a regular 9–5 work pattern. He was disappointed that he continued to have a problem getting off to sleep despite regularizing his bedtime.

Problem statement: Difficulty falling asleep due to tension and worry about sleep, leading to frustration, reluctance to go to bed, feeling tired during the day and napping early evening.

Goal:

- To get up at 7.30 each morning having had a rested night's sleep, at least five times a week.

Having established a problem statement and agreed a treatment goal, Roger was asked to keep a sleep diary for two weeks (included in 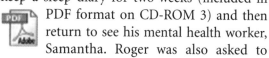 PDF format on CD-ROM 3) and then return to see his mental health worker, Samantha. Roger was also asked to complete the CORE-OM and the WSAS.

Sessions 2–4

At session 2 the following week, Roger returned with his completed measures. His CORE-OM scores were: Subjective well-being 3; Problems 19; Functioning 3; Risk 0. His WSAS scores were: Work 3; Home management 0; Social leisure 3; Private leisure 2; Relationships 4; Total = 12.

Sessions 2–4, which were held fortnightly and face-to-face, were used to educate Roger about good sleep hygiene and to encourage him to enhance his sleep environment. He cut out caffeine after 6pm and stopped napping in the chair. He also increased his physical activity earlier in the day. He removed the television from the bedroom and agreed that, if he did not fall asleep within a few minutes, he would get out of bed and engage in a quiet activity. Roger chose to sit in his easy chair and listen to relaxing music. He then returned to bed when he began to feel drowsy again.

Roger found it difficult to cut out the evening napping initially and found that, if he sat in his chair at his usual naptime, he could not help but fall asleep. It was therefore agreed that he would go for a gentle walk with the dog instead, at the times when he would usually have a nap. This increase in activity meant that he was not as sleepy on his return. He also found it difficult initially to reduce his tea intake, until he discovered that he had a liking for camomile and vanilla tea, which he drank from then on.

Getting out of bed in the middle of the night wasn't very easy for Roger at first either, but he soon got into a routine. By following the basic principles of good sleep hygiene and enhancing his sleep environment, Roger quickly noticed an improvement in his sleep.

Session 5

Three weeks later, Roger was seen for session 5. By now, he had re-established a good sleep regime. He was surprised at how easy it actually was to accomplish, after all this time, and that he had been able to do it without the help of any sleep medication which he had been particularly keen for his GP, Dr Hall, to prescribe. This session was spent on relapse prevention, and Roger and Samantha agreed to talk on the telephone in 6 weeks' time to review progress. Roger repeated the measures that he had completed at assessment. His CORE-OM scores were: Subjective well-being 0; Problems 6; Functioning 1; Risk 0. His WSAS scores were: Work 1; Home management 0; Social leisure 1; Private leisure 1; Relationships 0; Total = 3.

Follow-up call at 6 weeks

Roger was continuing to sleep well and, on the occasional times when he did have difficulty getting to sleep or had woken up during the night with difficulty returning to sleep, he reported experiencing no anxiety. Roger and Samantha decided that no further input was needed at this time and, therefore, no further contact was arranged. Table 11 summarizes the amount of contact time Samantha spent with Roger.

Table 11: Summary of Samantha's time spent in contact with Roger.

Type of session	Number spent	Time	Total time
Face-to-face	1 x 30min,	1hr 50min	
	4 x 20min		2hr
Telephone	1 x 10min	10min	

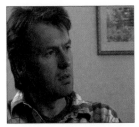

Ben (Anger)

Session 1

Assessment: Ben, 27, presented with irritability and angry outbursts, which mainly occurred whilst driving to and from work, but lasted beyond this. As a result, he was having difficulty unwinding when he got home in the evening, and was taking out his frustrations on his wife, Sue. He was keen to tackle his difficulties as he was aware that, with a baby due in the near future, this would only add to the stressors in his life and probably add to his frustrations.

Problem statement: Difficulty dealing with stressful situations, particularly traffic jams, due to low threshold of frustration leading to outbursts of anger at the time and irritability when I get home; putting a strain on my relationship with Sue.

Goals:
- To travel to and from work with minimal anger.
- To spend half an hour chatting with Sue about our respective days, with minimal irritability.

Ben was asked to keep a diary of anger episodes for a week (included in PDF format on CD-ROM 3). He was also given literature on anger to read and asked to complete the CORE-OM and WSAS for the next session.

Session 2–4

Sessions 2–4 were face-to-face contacts. At session 2, Ben returned with his completed measures. His CORE-OM scores were: Subjective well-being 5; Problems 17; Functioning 21; Risk 2. His WSAS scores were: Work 4; Home management 5; Social leisure 6; Private leisure 2; Relationships 7; Total = 24. Ben was introduced to strategies to reduce his anger. He learnt how to use relaxation strategies and began to use the nine-column thought diaries to enable him to evaluate his thoughts and to reduce his anger. Ben found the combination of relaxation to address the physical symptoms of anger and the thought diaries to tackle his angry thoughts and emotions to be very helpful, and quickly reported a reduction in his levels of anger. However, he was not symptom-free by this stage and he needed more practice with both strategies to further reduce his irritability and anger.

Sessions 5–7

These sessions were held fortnightly by telephone. Ben continued to use the strategies he learned in the earlier sessions and had begun to find that he was able to nip his anger in the bud by scanning his body for physical tension, and then using relaxation methods to release it. He was also using thought evaluation techniques to address his angry thoughts.

Session 8

In this face-to-face session two weeks later, Ben had improved significantly by this stage and felt ready to go it alone. He agreed to be telephoned by his mental health worker, Samantha, in a month's time to check progress. Ben repeated the measures he had completed at assessment. His CORE-OM scores were: Subjective well-being 1; Problems 8; Functioning 9; Risk 0. His WSAS scores were: Work 2; Home management 2; Social leisure 3; Private leisure 0; Relationships 3; Total = 10.

Follow-up call 4 weeks later

Ben reported that he was coping well and that, although not symptom-free, he had noticed a marked improvement in his problem and both he and Sue were pleased with how things were going. Ben and Samantha agreed to no further contact at that time, with the understanding that, should he experience any further difficulties, he would make an appointment to see Dr Hall. Table 12 summarizes the amount of contact time Samantha spent with Ben.

Table 12: Summary of Samantha's time spent in contact with Ben.

Type of session	Number spent	Time	Total time
Face-to-face	1 x 40min, 4 x 30min	2hr 40min	
			3hr 30min
Telephone	2 x 15min, 2 x 10min	50min	

In Summary

As you can see, most patients responded well to input from their mental health workers in the primary care setting. However, Julian was referred to secondary care and Andrew was 'stepped up' to specialist services, where he was offered CBT, to which he responded well.

Reference

National Institute for Health and Clinical Excellence (2004a). *Depression: management of depression in primary and secondary care.* London: National Institute for Health and Clinical Excellence.

Appendix

This section contains templates of documents referred to throughout the text for you to copy and use freely with your patients.

Activity Schedule

Instructions: Please write in each box for every of hour of the day: Activity, Achievement (A=0-10) and Pleasure (P=0-10)

Time	Monday	Tuesday	Wednesday	Thursday	Friday	Saturday	Sunday
6-7am							
7-8am							
8-9am							
9-10am							
10-11am							
11-12pm							
12-1pm							
1-2pm							
2-3pm							
3-4pm							
4-5pm							
5-6pm							
6-7pm							
7-8pm							
8-9pm							
9-10pm							
10-11pm							
11-12pm							
12-1am							

Anger Diary

Day/Date	Trigger	Level of anger 0-100%	Response

Exposure Practice Diary

Anxiety Scale

No Anxiety	Mild Anxiety	Moderate Anxiety	Severe Anxiety	Panic
0	25	50	75	100

Date/time	Activity	Anxiety Level

CLINICAL OUTCOMES in ROUTINE EVALUATION

OUTCOME MEASURE

Male ☐
Female ☐

Site ID — letters only
Client ID — numbers only

Age

Therapist ID — numbers only (1) — numbers only (2)

Sub codes

Date form given — D D / M M / Y Y Y Y

Stage Completed
S Screening
R Referral
A Assessment
F First Therapy Session
P Pre-Therapy (unspecified)
D During Therapy
L Last therapy session
X Follow up 1
Y Follow up 2

Stage
Episode

IMPORTANT - PLEASE READ THIS FIRST

This form has 34 statements about how you have been OVER THE LAST WEEK.
Please read each statement and think how often you felt that way last week.
Then tick the box which is closest to this.
Please use a dark pen (not pencil) and tick clearly within the boxes.

Over the last week

		Not at all	Only Occasionally	Sometimes	Often	Most or all the time	OFFICE USE ONLY
1	I have felt terribly alone and isolated	0	1	2	3	4	F
2	I have felt tense, anxious or nervous	0	1	2	3	4	P
3	I have felt I have someone to turn to for support when needed	4	3	2	1	0	F
4	I have felt O.K. about myself	4	3	2	1	0	W
5	I have felt totally lacking in energy and enthusiasm	0	1	2	3	4	P
6	I have been physically violent to others	0	1	2	3	4	R
7	I have felt able to cope when things go wrong	4	3	2	1	0	F
8	I have been troubled by aches, pains or other physical problems	0	1	2	3	4	P
9	I have thought of hurting myself	0	1	2	3	4	R
10	Talking to people has felt too much for me	0	1	2	3	4	F
11	Tension and anxiety have prevented me doing important things	0	1	2	3	4	P
12	I have been happy with the things I have done.	4	3	2	1	0	F
13	I have been disturbed by unwanted thoughts and feelings	0	1	2	3	4	P
14	I have felt like crying	0	1	2	3	4	W

Please turn over

Over the last week

		Not at all	Only Occasionally	Sometimes	Often	Most or all the time	OFFICE USE ONLY
15	I have felt panic or terror	0	1	2	3	4	P
16	I made plans to end my life	0	1	2	3	4	R
17	I have felt overwhelmed by my problems	0	1	2	3	4	W
18	I have had difficulty getting to sleep or staying asleep	0	1	2	3	4	P
19	I have felt warmth or affection for someone	4	3	2	1	0	F
20	My problems have been impossible to put to one side	0	1	2	3	4	P
21	I have been able to do most things I needed to	4	3	2	1	0	F
22	I have threatened or intimidated another person	0	1	2	3	4	R
23	I have felt despairing or hopeless	0	1	2	3	4	P
24	I have thought it would be better if I were dead	0	1	2	3	4	F
25	I have felt criticised by other people	0	1	2	3	4	F
26	I have thought I have no friends	0	1	2	3	4	P
27	I have felt unhappy	0	1	2	3	4	P
28	Unwanted images or memories have been distressing me	0	1	2	3	4	P
29	I have been irritable when with other people	0	1	2	3	4	F
30	I have thought I am to blame for my problems and difficulties	0	1	2	3	4	P
31	I have felt optimistic about my future	4	3	2	1	0	W
32	I have achieved the things I wanted to	4	3	2	1	0	F
33	I have felt humiliated or shamed by other people	0	1	2	3	4	F
34	I have hurt myself physically or taken dangerous risks with my health	0	1	2	3	4	R

THANK YOU FOR YOUR TIME IN COMPLETING THIS QUESTIONNAIRE

Total Scores

(W) → (P) → (F) → (R) → All items → All minus R

Mean Scores
(Total score for each dimension divided by
number of items completed in that dimension)

Stress Personality Types

Type A
- ☐ Must get things finished
- ☐ Never late for appointments
- ☐ Competitive
- ☐ Can't listen to conversations, interrupt, finish sentences for others
- ☐ Always in a hurry
- ☐ Don't like to wait
- ☐ Very busy, at full speed
- ☐ Trying to do more than one thing at a time
- ☐ Want everything perfect
- ☐ Pressured speech
- ☐ Do everything fast
- ☐ Hold feelings in
- ☐ Not satisfied with work/life
- ☐ Few social activities/interests
- ☐ If working, will often take work home

Type B
- ☐ Don't mind leaving things unfinished for a while
- ☐ Calm and unhurried about appointments
- ☐ Not competitive
- ☐ Can listen and let the other person finish speaking
- ☐ Never in a hurry even when busy
- ☐ Can wait calmly
- ☐ Easy going
- ☐ Take one thing at a time
- ☐ Don't mind things not quite perfect
- ☐ Slow and deliberate speech
- ☐ Do things slowly
- ☐ Express feelings
- ☐ Quite satisfied with work/life
- ☐ Many social activities/interests
- ☐ If in employment, limit time working to work hours

If most of your ticks are on the A side then you will be more prone to stress; if both As and Bs are ticked then you are a little prone to stress; if mainly Bs are ticked then you are less likely to suffer from stress. Those people who are more prone to stress may have to try harder to use some of the stress management approaches discussed later to tackle their natural tendency to stress.

PATIENT HEALTH QUESTIONNAIRE (PHQ-9)

NAME: _____   DATE:_____

Over the *last 2 weeks*, how often have you been
bothered by any of the following problems?
(use "✓" to indicate your answer)

	Not at all	Several days	More than half the days	Nearly every day
1. Little interest or pleasure in doing things	0	1	2	3
2. Feeling down, depressed, or hopeless	0	1	2	3
3. Trouble falling or staying asleep, or sleeping too much	0	1	2	3
4. Feeling tired or having little energy	0	1	2	3
5. Poor appetite or overeating	0	1	2	3
6. Feeling bad about yourself—or that you are a failure or have let yourself or your family down	0	1	2	3
7. Trouble concentrating on things, such as reading the newspaper or watching television	0	1	2	3
8. Moving or speaking so slowly that other people could have noticed. Or the opposite—being so fidgety or restless that you have been moving around a lot more than usual	0	1	2	3
9. Thoughts that you would be better off dead, or of hurting yourself in some way	0	1	2	3

add columns: _____ + _____ + _____

(Healthcare professional: For interpretation of TOTAL, please refer to accompanying scoring card).   TOTAL: _____

---

10. If you checked off *any* problems, how *difficult* have these problems made it for you to do your work, take care of things at home, or get along with other people?

Not difficult at all	_____
Somewhat difficult	_____
Very difficult	_____
Extremely difficult	_____

Problem Solving

Identify the problem

Write down as many solutions as possible

Consider the pros and cons of each possible solution

Select the best or most promising solution

Plan how to carry out the chosen solution

Resources needed

Main problems to be overcome

Steps to be undertaken

Put the plan into action

Review what happens

Sleep Diary

Day/Date	How long did it take you to get off to sleep?	Rate how difficult it was to fall asleep (0-100%)	Rate how tense you felt on going to bed (0-100%)	Number of times that you woke during the night	On each occasion that you woke up, how long were you awake?	What did you do during those waking periods?	Approximately how long did you sleep in total?	Rate the quality of your sleep (0-100%)	Significant events of the day	Medication, caffeine and alcohol consumption

4-Column Thought Diary

Date	Situation	Emotions Rate intensity 0-100%	Thoughts Rate belief 0-100%

9 Column Thought Diary

Date	Situation	Emotion Rate intensity 0-100%	Thought/ image Rate belief 0-100% and circle the hot thought	Evidence for the hot thought	Evidence against the hot thought	Alternative or balanced thought	Re-rate belief in hot thought and intensity of emotion	What to do next

Work and Social Adjustment Scale

Name_____   **Date**_____

Instructions: Circle a number that best describes your situation.

Work
Because of my problems my work is impaired

0	1	2	3	4	5	6	7	8

Home Management
Because of my problems my home management is impaired (paying bills, housework, shopping etc)

0	1	2	3	4	5	6	7	8

Social Life
Because of my problems my social life is impaired (outings, seeing friends, visiting parks etc)

0	1	2	3	4	5	6	7	8

Private Leisure
Because of my problems my private leisure is impaired (activities done alone)

0	1	2	3	4	5	6	7	8

Family
Because of my problems my family relationships are impaired

0	1	2	3	4	5	6	7	8

Reference: Mundt, J., Marks, I.M., Shear, M,K., & Griest, J.H. (2002). The work and social adjustment scale: a simple measure of impairment in functioning. British Journal of Psychiarty, 180, 461-464.

Glossary

Accountability: Being answerable for the consequences of what you do or omit to do.

Activity schedule: A type of diary used to monitor behaviours and moods, and to plan activity.

Adrenaline: A hormone that is secreted by the medulla (innermost part) of the adrenal gland in response to stress and emotional states such as fear and rage.

Advance directive: A decision made in advance by a person to refuse treatment, or state what treatment they would like.

Advocacy: A process of speaking and/or acting with, or on behalf of, a person or a group of people, with the aim of ensuring that their opinions, wishes, or needs are expressed and listened to. A key distinction to be kept in mind is between independent advocacy (which seeks to act with the service user and to empower them), and the more limited advocacy that healthcare professionals sometimes offer (as they may feel themselves constrained by perceived professional roles).

Affective symptoms: Symptoms concerned with mood and emotions (e.g. depressed mood).

Agenda: A detailed plan of what is to be covered in sessions.

Agoraphobia: Marked fear of being in places or situations from which escape might be difficult; fear of being out of control in a public place; fear of being in a situation in which help might not be available in the event of a panic attack.

Akathisia: Manifests as pacing and a total inability to sit still. If forced to sit still, the person experiences extreme anxiety and agitation. In severe cases, the anxiety and agitation may get worse even while the person is moving.

Alopecia: Loss of hair which can include all body hair as well as that on the scalp.

Anticholinergic: Drugs with an anticholinergic effect inhibit the secretion of acid in the stomach, slow the passage of food through the digestive system, inhibit the production of saliva, sweat, and bronchial secretions and increase the heart rate and blood pressure. Examples of drugs that have this effect include antidepressants and antipsychotics.

Antidepressant: A medicinal drug used for the treatment of depression.

Antiemetic: A drug used to control nausea and vomiting.

Anxiety: Characterised by fear, for example that something dreadful is going to happen. People become anxious when they face upsetting things like illness, unemployment, surgery or divorce. In severe cases, anxiety can become so extreme that fear affects an individual's ability to cope or function on a day-to-day basis. Feelings of anxiety can occur in response to all sorts of different situations, or about health. A person who is anxious may find that they have distressing physical symptoms, such as headaches, chest pains, feelings of tiredness and tension.

Arrhythmia: An irregular heart rhythm, or an abnormality in the timing or pattern of the heartbeat causing the heart to beat too rapidly, too slowly, or irregularly.

Arthritis: Inflammation of a joint or a state characterised by inflammation of joints.

Assertive: Confident and self-assured without being aggressive.

Assertive Outreach Team: Assertive Outreach Teams offer support for people with serious mental health problems, living across the locality, who require intensive interventions to engage and maintain contact with services.

Asthma: Disease of respiration marked by episodes of difficulty in breathing.

Atypicals: Usually a term referring to second-generation antipsychotic medication used to treat psychiatric conditions.

Autoimmune disorders: A group of diseases characterised by abnormal functioning of the immune system that causes the immune system to produce antibodies against its own tissues.

Avoidance: In this context, keeping away from something or a situation because the stimulus causes anxiety.

Behavioural Activation: A technique used to increase activity and access to reinforcement.

Best interests: Having the person's needs and interests at the heart of any decision.

Best value: The performance regime for all local government services, including Personal Social Services. Best value performance indicators are structured into five domains which, together, describe all aspects of performance: these are national priorities and strategic objectives; cost and efficiency; effectiveness of service delivery and outcomes; quality of services for users and carers; and fair access.

Bibliotherapy: A form of supportive psychotherapy in which carefully selected reading materials are used to assist an individual in solving personal problems or for other therapeutic purposes.

Bipolar Affective Disorder: A mood disorder characterised by episodes of mania (exaggerated feeling of well-being) and depression, formerly known as Manic Depressive Disorder.

Blood dyscrasias (Neutropenia): An abnormal decrease in the number of neutrophils (granular white blood cells) in the blood.

Bronchitis: A lung disease characterised by inflammation of the bronchial mucous membrane.

Caldicott Guardian: Each NHS Trust and Board has appointed a Caldicott Guardian. This is normally a senior health professional, for example the Medical Director. The Guardian's key responsibilities are to oversee how staff use personal health information and ensure that patients' rights to confidentiality are respected.

Capacity: A legal term to define a person's ability to make decisions, sometimes referred to as competence. Everyone must be presumed to have capacity unless proven otherwise.

Cardiac disease: Disease related to the heart.

Cardiotoxic side-effects: The unintended actions of a drug which result in a toxic effect on the heart.

Cardiovascular: Refers to the circulatory system (the heart and blood vessels).

Carer: A person, usually a relative or friend, who provides care on a voluntary basis.

Care Programme Approach (CPA): The formal and written process (integrated with Case management) of recording and reviewing an individual's needs, usually prior to and after discharge from hospital. The acronym CPA is increasingly being replaced by ECC – Effective Care Coordination.

Care Services Improvement Partnership (CSIP): A body commissioned by the Department of Health and other agencies in 2005 to help services implement national policies for local benefit.

Case management: A process whereby a patient's healthcare needs are identified, and a plan, which efficiently utilises healthcare resources, is designed and implemented to achieve the optimum outcome for the patient in the most cost-effective way.

Catatonia: A form of schizophrenia characterised by a tendency to remain in a fixed stuporous state for long periods; the catatonia may give way to short periods of extreme excitement.

Cerebrovascular disease: A disease affecting any artery supplying blood to the brain; may cause blockage or rupture of a blood vessel, leading to a stroke.

Cholesterol: A fat-like substance manufactured in the liver that is important for the metabolism and transport of fatty acids, and in the production of hormones and vitamin D. Too much cholesterol in the bloodstream can be unhealthy and lead to coronary heart disease.

Cholinergic rebound: A side-effect that may be experienced with the withdrawal of some psychiatric drugs. Symptoms include profuse sweating, headache, nausea, vomiting and diarrhoea.

Chronic Fatigue Syndrome: An illness characterised by prolonged, debilitating fatigue and multiple non-specific symptoms such as headaches, recurrent sore throats, muscle and joint pains, and memory and concentration difficulties. Profound fatigue can come on suddenly or gradually and persists or recurs throughout the period of illness. Symptoms can linger for at least six months, and often for years. The cause of Chronic Fatigue Syndrome remains unknown.

Clinical Governance: A framework through which NHS organisations are accountable for continuously improving the quality of their services and safeguarding high standards of care, by creating an environment in which clinical care will improve. The NHS Modernisation Agency has a website dedicated to clinical governance at www.cgsupport.nhs.uk.

Clinical supervision: 'A formal process of professional support and learning which enables individual practitioners to develop knowledge and competence, assume responsibility for their own practice and enhance consumer protection and safety in complex situations' (Department of Health).

Codes of Professional Conduct: Each health profession has its own Code of Conduct which governs its professional practice. Codes of Professional Conduct set standards for professional practice and must be adhered to.

Cognitive Behavioural Therapy (CBT): CBT is an effective talking therapy that aims to break the vicious cycle between thoughts, feelings and behaviours by helping people with mental health problems to learn more functional ways of thinking and coping. Treatment tends to be highly active, brief, structured, and problem oriented.

Colitis: Inflammation of the large intestine.

Collaborative approach: A way of working in partnership, within an open and explicit relationship, whereby the clinician and patient work together on defining the problem and working on solving it.

Commission for Healthcare and Audit Inspection (CHAI): *See* Healthcare Commission.

Commission for Health Improvement (CHI): CHI ceased to exist on 31st March 2004 and was replaced by the Commission for Healthcare and Audit Inspection (CHAI).

Commission for Patient and Public Involvement in Health (CPPIH): An independent body that appoints and performance-manages all Patient and Public Involvement Forums (PPIFs), submits reports to the Secretary of State on how the system is working and carries out national reviews of services from the patient perspective.

Common law: Contrary to statute law, common law is based either upon past legal judgements (precedents) or, where no sufficiently close precedent exists, upon the interpretation of a judge. In this way, common law (sometimes called 'case law') remains in harmony with the community to which it applies.

Common mental health problems: Covers a very wide spectrum of distress, from the worries and grief we all experience as part of everyday life, to severe and disabling depression and anxiety that affects an individual's ability to cope or function on a day-to-day basis. Common mental health problems are those mental health difficulties that are more frequently seen within the population.

Community Mental Health Team (CMHT): A team made up of a number of different mental health professionals who, together, offer a wide range of expertise and support. Their role is to provide assessment and treatment for those people who have mental health problems and/or who have social care needs.

Concordance: Concordance is based on the notion that the work of the healthcare worker and the patient is a negotiation between equals and, therefore, the aim is a therapeutic alliance between them.

Confidential information: Information (that could identify a person) entrusted by one individual to another in confidence and where there is a legitimate expectation that it will remain in confidence unless consent to reveal is sought and given.

Congestive heart failure: A condition in which the heart cannot pump out all of the blood that enters it, which leads to an accumulation of blood in the vessels and fluid in the body tissues.

Consent: To give permission, or agreement, to do something; to allow. *See* Lawful consent.

Contraindications: Factors that render inadvisable the administration of a drug or the carrying out of a medical procedure.

Controlled breathing: A technique used to slow down breathing when a person is over-breathing, perhaps because of a panic attack.

Convention Rights: Rights and fundamental freedoms set out in the Human Rights Act 1998.

CORE-OM: The Clinical Outcomes in Routine Evaluation – Outcome Measure is a 34-item self-completed questionnaire measuring subjective well-being (4 items), problems (12 items), functioning (12 items) and risk (6 items: 4 risk-to-self items and 2 risk-to-others items).

Corticosteroids: A group of anti-inflammatory drugs, similar to the natural corticosteroid hormones produced by the adrenal glands.

Crisis Resolution Teams: Teams offering support to people in their own homes on a 24-hour basis – through counselling, practical help, monitoring, and liaison with other services.

Cultural awareness: A level of awareness of cultural diversity and of communicating effectively across cultures.

Deaf awareness: Awareness of the communication challenges facing deaf and hard of hearing people and the identification of some ways in which hearing people can improve their communication skills.

Delirium: A state of partial consciousness, accompanied by confusion, loss of attention, disordered thinking, and disturbed sleep–wake cycle.

Delusion: An erroneous belief that usually involves a misinterpretation of perceptions or experiences.

Dementia: An organic disease that affects older people, characterised by deterioration in mental capacity and leading to a gradual decline of memory and other mental abilities resulting in confused behaviour. The disease is chronic, incurable and often worsens over a period of time.

Depot injection: Antipsychotic medication that is injected into the patient.

Depression: Used to describe feelings of low mood, often in response to experiences that are upsetting, stressful or difficult. When a patient is said to have a depressive illness, they are experiencing long-lasting intense feelings of persistent sadness, with, for example, thoughts of helplessness and hopelessness often accompanied by physical symptoms such as sleeplessness, loss of energy, or physical aches and pains.

Dermatitis: Inflammation of the skin.

Diabetes: A disease characterised by excessive urination. Diabetes Mellitus is caused by insufficient insulin production or lack of responsiveness to insulin, resulting in hyperglycaemia (high blood glucose levels). There are two primary types of Diabetes Mellitus: Type I (insulin-dependent or juvenile-onset), which may be caused by an autoimmune response; and Type II (non-insulin-dependent or adult-onset).

Disorientation: Confusion about the time of day, date, or season (time), where one is, or who one is.

Doctrine of necessity: A legal doctrine that permits medical intervention without consent in order to save a person's life.

Dopamine: A neurotransmitter found in the brain and essential for the normal functioning of the central nervous system.

DSM-IV-TR: Diagnostic Statistical Manual of Mental Disorders (4th edition, Text Revision), published by the American Psychiatric Association. The main diagnostic reference of mental health professionals in the USA and the UK.

Duty of care: The duty owed by one party to another.

Early Intervention Teams: Teams intended to provide intensive support for people suffering acute mental health crises, often for the first time, with the aim of reducing the longer-term impact of an episode and the likelihood of its recurrence. The team is usually comprised of mental health nurses, social workers, support staff and medical input. They operate on a 24-hour, seven-day-a-week, basis.

Early warning signs: Symptoms that are early indicators of relapse and alert the person to take action in an attempt to prevent further deterioration.

Eczema: A non-contagious inflammation of the skin, characterised by the presence of itching and sometimes accompanied by scaling and blisters.

Effective Care Coordination (ECC): *See* Care Programme Approach (CPA).

Electroconvulsive Therapy (ECT): A treatment where convulsions and loss of consciousness are produced by the passage of an electric current through the brain to an anaesthetised patient, sometimes used as a treatment for severe depression if it has been unresponsive to other more conventional treatments.

Empathy: The act of understanding and fully appreciating another person's perspective sufficiently well to be able to acknowledge their feelings.

Empowerment: The concept of empowerment in healthcare is not just related to (for example) legislative change that might secure or enlarge the rights of any individual or group. Also involved is the process of learning (and putting into practice) competencies by which an individual or group can intensify their ability to act in pursuit of their own interests. A necessary complement to the development of specific knowledge or resources is a healthcare system, which can respond and make changes where necessary.

Ephedrine: A white odourless powdered or crystalline compound from the plant Ephedra, or made synthetically, used to treat bronchitis and asthma.

Epidemiology: The branch of medicine that deals with the study of the causes, distribution and control of disease in populations.

Epilepsy: A disorder associated with disturbed electrical discharges in the central nervous system, causing convulsions. *See* Seizure.

Evidence-based: In this context, an approach that promotes the results of research on the effectiveness of healthcare interventions and uses the findings to influence practice.

Expert Patient: A person who has a long-term condition and who acts as advisor to people with similar conditions on topics such as diet, exercise, managing pain and medication, and communication with healthcare professionals.

Fight or flight: The body's natural reaction to unexpected threat. The reaction is to stay and confront the source of the threat or to run away, hence the term. The person will experience an increase in blood flow to the muscles, increase in blood pressure, heightened muscle strength and mental ability, which all help prepare the body for a confrontation or a fast escape.

Flashback: An unexpected but vivid reliving of a past experience, a symptom commonly experienced in Post Traumatic Stress Disorder.

Food Standards Agency: This is a government agency that is responsible for protecting public health in relation to food throughout the UK.

Foreseeability: In legal terms, actions or omissions that you know could have harmful consequences to another person

Functional impairment: A negative effect on a person's ability to perform at their normal level of functioning.

Gateway Workers: These workers operate at a general practice level, although they are managed by Community Mental Health Teams (CMHTs). Their role is to improve access to appropriate specialised mental health services for service users accessing the health service from any point of first contact (such as A&E departments, NHS Direct and primary care teams).

Generalized Anxiety Disorder (GAD): A condition, unlike phobic anxiety, in which the main symptoms are chronic, with persistent apprehension and tension that are not related to any situation in particular. There may be many unspecific physical reactions, such as trembling, jitteriness, sweating, lightheadedness and irritability.

Genuineness: A state of being undisputedly natural and genuine.

Gillick Competence: Sufficient level of under-standing and intelligence in a child to enable them to understand fully what is proposed.

Glaucoma: A disease of the eye marked by increased pressure within the eyeball. If left untreated, glaucoma can damage the optic nerve and cause loss of vision.

GP Fund Holding: Family doctors controlled their own budget and purchased healthcare independently.

Graded exposure: Facing a feared situation in preplanned steps of increasing difficulty. Progress from each step to the next is usually delayed until the previous step can be performed with relative ease.

Grandiose: Characterised by feigned or affected greatness; pompous; with an inflated sense of self-importance.

Habituation: The waning of a response, such as anxiety, to repeated presentations of the same stimulus.

Hallucination: A false perception with no basis in reality; may be visual (sight), auditory (sound), tactile (touch), olfactory (smell) or gustatory (taste).

Healthcare Commission: An independent body covering England and Wales, whose aims are to provide independent scrutiny of local efforts to assure and improve quality in the NHS, to help tackle local service problems, and to monitor the NHS's efforts to address inappropriate variations in service standards. Its proper name is the Commission for Healthcare Audit and Inspection (CHAI). It was created by the Health and Social Care Act (2003) and began operation on 1 April 2004, replacing the Commission for Health Improvement (CHI).

Health Improvement Programme (HimP): Overarching strategic documents which set out local health strategies for a health and social care system within a local area.

Health promotion: The process of enabling individuals to gain control over and improve their health. It involves the population as a whole in the context of their everyday lives, rather than focusing on people at risk for specific diseases, and is directed towards action on the determinants or causes of health.

Hepatic impairment: Liver abnormality.

Her Majesty's Stationary Office (HMSO): A department of the British Government that prints many official documents.

Herpes: A viral disease characterised by eruptions of the skin or mucous membrane.

Hierarchy: Ranking of feared situations in order of levels of difficulty.

Hot thought: A negative automatic thought that is most connected to adverse emotion.

Hypertension: Arterial disease in which chronic high blood pressure is the primary symptom.

Hypertensive crisis: A critical elevation in blood pressure in which diastolic pressure exceeds 120mm HG.

Hyperthyroidism: A disorder caused by excessive production of thyroxine by the thyroid gland, characterised by increased metabolic rate, enlargement of the thyroid gland, rapid heart rate, high blood pressure and protruding eyes.

Hyperventilation: Abnormally deep or rapid breathing, frequently seen in someone who is anxious.

Hypervigilance: Being overly watchful and careful.

Hypomania: A mild form of Mania, with similar yet less severe symptoms and less overall impairment. The individual may have an elevated mood, feel better than usual and be more productive.

Hyponatraemia: Low sodium level in the blood.

Hypothalamus: The region of the brain that contains several important centres which control body temperature, thirst, hunger, water balance and sexual function. It is closely connected with emotional activity and functions as a centre for the integration of hormonal and autonomic nervous activity.

ICD-10: The International Statistical Classification of Diseases and Related Health Problems (10th Revision) is published by the World Health Organisation and is used worldwide for morbidity and mortality statistics. Every disease (or group of related diseases) is described with its symptom list and given a unique code.

Incapacity Benefit: A state benefit payable after the expiry of state sickness benefit if a person is still unfit to work. This replaces the former invalidity benefit and, as such, is a reduced level of benefit.

Independent Complaints Advocacy Service (ICAS): An independent body designed to help people who wish to make a complaint about their NHS care or treatment. Primary Care Trust Patients' Forums are responsible for commissioning and/or providing ICAS for their local population.

Infant mortality: A measure of the number of children who die before they reach the age of 5.

Informed consent: *See* Lawful consent.

Insomnia: Inability to sleep.

Internal market: This was the Conservative Government's attempt to address problems such as growing hospital waiting lists in the early 1990s. Purchasers of healthcare were given a budget to buy healthcare from providers.

Interpersonal therapy: A brief and highly structured, manual-based psychotherapy that addresses interpersonal issues in depression.

Irritable Bowel Syndrome (IBS): Recurrent abdominal pain and diarrhoea, often alternating with periods of constipation, and frequently associated with emotional stress.

Ischaemic heart disease: A disease of the heart caused by narrowing of the coronary arteries and decreased blood flow to the heart.

Job Seekers' Allowance: Job Seekers' Allowance (Income Based) – JSA(IB) – is based on the need for a minimum level of income; but in order to qualify, the person claiming must be available for work (and actively seeking work).

Joint Investment Plans (JIPs): Agreed between health and local authorities, JIPs are detailed three-year rolling plans for investment and reshaping of services.

Knowledge Community: A shared space provided by the National Institute for Mental Health in England (NIMHE), where people can exchange knowledge, information and experiences relating to any aspect of mental health in order to contribute to the improvement of mental health services. This can be found at http://kc.nimhe.org.uk.

Law: The body of rules, whether formally enacted or customary, which a state or community recognises as binding on its members or subjects.

Lawful consent: Consent is only lawful if it is 'true' or 'real', when a person has been informed in broad terms of the treatment or procedure and has indicated their acceptance of it. This must now include an explanation of the consequences and risks of the treatment and what would happen if treatment was not given. This is often called 'informed consent', although consent has to be informed by definition.

Learning disability: Any of various cognitive, neurological or psychological disorders that impede the ability to learn, especially one that interferes with the ability to learn mathematics or develop language skills.

Liability: Legal responsibility for one's acts or omission

Libido: Sexual drive.

Limbic system: A group of interconnected deep brain structures, common to all mammals, and involved in the regulation of emotion, memory, motivation, behaviour, etc.

Local authorities: Regional councils or territorial local authorities.

Local Mental Health User Forums: These offer support and guidance on issues that affect service users across a locality, and provide a voice for those who use mental health services to contribute to the way these are planned and developed by liaising with service providers.

Makaton: A proprietary name for a language programme integrating speech, manual signs and graphic symbols, developed to help people for whom communication is very difficult, especially those with learning disabilities.

Mania: An elevation of mood that is often characterised by grandiose ideas. The person with mania may also become very irritable.

Medication management: The process of supporting patients taking medication, and troubleshooting any difficulties they may be experiencing.

Menopause: The cessation of menstruation. Natural menopause typically occurs between 45 and 60 years of age.

Mental health: The diagnosis and definition of mental health is a controversial area. A variety of clinical and social models are used by mental health organisations: service users may eschew definitions based around mental disorder, and equate the concept more with what people would aspire to for themselves and associate it with a recovery model. The mental health charity Rethink sees the idea of mental health as encompassing emotional, psychological and spiritual well-being (http://www.rethink.org/publications/Glossary).

Mental Health Act 1983: Makes provision for the compulsory detention, assessment and treatment in hospital of those with mental disorder.

Mental health promotion: Mental health promotion can be seen as a kind of immunisation, working to strengthen the resilience of individuals, families, organisations and communities – as well as to reduce conditions that are known to damage well-being in everyone, whether or not they have a mental health problem.

Meta analysis: A statistical technique for quantitatively combining and integrating the results of multiple studies focusing on the same area of interest.

Migraine: A vascular headache caused by blood flow and chemical changes in the brain, leading to constriction of the arteries supplying blood to the brain and often causing severe pain.

MIND: The leading mental health charity in England and Wales, which works to create a better life for everyone with experience of mental distress.

Modernisation Agency (MA): This agency is envisaged as a resource of current thinking, practical advice and tips for everyone involved in improving patient care and experience. Its website is at http://www.modern.nhs.uk/home.

Modernisation Board: Nationally, The Modernisation Board is a 30-member advisory panel of health and social care professionals, including frontline staff and patient representatives, which provides independent advice to Ministers on the way forward for the NHS. There are also local Modernisation Boards.

Monitoring diaries: Diaries that are used to monitor activities or moods.

Monoamine Oxidase Inhibitors (MAOIs): A

type of antidepressant that is usually tried when other antidepressants have been ineffective. MAOIs elevate mood by blocking the actions of a chemical in the brain (monoamine oxidase), which normally breaks down the neurotransmitters that stimulate the brain .

Monoamines: An amine compound containing one amino group, especially a compound that functions as a neurotransmitter.

Morbidity: In clinical usage, any disease state, including diagnosis and complications, is referred to as morbidity.

Motor tension: Bodily symptoms such as restless fidgeting, jumpiness, trembling and inability to relax.

Movement disorders: Neurological conditions characterised by abnormalities of movement and posture.

Multiple sclerosis: A disease in which there are foci of demyelination (loss of the myelin sheath around nervous tissue) throughout the white matter of the central nervous system. Typically, the symptoms of lesions of the white matter are weakness, lack of coordination, loss of function, speech disturbances, and visual complaints. The course of the disease is usually prolonged, so that the term also includes remissions and relapses that may occur over a period of many years.

Myocardial infarction: More commonly known as a heart attack, occurring when one or more regions of the heart muscle experience a severe or prolonged decrease in oxygen supply, caused by a blocked blood flow to the heart muscle.

Narcolepsy: A sleep disorder characterised by excessive sleepiness, where the person has an abnormal tendency to pass directly from full wakefulness into REM sleep.

National Institute for Health and Clinical Excellence (NICE): Established to provide guidance on new and existing technologies, and to develop clinical guidelines and clinical audit. It functions as a Special Health Authority that promotes clinical excellence and the effective use of resources in the health service.

National Institute for Mental Health in England (NIMHE): Promotes research and advises on evidence-based best practice. It aims to develop partnerships – between government and other agencies, service users, carers, professionals and managers – and to be the development arm for national mental health policy.

National Primary Care Development Team: Developed to support organisations in programmes of work that will help them deliver rapid, systematic and sustainable care for patients and communities.

National Service Frameworks (NSFs): Sets of national standards produced by the Department of Health for care in certain medical areas. They set out service models to which all NHS organisations must comply; set up programmes to support the implementation of the agreed standards; and establish performance measures against which progress within an agreed time-scale is measured. NSFs are developed at the rate of two per year. So far, they cover coronary heart disease, cancer, older people, mental health, diabetes, paediatric intensive care, and children's services etc.

Negative symptoms: These are symptoms experienced in psychotic illness and include: social withdrawal, difficulty expressing emotions, poor self-care, inability to feel pleasure.

Negligence: Lack of proper care or attention. Negligence in healthcare law terms is the failure to do something the 'ordinary skilled man exercising the ordinary skill of that particular art' would do.

Neurological: Relating to the nervous system.

Neurosis: A psychological or behavioural disorder, where psychotic symptoms are not present.

New Public Health: The strategies for developing health promoting policies and working in partnership with communities that date from the 1980s.

NHS Centre for Reviews and Dissemination: Proactively commissions or carries out reviews on behalf of the NHS. The reviews focus on specific questions of importance to the NHS, principally in areas of effectiveness and cost-effectiveness of healthcare interventions, management and organisation of health services.

NHS Plan: Sets out how the government intends to reform the NHS so that services are redesigned around the needs of the patient. It gives proposals for monitoring national standards to provide a health service fit for the 21st century.

Non-verbal cues: Signs that a person is listening and which give the person confidence to continue, e.g. nodding.

Noradrenaline, norepinephrine: A neurotransmitter found mainly in areas of the brain that are involved in governing autonomic nervous system activity, it is implicated in depression.

Occupational impairment: A negative effect on a person's ability to work at their normal level of functioning.

Oedema: Swelling from excessive accumulation of serous fluid in tissue.

Office of National Statistics (ONS): The government agency responsible for compiling, analysing and disseminating many of the United Kingdom's economic, social and demographic statistics.

One-stop centres: Bring together primary and community services in one location. They are envisaged to include social services.

Overgeneralization: Seeing a single negative event as a never-ending pattern of defeat.

Overview and Scrutiny Committee (OSC): A body that is part of a local authority (which has social service responsibilities). OSCs have the power to scrutinise health services, giving local authorities a stronger role in the monitoring of local healthcare.

Panic attack: An episode of extreme anxiety with physical symptoms such as palpitations, shakiness, dizziness and racing thoughts.

Panic Disorder: An anxiety disorder characterised by panic attacks, with or without Agoraphobia. Common symptoms include palpitations, overbreathing, sweating and dizziness, and a fear that something catastrophic is about to happen (e.g. a heart attack).

Paraphrasing: To express the meaning of something in other words.

Pathway of care: An outline of anticipated care to help a patient with a specific condition or set of symptoms to move progressively through a clinical intervention to positive outcomes.

Patient Advice and Liaison Service (PALS): A locally-based service which is concerned with resolving problems on the spot before they become major problems. They also provide information about local health services, put people in touch with local support groups, inform people about complaints procedures, and act as an early warning system for Trusts and Patient Forums by monitoring trends.

Patient and Public Involvement Forum (PPIF): A body within an NHS Trust or a Primary Care Trust which monitors and reviews services from the patient's perspective. It seeks to promote the involvement of the public by canvassing the views of patients receiving services, inspects premises where NHS services are delivered, provides training and support to empower local communities, and reviews how well the NHS is meeting its duty to involve and consult the public.

Performance Assessment Frameworks (PAFs): PAFs are designed to give a general picture of NHS and social care performance. Six areas are covered for the NHS: health improvement; fair access to services; effective delivery of healthcare; efficiency; patients and carer experience; and the health outcomes of NHS care.

Personal Social Services (PSS): Personal care services for vulnerable people (including those with special needs because of old age or physical disability). Examples of services are residential care homes, home helps, and social workers who provide help and support for a wide range of people.

Personality disorder: A disorder characterised by enduring and disturbed patterns of perceiving, relating to, and thinking about oneself and the environment. The individual consequently uses inflexible and maladaptive behaviour patterns, often at the expense of self, others and society in general.

Phaeochromocytoma: A vascular tumour of the adrenal gland.

Pharmacological: Relating to medication.

Phenomenology: A philosophical doctrine based on the study of human experience.

PHQ-9: The Patient Health Questionnaire (9 items) is a self-completed questionnaire which scores each of the nine DSM-IV criteria for depression.

Pneumonia: Inflammation of the lungs.

Positive symptoms: Symptoms experienced in psychotic illness that include: hearing voices, suspiciousness, feeling under constant surveillance, delusions, and making up words without meaning.

Post Traumatic Stress Disorder: An anxiety disorder that occurs after someone has experienced or witnessed a traumatic event such as war, an accident, rape, etc. The person may experience flashbacks and nightmares, along with depression, anger and sleep problems.

Postural hypotension: Low blood pressure occurring in some people when they stand up.

Power of Attorney: Power of Attorney is a legal instrument that is used to delegate legal authority to another

Praxis: Originally from the work of Karl Marx. It has two closely related meanings: it suggests action rather than philosophical speculation – or the direct translation of ideology into action; it implies that the fundamental characteristic of human society is material production to meet human need, i.e. people work and then, only secondarily, think about it.

Precedent: A taught body of instruction, which takes previous cases as an example for subsequent cases.

Prejudices: An attitude or belief system that prevents objective consideration of an issue or situation.

Premenstrual syndrome (PMS): A syndrome that occurs in many women from 2 to 14 days before onset of menstruation, often characterised by a wide range of physical or emotional symptoms.

Prevalence: General occurrence of something, in this case a psychological disorder.

Primary care: Services provided by family doctors, dentists, pharmacists, optometrists and ophthalmic medical practitioners, together with district nurses and health visitors, along with their administrative support.

Primary Care Groups: Precursors to Primary Care Trusts.

Primary Care Trust: A grouping of primary care teams, with responsibility for commissioning specialist services as well as for providing primary care (working closely with social services).

Prison In-reach Staff: Multi-disciplinary teams, similar to CMHTs, which offer to prisoners the same sort of specialised care as that which they would have if they were in the community. While they may provide for prisoners with a wide range of mental health needs, their principal focus is likely to be on those with severe and enduring mental illness.

Problem solving: An approach used to find practical solutions to problems.

Prognosis: A forecast of the probable course of disease.

Protective factors: In this context, reasons why the patient has a reduced likelihood of acting on suicidal thoughts.

Provider: To become providers in the internal market, health organisations became NHS Trusts, independent organisations with their own management systems which provided healthcare. Providers were primarily acute hospitals, organisations providing care for the mentally ill, people with learning disabilities and the elderly.

Proximity: In legal terms, closeness to people who will be directly affected by your actions

Pseudoephedrine: A substance derived from ephedrine, used primarily as a decongestant.

Psychoactive substance: A drug that can produce mood changes and distorted perceptions.

Psycho-education: Provision to patients of information about their disorder, and evidence-based approaches to overcome their difficulties.

Psychomotor disturbance: Impairment of the ability to carry out complex sequences of actions that require perceptual information and control of the muscles.

Psychopathology: The branch of medicine dealing with causes and nature of mental illness.

Psychosis: Severe mental health problem, with or without organic damage, characterised by loss of contact with reality and causing deterioration of normal social functioning.

Psychosocial support: Interventions by health professionals using psychological methods intended to improve the psychological and emotional well-being of the patient.

Psychotherapy: While there are many different types of psychotherapy, with differing theoretical underpinnings, what they have in common is that they are talking therapies with the aim of helping people to overcome stress, emotional problems, relationship problems or troublesome habits.

Psychotic disorder: Where a patient experiences unusual perceptions, such as hearing voices (hallucinations), or unusual beliefs (delusions).

Psychotic symptoms: Experiences related to a psychotic illness, such as schizophrenia (e.g. delusions and hallucinations).

Purchaser: After the establishment of the internal market, health authorities and some family doctors were given budgets to buy healthcare from providers. They were known as purchasers.

Rapport: A state of mutual understanding or trust and agreement between people.

Records: Any permanent form of information recorded about a patient or client.

Reflection: The act of mirroring back what someone has said.

Reflection-in-action: The process of thinking about doing something whilst we are doing it.

Reflection-on-action: The process of looking back at what we have done after the event, making sense of experience, exploring understanding and knowledge.

Relapse prevention: Help to train patients to cope more effectively and to overcome the stressors or triggers in their environments that may cause relapse.

Renal: Pertaining to the kidneys.

Representativeness: When users and carers are actively involved, their 'representativeness' may be called into question: as individuals, they may not be seen to represent the views held by their peers. This objection can work as a strategy for sidelining users' and carers' views; other individuals (such as clinicians) may not be subject to the same requirement always to represent a wider group. User and carer involvement is more about valuing previously under-represented viewpoints derived from personal experience than about claiming universality.

Respect: To treat with consideration; a key ingredient to successful relationships.

Ruminating: Turning a matter over and over in the mind.

Safety behaviours: Actions that a person takes to decrease their anxiety and that can be very subtle.

Scheduled contact: In this context, sessions either face-to-face or by telephone that are pre-arranged.

Scheduling activities: The planning of actions that a person will take.

Schizophrenia: A serious mental health problem that causes a separation between the thought processes and the emotions. Sufferers may experience confusion of reality with hallucinations and/or delusions and may become paranoid.

Secondary care: Healthcare services provided by practitioners who do not have first contact with patients (e.g. psychiatrists, CBT nurse therapists, cardiologists, urologists, etc.).

Sedative: An agent that calms nervous excitement; used to treat agitation.

Seizure: A sudden attack or convulsion, due to involuntary electrical activity in the brain, that can result in a wide variety of clinical manifestations such as: muscle twitches, staring, tongue biting, urination, loss of consciousness and total body shaking. *See* Epilepsy.

Selective Serotonin Re-uptake Inhibitor (SSRI): A class of antidepressant drugs that act by blocking the re-uptake of serotonin so that more serotonin is available to act on receptors in the brain.

Self-disclosure: The sharing of private information about oneself with another person.

Self-efficacy: The extent to which an individual believes themself capable of making a change in their behaviour, using the skills and behaviours that are proven to be helpful in a given condition. Within Chronic Disease Self-Management Programmes, these skills are taught and modelled by someone who shares similar difficulties.

Serious mental illness: The term which groups together Schizophrenia and Bipolar Affective Disorder, where the individual has extreme difficulties with their thoughts or perceptions to such an extent that it affects their ability to cope or function on a day-to-day basis.

Serotonin: A neurotransmitter involved in the processes of sleep and memory, as well as other neurological functions; it is implicated in all affective disorders.

Service and Financial Frameworks (SAFFs): SAFFs make explicit levels of NHS activity and the resources needed to support the local contribution to the national and local priorities, as set out in the NHS Plan and in local Health Improvement Programmes.

Setback: A reverse in progress.

Sexual dysfunction: Difficulty in having sexual intercourse, which may be caused by physical illness (e.g. diabetes) or emotional factors (e.g. depression).

Shared decision-making: Allowing patients to share the decision about which treatment option is best for them by informing them about likely outcomes, providing supporting evidence for the treatment options and working with them in deciding which choice is best for them, bearing in mind their preferences, values and lifestyle.

Shingles: Disease in adults, caused by the varicella zoster virus (Herpetoviridae) that in children causes chicken pox. *See* Herpes.

Signposting: The act of directing the patient towards other organisations that can provide more expert advice on their difficulties (e.g. local support groups, voluntary agencies, etc.).

Sleep apnoea: A sleep disorder in which a person has irregular breathing during sleep, when the upper airway collapses repeatedly at irregular intervals, and can result in the airway becoming blocked completely, cutting off the flow of air.

Sleep hygiene: Refers to activities that either promote sleep (good sleep hygiene) or hinder sleep (poor sleep hygiene).

Smoking Cessation Groups: Self-help groups providing help to smokers who wish to stop.

Social Care Institute for Excellence (SCIE): The organisation responsible for promoting good practice in social care.

Social exclusion: Multidimensional disadvantage which is of substantial duration and which involves dissociation from the major social and occupational environment of society. Key risk factors for social exclusion include: mental health problems; low income; family conflict; being in care; school problems; being an ex-prisoner; being from a minority ethnic group; living in a deprived neighbourhood in urban and rural areas; age and disability.

Social impairment: Negative effects on a person's ability to function at work, in their home life, leisure activities and in relationships with others.

Social inclusion: Strategies to increase the participation of communities marginalised by lack of economic opportunity, educational achievement or other barriers.

Social Phobia: A marked and persistent fear of one or more social or performance situations in which the person is exposed to possible scrutiny by others.

Social Services Inspectorate (SSI): The SSI is a division within the Department of Health. It provides policy advice, manages the Department's links with social services and inspects the quality of social care.

Social stratification: The process that occurs when individual inequalities, be they of strength, wealth or power, become systematic. Social stratification necessarily involves social inequality.

Somatic symptoms: Physical symptoms.

Special Health Authorities: Set up to provide a national service to the NHS or the public, under Section 11 of the NHS Act (1977). They are independent, but can be subject to ministerial direction like other NHS bodies.

Specialist Resistant Services: Services that provide treatment to patients who have not responded to lower-intensity treatments.

Specific Phobia: Marked and persistent fear that is excessive or unreasonable, cued by the presence or anticipation of a specific object or situation (e.g. insects, heights, animals, flying, etc.).

Statute: Statute laws are Acts of Parliament, which are written down and govern the behaviour of people and organisations.

Stepped Care: A model of healthcare in which there are two main features: the first-line treatments offered to the patient are the least intensive of those available, yet are still expected to bring about positive outcomes; the outcomes of interventions and decisions about treatment provision are monitored systematically, and changes made (this is called 'stepping up') if the interventions the patient is currently receiving are not resulting in significant improvement.

Stepping up: The process of moving up to a more involved treatment than that currently provided in response to patient need.

Stigma: Broadly refers to a construction of difference – for example, between people with mental health problems and others.

Stigma can result in social exclusion for those subjected to stigmatising attitudes. Related terms include 'discrimination' and 'otherness'.

Strategic Health Authority: Strategic Health Authorities are in effect responsible for managing the NHS on behalf of the Department of Health. Their three fundamental functions are: creating a coherent strategic framework; agreeing annual performance agreements and performance management; building capacity and supporting performance improvement.

Stress: A state of emotional or mental strain experienced by a person when they perceive that the demand placed on them is beyond their ability to cope.

Stroke: A sudden loss of consciousness resulting when the rupture or occlusion of a blood vessel leads to a lack of oxygen in the brain, resulting in loss of brain function in the area affected.

Subclinical: The stage in the development of a disorder or disease before symptoms are observable.

Sub-therapeutic dose: An amount taken of a drug that is too low to expect any therapeutic benefit.

Summarizing: Reiterating briefly and succinctly.

Support, Time and Recovery Workers (StaR workers): Key mental health workers who give direct support to users of mental health services by spending time with them. They are accessible to service users and help them to get access to other appropriate staff and services. They focus on respecting the person's own perspective of their needs, enabling independence and working towards recovery.

Symptomatology: The branch of medicine concerned with the study and classification of the symptoms of disease.

Tackling Health Inequalities Programme: A Department of Health initiative which lays the foundations for meeting the government's target to reduce the health gap in infant mortality and life expectancy by 2010.

Therapeutic alliance: The relationship between patient and health practitioner.

Thyroid disease: Disease of the thyroid gland.

Tokenism: The practice of making only a perfunctory or symbolic effort, especially by recruiting a single individual or too small a number of people from an under-represented group.

Tolerability: Measure of how much something is capable of being tolerated or is endurable.

Tort: A wrongful act, whether intentional or accidental, from which injury occurs to another

Toxicity: Measure of how much something is poisonous or harmful; often used to refer to side-effects of medication.

Tricyclic antidepressants (TCA): A class of antidepressant drugs that act by blocking the re-uptake of noradrenaline (norepinephrine) and serotonin, to varying degrees, and thus make more of those substances available to act on receptors in the brain .

Tyramine: An amino acid, derived from tyrosine, found in chocolate, cola drinks, ripe cheese and beer. Patients taking MAOIs should avoid foods containing tyramine.

Urinary retention: Holding urine in the bladder.

Vegetative state: A condition experienced by some patients with severe depression, where there is minimal physical activity and a vastly reduced response to stimulation.

Vertigo: The sensation of spinning or whirling that occurs as a result of a disturbance in balance. It also refers to feelings of dizziness, lightheadedness, faintness and unsteadiness.

Vicarious liability: The liability of an employer for the negligent acts or omissions of their employee.

Vicious circle: When one symptom leads to another that aggravates the first, and so on.

Watchful waiting: Close monitoring of a patient by a healthcare professional, instead of immediate treatment.

Workforce Action Team (WAT): The aim of WATs is to enable mental health services to ensure that their workforce is sufficient and skilled, well led and supported, so as to deliver high-quality mental healthcare. Their work is not just confined to the statutory sector, and they comprise members of many organisations in health and social services.

Workforce Development Directorate (WDD): Formerly known as Workforce Development Confederations, WDDs gave a clear leadership and direction to workforce planning and development, and manage the multi-professional education and training budget (and other relevant budgets). They brought together local NHS and non-NHS employers to plan and develop the whole healthcare workforce. The responsibilities of WDDs have now been subsumed within Strategic Health Authorities.

World Health Organisation (WHO): The United Nations specialized agency for health, acting as a coordinating authority on international health matters.

Work and Social Adjustment Scale (WSAS): A self-completed measure which assesses how five key areas in a person's life are affected by their problem. These areas are: ability to work; home management; social leisure activities; private leisure activities; and ability to form and maintain close relationships with others.

Reading List

Allebeck, P. (1989). Schizophrenia: A Life Shortening Disease. *Schizophrenia Bulletin*, 15, 1, 81-89.

American Psychiatric Association (2000). *Diagnostic and Statistical Manual of Mental Disorders: DSM-IV-TR: Fourth Edition Text Revision.* Washington DC: American Psychiatric Association.

Anon. (1999). Withdrawing Patients from Antidepressants. *Drugs and Therapeutics Bulletin.* 37, 49-52.

Ashenden, R., Silagy, C. and Weller, D. (1997). A systematic review of effectiveness of promoting lifestyle change in general practice. *Family Practice*, 14, 160-175.

Association of the British Pharmaceutical Industry (1999). *The Expert Patient – Survey October 1999*, London: ABPI, available on www.abpi.org.uk.

Audit Commission (2001). *Change Here! Managing Change to Improve Local Services.* London: Audit Commission. Also available on www.audit-commission.gov.org.

Badamgarav, E., Weingarten, S.R., Henning, J.M., Knight, K., Hasselblad, V., Ganto, A. and Ofman, J. (2003). Effectiveness of disease management programs in depression: A systematic review. *The American Journal of Psychiatry*, 160 2080-2090.

Barker, P. (1997). *Assessment in psychiatric and mental health nursing: In search of the whole person.* Cheltenham: Stanley Thornes Ltd.

Barkham, M., Rees, A., Stiles, W., Shapiro, D., Hardy, G. and Reynolds, S. (1996). Dose-effect relations in time-limited psychotherapy for depression. *Journal of Consulting and Clinical Psychology*, 64, 927-935.

Barnes D, Brandon T and Webb, T. (2002). *Independent Specialist Advocacy in England and Wales: Recommendations for Good Practice.* Durham: University of Durham.

Also available from Department of Health website, www.dh.gov.uk/Home/fs/en.

Barnes, M. and Bowl, R. (2001). *Taking Over the Asylum: Empowerment and Mental Health.* Basingstoke: Palgrave.

Barnes, M. and Shardlow, P. (1997). From passive recipient to active citizen: participation in mental health user groups. *Journal of Mental Health*, 6 (3), 289-300.

Bartley, M. (2004). *Health Inequality: Theories, Concepts and Methods.* Oxford: Polity.

Bazire, S. (2003/4). *Psychotropic Drug Directory.* Wiltshire: Quay Books.

Bearpark, H. (1994). *Overcoming insomnia.* Rushcutters Bay, Sydney: Gore and Osment Publications.

Beck, J.S. (1995). *Cognitive Therapy. Basics and Beyond.* New York: Guildford Press.

Bootzin, R.R. and Perlis, M.L (1992). Nonpharmacological treatments of insomnia. *Journal of Clinical Psychiatry*, 53 (Suppl.) 37-41.

Bower, P., Richards, D. and Lovell, K. (2001). The clinical and cost-effectiveness of self-help treatments for anxiety and depression disorders in primary care: a systematic review. *British Journal of General Practice*, 51 (471) 838-845.

Bowles, N. and Bowles, A. (1999). Transformational leadership. *Nursing Times (Learning Curve Supplement)* 3 (8), 2-5.

Bowman, C. and Asch, D. (1999). *Strategic Management.* London: Macmillan.

Bowman, D., Scogin, F. and Brenda, L. (1996). The efficacy of self-examination and cognitive bibliotherapy in the treatment of moderate depression. *Psychotherapy Research*, 5, 131-140.

Bradshaw, T. (in press) A Systematic review of the efficacy of healthy living interventions for adult with a diagnosis of schizophrenia a schizo-affective disorder. *Journal of Advanced Nursing.*

British Medical Association and Royal Pharmaceutical Society of Great Britain (2004). *British National Formulary.* London: British Medical Association and Royal Pharmaceutical Society of Great Britain.

British Medical Journal (2003). 'The Patient Issue', Volume 326 (14 June).

British Psychological Society (1993). *Code of Conduct, Ethical Principles and Guidelines,* The British Psychological Society.

British Psychological Society (2000). *Recent advances in understanding mental illness and psychotic experiences.* Leicester: The British Psychological Society.

Brooker, C. (1990). The health education needs of families caring for a schizophrenic relative and the potential role for community psychiatric nurses. *Journal of Advanced Nursing,* 15 (9), 1092-1098.

Brown, S. (1997). Excess mortality of Schizophrenia: A meta-analysis. *British Journal of Psychiatry,* 171, 12, 502-508.

Brown, S., Inskip, H. and Barrowclough, B. (2000). Causes of the excess mortality of schizophrenia. *British Journal of Psychiatry,* 177, 212-217.

Burns, D.D. (2005) (3rd Edition). *Feeling Good. The New Mood Therapy.* New York: Penguin.

Burns, D.D. and Spangler, D.L. (2000). Does psychotherapy homework lead to improvements in depression in C.B.T. or does improvement lead to increased homework concordance. *Journal of Consulting and Clinical Psychology,* 68, 1, 46-56.

Butler, G. (1999). *Overcoming Social Anxiety and Shyness. A self-help guide using Cognitive Behavioural Techniques.* London: Robinson.

Butterworth, T. and Woods, D. (1998). *Clinical governance and Clinical Supervision Working Together to Ensure Safe and Accountable Practice.* Manchester: School of Nursing, Midwifery and Health Visiting, University of Manchester.

Campbell, P. (2001). From petitions to professionals. *Openmind,* 107 Jan/Feb, p10.

Car, J. and Sheikh, A. (2003). Telephone consultations. *British Medical Journal,* 326, 966-969.

Carey, P. (2002). 'Community Health and Empowerment' in Kerr J (ed) *Community Health Promotion.* London: Bailliere Tindall.

Carroll, M. and Holloway, E. (1999). *Counselling Supervision in Context.* London: Sage.

Chadwick, P.D.J. and Birchwood, M. (1994). The omnipotence of voices: A cognitive approach to auditory hallucinations. *British Journal of Psychiatry,* 164, 190-201.

Church, K. (1996). Beyond 'Bad Manners': the Power Relations of Consumer Participation in Ontario's Mental Health System. *Canadian Journal of Community Mental Health,* 15 (2), 27-44.

Clark, D.M. (1986). A cognitive model of panic. *Behaviour Research and Therapy,* 24, 461-470.

Cohen, A. and Hove, M. (2001). *Physical health of the Severe and Enduring Mentally Ill: A Training Pack for GP Educators.* London: Sainsbury Centre for Mental Health.

Commission for Health Improvement (CHI). (2004). *Unpacking the Patients' Experience: Variations in the NHS patient experience in England.* London: CHI. Also available at www.chai.nhs.uk.

Consumers in NHS Research Support Unit (2000). *Involving Consumers in Research and Development in the NHS: Briefing Notes for Researchers.* Eastleigh, Hampshire: CNHSR Support Unit.

Cook, M. (1999). Improving care requires leadership in nursing. *Nurse Education Today,* 19, 306-312.

Cooper, C. (1994). Finding the solution – primary prevention: identifying the causes and preventing mental ill health in the workplace, in *Mental Health in the Workplace.* London: HMSO.

Crowther, R., Bond, G., Huxley, P. and Marshall, M. (2000). Vocational training for people with severe mental disorders (Protocol for a Cochrane Review). *The Cochrane Library,* Issue 3, Oxford.

Curran, C. and Grimshaw, C. (2000). Advocacy. *Openmind,* 101, Jan/Feb p28.

Darbisher, L. and Glenister, G. (1998). *The Balance for Life Scheme: mental health benefits of GP recommended exercise in relation to depression and anxiety.* Colchester: The University of Essex: Health and Social Services Unit.

Davies, W. (2000). *Overcoming Anger and Irritability. A self-help guide using Cognitive Behavioural Techniques.* London: Robinson.

Demyttenaere, K. (2003). Risk factors and predictors of concordance in depression. *European Neuropsychopharmacology*, 13, 69-75.

Department of Health (1989). *Working for Patients.* London: HMSO.

Department of Health (1990). *The NHS and Community Care Act.* London: HMSO.

Department of Health (1992). *Health of the Nation White Paper.* London: HMSO. www.dh.gov.uk.

Department of Health (1993). *A Vision for the future: The Nursing, Midwifery and Health Visiting Contribution to Health and Health Care.* London: HMSO.

Department of Health (1997a). *The New NHS: Modern, Dependable.* London: HMSO.

Department of Health (1997b). *The NHS (Primary Care) Act 1997.* London: HMSO.

Department of Health (1997c). *The Caldicott Committee: Report on the Review of Patient-Identifiable Information.* London: HMSO.

Department of Health (1998a). *A first class service: quality in the NHS.* London: HMSO.

Department of Health (1998b). *Modernising Mental Health Services.* London: HMSO.

Department of Health (1998c). *Modernising Social Services.* London: HMSO.

Department of Health (1999a). *A National Service Framework for Mental Health: Modern standards and service models.* London: HMSO.

Department of Health (1999b). *The Future Organisation of Prison Health Care.* London: HMSO.

Department of Health (1999c). *Clinical governance: quality in the new NHS.* HSC 1999/065, London: HMSO.

Department of Health (1999d). *Managing Dangerous People with Severe Personality Disorder.* London: HMSO.

Department of Health (1999e). *The Health Service Circular: Using Electronic Patient Records in Hospitals: Legal requirements and Good practice.* HSC 1998/153 London: HMSO.

Department of Health (1999f). *Saving Lives: Our Healthier Nation.* London: HMSO.

Department of Health (2000a). *The NHS Plan: A Plan for Investment, A Plan for Reform.* London: HMSO.

Department of Health (2000b). *Reforming the Mental Health Act, Part I, The New Legal Framework.* London: HMSO.

Department of Health (2000c). *Reforming the Mental Health Act, Part II, High Risk Patients.* London: HMSO.

Department of Health (2000d). *NHS Implementation Programme.* London: HMSO.

Department of Health (2001a). *Treatment Choice in Psychological Therapies and Counselling.* London: Department of Health Publication. www.dh.gov.uk.

Department of Health (2001b). *Shifting the Balance of Power within the NHS. Securing Delivery,* London: HMSO.

Department of Health (2001c). *The Journey to Recovery: The Government's Vision for Mental Health Care.* London: HMSO.

Department of Health (2001d). *The Expert Patient: A New Approach to Chronic Disease Management for the 21st Century.* London: HMSO.

Department of Health (2001e). *The Mental Health Policy Implementation Guide.* London: Department of Health.

Department of Health (2001f). Office of National Statistics: Psychiatric Morbidity Among Adults Living in Private Households, 2000. London: HMSO.

Department of Health (2001g). *Choosing Talking Therapies?* London: Department of Health.

Department of Health (2001h). *Safety First: Five-year report of the National Confidential Inquiry into Suicide and Homicide by People with Mental Illness.* London: HMSO.

Department of Health (2001i). *Making it Happen: A Guide to Delivering Mental Health Promotion.* London: HMSO.

Department of Health (2001j). *National Service Framework for Older People: Modern Standards and Service Models.* London: Department of Health.

Department of Health (2002a). *Fast Forwarding*

Primary Care Mental Health: 1000 New Graduate Workers to Support Primary Care Mental Health. London: Department of Health.

Department of Health (2002b). *Improvement, Expansion and Reform: The Next Three Years.* London: HMSO.

Department of Health (2002c). *Women's Mental Health: Into the Mainstream - Strategic Development of Mental Health Care for Women.* London: HMSO.

Department of Health (2002d). *A Sign of the Times: Modernising Mental Health Services for People who are Deaf.* London: HMSO.

Department of Health (2003a). *Mental Health Policy Implementation Guide: Support, Time and Recovery (STR) Workers.* London: HMSO.

Department of Health (2003b). *The NHS Confidentiality Code of Practice; Guidelines on the use and protection of patient information.* London: HMSO.

Department of Health (2003c). *Self-Help Interventions for Mental Health Problems.* London: Department of Health.

Department of Health (2003d). *Tackling Health Inequalities: A Programme for Action.* London: HMSO.

Department of Health (2003e). *Delivering Investment in General Practice: Implementing the new GMS Contract.* London: HMSO.

Department of Health (2004a). *Patient and Public Involvement in Health: The Evidence for Policy Implementation.* London: HMSO.

Department of Health (2004b). *The General Medical Services Contract.* London: HMSO.

Department of Health (2004c). *Making Partnership Work for Patients, Carers and Service Users.* London: HMSO.

Department of Health (2004d). Regulation of Health Care Staff in England and Wales: A consultation document. London: HMSO.

Department of Health (2005). "*12 key points on consent: the law in England*" (online) www.dh.gov.uk/assetRoot/ 04/01/91/86/04019186.pdf [15th January 2005]

Disability Discrimination Act (1995). Available on www.disability.gov.uk/dda/

Doran, C.M. (2003). *Prescribing mental health medication: The Practitioner's Guide.* New York: Routledge.

Driscoll, J. (2000). *Practising Clinical Supervision: A Reflective Approach.* London: Balliere Tindall.

Dryden, W (1996). *Overcoming Anger.* London: Sheldon Press.

Duarri, W. and Kendrick, K. (1999). Implementing Clinical Supervision. *Professional Nurse,* 14, 12, 849-842.

Eaton, L. (2002a). The road to consensus. *Health Service Journal,* 12 (5789) 24 January, 16-17.

Eaton, L. (2002b). A third of Europeans and almost half of Americans use internet for health information. *British Medical Journal,* 325, p989.

Eccles, T. (1994). *Succeeding with Change: Implementing Action-Driven Strategies.* London: McGraw Hill.

Egan, G. (2001). *The Skilled Helper: A systematic approach to effective helping (seventh edition).* California: Brooks/Cole.

Epstein, R.S. (1994). *Keeping boundaries – Maintaining safety and integrity in the psychotherapeutic process.* Arlington, VA: American psychiatric publishing inc.

Evans, K., Tyrer, P., Catalan, J., Schmidt, U., Davidson, K., Dent, J., Tata, P., Thornton, S., Barber, J. and Thompson, S. (1999). Manual-assisted cognitive behaviour therapy (MACT): a randomised controlled trial of a brief intervention with bibliotherapy in the treatment of self-harm. *Psychological Medicine,* 29, 19-25.

Faugier, J. (1992). The supervisory relationship. In Butterworth, T. and Faugier, J. (eds). *Clinical Supervision and Mentorship in Nursing.* London: Chapman and Hall.

Felker, B., Yazel, J.J. and Short, D. (1996). Mortality and medical co-morbidity among psychiatric patients: A review. *Psychiatric Services,* 47, 12, 1356-1363.

Fennel, M. (1999). *Overcoming Low Self-Esteem. A self-help guide using Cognitive Behavioural Techniques.* London: Robinson.

Freedman, D.B. (2002). Clinical governance – bridging management and clinical approaches to quality in the UK. *Clinica Chimica Acta,* 319, 133-141.

Fritzler, B., Hecker, J. and Loose, M. (1997). Self-directed treatment with minimal therapist contact: preliminary findings for obsessive-compulsive disorder. *Behavioural Research and Therapy,* 35, 627-631.

Frude, N.J. (2004a). A book prescription scheme in primary care. *Clinical Psychology,* 39, 11-14.

Frude, N.J. (2004b). Bibliotherapy as a means of delivering psychological therapy. *Clinical Psychology,* 39, 8-10.

Furukawa, T., McGuire, H. and Barbui, C. (2002). Meta-analysis of effects and side effects of low dosage tricyclic antideressants in depression: systematic review. *British Medical Journal,* 325, 991-1001.

Gabe, J., Bury, M. and Elston, M.A. (2004). *Key Concepts in Medical Sociology.* London: Sage.

Gamble, C. and Brimblecombe, N. (2005). *Key Skills in Community Mental Health Nursing.* London: Quay Books.

Gilbert, P (1997). *Overcoming Depression. A self-help guide using Cognitive Behavioural Techniques.* London: Robinson.

Gilbody, S., Whitty, P., Grimshaw, J. and Thomas, R. (2002). *Improving the recognition and management of depression in primary care.* The University of York: *Effective Healthcare Bulletin.*

Gilbody, S., Whitty, P., Grimshaw, J. and Thomas, R. (2003). Educational and Organizational Interventions to Improve the Management of Depression in Primary Care. *The Journal of the American Medical Association (JAMA),* 289 3145-3151.

Glasgow Media Group (2001). 'Media and Mental Illness' in Davey, B., Gray, A. and Seale, C. (eds), *Health and Disease; A Reader.* Buckingham: Open University Press.

Goffman, E. (1963). *Stigma: Notes on the Management of Spoiled Identity.* New Jersey: Prentice Hall.

Goldberg, D. and Huxley, P. (1992). *Common Mental Disorders: A biosocial module.* London: Routledge.

Greenberger, D. and Padesky, C.A. (1995). *Mind Over Mood, A Cognitive Therapy Treatment Manual for Clients.* London: Guildford Press.

Greenwood, J. (1993). Reflective Practice: a critique of work of Argyris and Schön. *Journal of Advanced Nursing,* 18, 8, 1183-1187.

Gutheil, T.G. and Gabbard, G.O. (1993). The concept of boundaries in clinical practice: theoretical and risk-management dimensions. *American Journal of Psychiatry,* 150, 2, 188-196.

Ham, C. and Alberti, K. (2002). The Medical Profession, the Public and the Government. *British Medical Journal,* 324, 838-842.

Ham, C. (2004). *Health Policy in Britain* (Fifth Edition). London: Macmillan.

Handy, C. (1995). *Beyond Certainty.* London: Hutchinson.

Harbin, T.J. (2000). *Beyond Anger: a Guide for Men: How to Free Yourself from the Grip of Anger and Get More Out of Life.* New York: Marlowe and Co.

Hawkins, P. and Shohet, R. (1989). *Supervision in the helping professions.* Milton Keynes: Open University Press.

Haynes, R. B, McDonald H, Gang, A.X. and Montague, P. (2004). *Interventions for Helping patients to follow prescriptions for medications.* Chichester: Cochrane Database of Systematic Reviews.

Health Advisory Service (1995). *With Care in Mind, Secure.* London: HMSO.

Health Professions Council (2003). *Standards of Conduct, Performance and Ethics. Your Duties as a Registrant:* London: Health Professions Council.

Hegel, M., Imming, J., Cyr-Provost, M., Noel, P., Arean, P. and Unutzer, J. (2002). Role of Behavioural Health Professionals in a Collaborative Stepped Care Treatment Model for Depression in Primary Care: Project IMPACT. *Families, Systems and Health,* 20, 3, 265-277.

Henderson, R. and Pochin M. (2001) *Right Result? Advocacy, Justice, and Empowerment.* Bristol: Policy Press.

Heron, J. (2000). *Helping the client: A creative practical guide (fifth edition).* London: Sage.

Herrman, H.E., Baldwin, J.A. and Christie, D. (1983). A record-linkage study of mortality and general hospital discharge in patients diagnosed as schizophrenic. *Psychological*

Medicine, 13, 581-593.

Hiller, W., Zaudig, M. and Mombour, W. (1996). *ICD-10 Psychodiagnostic Checklists.* Hogrefe and Huber, Cambridge, MA.

Hollon, S.D. (2001). Behavioural activation treatment for depression: a commentary. *Clinical Psychology: Science and Practice,* 8 (3) 271-274

Hollon, S., DeRubeis, R. and Evans, M, D. (1987). Casual mediation of change in treatment for depression: Discriminating between nonspecificity and noncausality. *Psychological Bulletin,* 102, 1, 139-149.

Hunkeler, E.M., Meresman, J.F., Hargreaves, W.A. et al. (2000). Efficacy of nurse telehealth care and peer support in augmenting treatment of depression in primary care. *Archives of Family Medicine,* 9, 700-708.

Iles, V. and Sutherland, K. (2001). *Managing Change in the NHS: Organisational Change.* London: National Co–coordinating Centre for NHS Service Delivery and Organisation RandD. www.sdo.lshtm.ac.uk

Inskipp, F. and Proctor, B. (1993). *The art, craft and tasks of supervision: making the most of supervision.* London: Cascade.

Inskipp, F. and Scaife, J. (2001). *Supervision in the Mental Health Professions: A Practitioner's Guide.* Hove: Philadelphia Taylor Francis.

International Council of Nurses (2001). Mental Health: Stop exclusion – Dare to care. *Nursing Matters,* Retrieved August 2004.

Jacobsen, E. (1938). *Progressive relaxation.* Chicago: University of Chicago Press.

Jacobson, N., Martell, C.R. and Dimidjian, S. (2001). Behavioural activation treatment for depression: Returning to contextual roots. *Clinical Psychology: Science and Practice* 8 (3) 255-270.

Jafri, T., Jones, R., Taylor, D. and Wakeling, M. (2003). *Future Partnerships: Primary Care in 2020?* University of London: The School of Pharmacy.

Johns, C. (2000). *Becoming a reflective practitioner. A reflective and holistic approach to clinical nursing practice development and clinical supervision.* London: Blackwell Science.

Jones, J.R., Huxtable, C.S., Hodgson, J.T., Price, M.J. (2003). *Self-reported work-related illness in 2001/02.* Caerphilly: Health and Safety Executive.

Katon, W., Robinson, P., Von Korff, M., Lin, L., Bush, T., Ludman, E., Simon, G. and Walker, E. (1996). A multifaceted intervention to improve treatment of depression in primary care. *Archives of General Psychiatry,* 53, 924-932.

Katon, W. Von Korff, M., Lin, E., Simon, G., Walker, E. and Unutzer, J. (1999). Stepped collaborative care for primary care patients with persistent depression: A randomised trial. *Archives of General Psychiatry.* 56, 1109-1115.

Katon, W., Von Korff, M., Lin, E., Unutzer, J., Simon, G., Walker, E., Ludman, T. and Bush, T. (1997). Population Based Care of Depression: Effective Disease Management Strategies to decrease prevalence. *General Hospital Psychiatry, 19:169-178.*

Katon, W., Von Korff, M., Lin, E., Walker, E., Simon, G.E., Bush, T., Robinson, P. and Russo, J. (1995). Collaborative Management to achieve treatment guidelines: Impact on depression in primary care. *JAMA,* 273 (13), 1026-1031.

Kazantzis, N., (2000). Power to detect homework effects in psychotherapy outcome research. *Journal of Consulting and Clinical Psychology,* 68, 1, 166-170.

Kazantzis, N., Deane, F.P. and Ronan, K.R. (2000). Homework assignments in cognitive and behavioural therapy: A Meta-Analysis. *Clinical Psychology: Science and Practice,* 7, 2, 189-202.

Kelly, C. and McCreadie, R.G. (1999). Smoking habits, current symptoms and premorbid characteristics of schizophrenic patients in Nithsdale, Scotland. *American Journal of Psychiatry,* 156, 11, 1751-1757.

Kemshall, H. and Pritchard, J. (1996). *Good Practice in Risk Assessment and Risk Management 1.* London: Jessica Kingsley.

Kendrick, T., Burns. T., Freeling, P. and Sibbard, B. (1994). Provision of care to General Practice patients with a disabling long-term illness: a survey in 16 practices. *British Journal of General Practice,* 44: 301-309.

Kennerley, H. (1997). *Overcoming Anxiety. A*

self-help guide using Cognitive Behavioural Techniques. London: Robinson.

Korff, M. and Golberg, D. (2001). Improving outcomes in depression: the whole process of care needs to be enhanced. *British Medical Journal,* 323, 948-949.

Kubler-Ross, E. (1970). *On Death and Dying.* London: Tavistock Publications.

Lacks, P. (1987). *Behavioural treatment for persistent insomnia.* Oxford: Pergamon Press.

Lacks, P. and Morin, C.M. (1992). Recent advances in the assessment and treatment of insomnia. *Journal of Consulting and Clinical Psychology,* 60, 586-594.

Lam, H.L., Jones, S.H., Hayward, P. and Bright, J.A. (1999). *Cognitive Therapy for Bipolar Disorder.* Chichester: Wiley.

Leader, A. and Crosby, K. (1998). *Power Tools - Resource Pack for Mental Health Advocacy.* Brighton: Pavillion.

Leeder, S. and Dominello, A. (1999). Social Capital and its relevance to health and family policy. *Australian and New Zealand Journal of Public Health,* 23 (4), 424-429.

Lin, E.H., Von Korff, M., Ludman, E.J., Rutter, C., Bush, T.M., Simon, G.E., Unutzer, J., Walker, E. and Katon, W.J. (2003). Enhancing adherence to prevent depression relapse in primary care. *General Hospital Psychiatry,* 25 (5), 303-310.

Lin, E.H., Von Korff, M., Russo, J., Katon, W., Simon, G.E., Unutzer, J., Bush, T., Walker, E. and Ludman, E. (2000) Can depression treatment in primary care reduce disability? A stepped care approach. *Archives of Family Medicine,* 9, 1052-1058.

Looker, T. and Gregson, O. (2003). *Managing Stress.* London: Teach Yourself Books.

Lord, J., Ochoka, J., Czarny, W. and MacGillivary, H. (1998). Analysis of change within a mental health organisation: a participatory process. *Psychiatric Rehabilitation Journal,* 21 (4), 327-29.

Lorig, K.R., Holman, H.R., Sobel, D.S., Laurent, D.D., González, V.M. and Minor, M.A. (2000). *Living a Healthy Life With Chronic Conditions* (Second Edition). Boulder: Bull.

Lorig, K.R., Ritter, P., Stewart, A.L., Sobel, D.S., Brown, B.W., Bandura, A., González, V.M.,

Laurent, D.D. and Holman, H.R. (2001). Chronic Disease Self-Management Program: 2-Year health status and health care utilisation outcomes. *Medical Care,* 39 (11), 1217-1223.

Lovell, K. and Richards, D. (2000). Multiple access points and levels of entry (MAPLE): ensuring choice, accessibility and equity for CBT services. *Behavioural and Cognitive Psychotherapy,* 28, 379-391.

Lovell, K., Richards, D.A. and Bowers, D. (2003). Improving access to primary care mental health: uncontrolled evaluation of a pilot self-help clinic. *British Journal of General Practice.* 53, 133-135.

Lucock, M.P., Olive, R.E., Sinha, A., Horner, C. and Hames, R. (2003). Graduate primary care mental health workers providing safe and effective client work – what is realistic? *Primary Care Mental Health,* 2, 37-46.

Ludman, E., Simon, G., Von Korff, M., Bush, T., Lin, E., Katon, W. and Walker, E. (2002). Multifaceted interventions to improve the management of depression in primary care: an overview. *Journal of Affective Disorders,* 68-98.

McKeown, C. and Thompson, J. (2001). Implementing Clinical Supervision. *Nursing Management,* 8, 6, 10-13.

Margo, A., Hemsley, D. and Slade, P. (1981). The effects of varying auditory input on schizophrenic hallucinations. *British Journal of Psychiatry.* 139, 122-127.

Marks, I.M. (2001). *Living With Fear, 2nd edition,* London: McGraw-Hill.

Martell, C.R., Addis, M.E. and Jacobson, N.S. (2001). *Depression in Context: Strategies for Guided Action.* New York: Norton.

Mason, T. and Mercer, D. (1998). *Critical Perspectives in Forensic Care: Inside Out.* London: Macmillan.

Maxmen, J. and Nicholas, G. (1995). Schizophrenia and Related Disorders. In *Essential Psychopathology and Its Treatment,* (second edition) New York: W.W. Norton.

Mead, N. and Bower, P. (2000). Patient centredness: a conceptual framework and review of the empirical literature. *Social Science and*

Medication, 51, 1087-1110.

Melzer, H., Gill, B., Petticrew, M. and Hinds, K. (1995). *The prevalence of psychiatric morbidity among adults living in private households.* London: HMSO.

Mentality (2002). *Mental Health Improvement: What Works? A Briefing for the Scottish Executive.* Edinburgh: Scottish Development Centre for Mental Health.

Mentality (2004). *Participation promotes mental health,* London: Sainsbury Centre for Mental Health. www.mentality.org.uk.

Milewa, T. (1999). Community participation and citizenship in British health care planning: narratives of power and involvement in the British welfare state. *Sociology of Health and Illness,* 21 (4), 445-465.

MIND (2000). *Counting the Cost.* London: MIND.

Morrison, A. and Haddock, G. (1997). Cognitive factors in source monitoring and auditory hallucinations. *Psychological Medicine.* 27, 3, 669-679.

Murie, J. (2004). Contract will address needs of patients with severe mental illness. *Guidelines in Practice,* 7, 3, 35-42.

Mynors-Wallis, L.M., Gath, D.H., Day, A. and Baker, F. (2000). Randomised controlled trial of problem solving treatment, antidepressant medication, and combined treatment for major depression in primary care. *British Medical Journal,* 320, 26-30.

Naidoo, J. and Wills, J. (2000). *Health Promotion: Foundations for Practice* (Second Edition). London: Bailliere Tindall.

Naish, S. and Clark, S. (1996). *Profoundly Deaf Patients and General Practitioners: A Qualitative Study Looking at Communication and its Difficulties.* Unpublished document, University of Birmingham: quoted in Department of Health (2002c).

National Health Service Information Authority (2003). *The NHS Model of Data Protection.* Information Governance Toolkit. NHSIA.

National Institute for Health and Clinical Excellence (2004). *Anxiety: Management of anxiety (panic disorder, with or without agoraphobia, and generalised anxiety disorder) in adults in primary, secondary and community care.* London: National Institute for Health and Clinical Excellence. www.nice.org.uk.

National Institute for Health and Clinical Excellence (2004). *Depression: the management of depression in primary and secondary care.* London: National Institute for Health and Clinical Excellence. www.nice.org.uk.

National Institute for Health and Clinical Excellence (2002). *Guidance on the use of computerised cognitive behavioural therapy for anxiety and depression.* National Institute for Health and Clinical Excellence.

National Institute for Mental Health in England (NIMHE) (2003). *Self-help interventions for mental health problems.* London: National Institute for Mental Health in England.

National Institute for Mental Health in England (NIHME) and Department of Health (2003a). *Fast-Forwarding Primary Mental Health: Graduate Primary Care Mental Health Workers – Best Practice Guidance.* London: HMSO.

National Institute for Mental Health in England (NIMHE) and Department of Health (2003b). *Inside Outside – Improving Mental Health Services for Black and Minority Ethnic Communities in England.* London: HMSO.

National Institute for Mental Health in England North West Development Centre (2004a). *Enhanced Services for Depression under the new GP Contract: A Commissioning Handbook.* Hyde: NIMHE North West Development Centre.

National Institute for Mental Health in England North West Development Centre (2004b). *Primary Care Graduate Mental Health Workers – a practical guide.* Hyde: NIMHE North West Development Centre.

National Institute for Mental Health in England (NIMHE), National Health Service University and Sainsbury Centre for Mental Health (2004). *The Ten Essential Shared Capabilities: A framework for the whole of the mental health workforce.* London: Department of Health.

Newell, R and Gourney, K. (2000). *Mental Health Nursing: An Evidenced-based Approach.* London: Churchill Livingstone.

Newman, J. and Clarke, J. (1994). 'Going about

our Business? The Managerialisation of Public Services' in Clarke, J., Cochrane, A. and McLaughlin, E. (eds). *Managing Social Policy.* London: Sage.

NHS Centre for Reviews and Dissemination (2002). Improving the recognition and management of depression in primary care. *Effective Health Care Bulletin*, 7, 5, 1-12.

NHS Confederation and British Medical Association (2003). *New GMS Contract 2003 – Investing in general practice.* London: NHS Confederation and BMA.

NHS Executive (1999). *Leadership for Health: the Health Authority Role.* Leeds: NHS Executive.

Norman, I. and Ryrie, I. (2004). *Art and Science of Mental Health Nursing: A Textbook of Principles.* Maidenhead: Open University Press.

North East Public Health Observatory (2004). *Occasional Paper 2: Scoping Study of Mental Health Data: Key Messages,* available on www.nepho.org.uk.

Nursing and Midwifery Council (2002a). *Code of professional Conduct.* London: Nursing and Midwifery Council.

Nursing and Midwifery Council (2002b). *Guidelines for records and record keeping.* London: Nursing and Midwifery Council.

Nursing and Midwifery Council (2004). Too much information: When to tell and what not to tell about your patients. *NMC News,* July 2004.

Ost, L.G. (1987). Applied relaxation: description of a coping technique and review of controlled studies. *Behaviour Research and Therapy* 25, 397-410.

Palmer, S. (2003). Whistle-stop tour of the theory and practice of stress management and prevention: Its possible role in postgraduate health promotion. *Health Education Journal,* 62 (2), 133-142.

Payne, F., Harvey, K., Jessopp, L., Plummer, S., Tylee, A. and Gournay, K. (2002). Knowledge, confidence and attitudes towards mental health of nurses working in NHS Direct and the effects of training. *Journal of Advanced Nursing,* 40, 549-559.

Peet, M. (2004). *Nutrition and mental health.*

Northern Centre for Mental Health.

Perkins, R., Buckfield, R. and Choy, D. (1997). Access to employment: a supported employment project to enable service users to obtain jobs within mental health teams. *Journal of Mental Health,* 6(3), 307-318.

Peters, T. (1990). Get innovative or get dead. *California Management Review,* Fall, 9-26.

Peveler, R., George, C., Kinmonth, A-L., Campbell, M. and Thompson, C. (1999). Effect of antidepressant drug counselling and information leaflets on adherence to drug treatment in primary care: randomised controlled trial. *British Medical Journal,* 319, 612-615.

Pilgrim, D. and Waldron, L. (1998). User involvement in mental health service development: how far can it go? *Journal of Mental Health,* 1, 95-104.

Pyne, J., Rost, K., Zhang, M., Williams, K., Smith, J., Fortney, J. (2003). Cost-effectiveness of a primary care depression intervention. *Journal of General Internal Medicine,* 18 (6): 432-41.

Race, P. (2001). *The Lecturers Toolkit.* (second edition) London: Routledge Falmer.

Rainford, L., Mason, V. and Hickman, M. (2000). *Health in England 1998: Investigating the Links between Social Inequalities and Health.* London: HMSO.

Readhead E and Briel R (2001). *Review of the Mental Health Training Process.* Durham: Northern Centre for Mental Health.

Reite, M.L., Ruddy, J.R., Nagel, K.E. (1990). *Concise Guide to the Evaluation and Management of Sleep Disorders.* Washington: American Psychiatric Press

Richards, D.A. (2004). Self-Help: Empowering service users or aiding cash strapped mental health services? *Journal of Mental Health,* 13, 2, 117-123.

Richards, D.A., Lovell, K. and McEvoy, P. (2003). Access and effectiveness in psychological therapies: self-help as a routine health technology. *Health and Social Care in the Community.* 11, 175-182.

Richards, D., Richards, A., Barkham, M., Williams, C. and Cahill, J. (2002). PHASE: a health technology approach to psychological treatment in primary mental health care. *Primary Health Care Research and Developments.* 3: 159-168.

Ritchie, J. (1994) *The report of the inquiry into the case and treatment of Christopher Clunis.* London: The Stationery Office.

Roberts, S.E. (1992). *Healthy Participation: an Evaluative Study of the Hartcliffe Health and Environmental Action Group, a Community Development Project in Bristol.* Bristol: University of the West of England (unpublished MSC Dissertation).

Robins, C.J. and Hayes, A.M. (1993). An appraisal of cognitive therapy. *Journal of Consulting and Clinical Psychology,* 61, 2, 205-214.

Rogers, A., Flowers, J. and Pencheon, D. (1999). Improving access needs a whole systems approach. *British Medical Journal,* 319, 866-7.

Rogers, A. and Pilgrim, D. (1991). Pulling down churches: accounting for the British mental health users movement. *Sociology of Health and Illness,* 13 (2), 129-148.

Rogers, A., Pilgrim, D. and Lacey, R. (1993). *Experiencing Psychiatry: Users' Views of Services.* Hampshire: McMillan.

Rollnick, S., Mason, P. and Butler, C. (1999). *Behaviour Change: A Guide for Healthcare Professionals.* Edinburgh: Churchill Livingstone.

Ross, M. (1995). *Community Organisations: Theories and Principles.* New York: Harper.

Rost, K., Nutting, P., Smith, J. and Werner, M. (2000). Designing and implementing a primary care intervention trial to improve the quality and outcome of care for major depression. *General Hospital Psychiatry,* 22, 66-77.

Roth, A. and Fonagy, P. (1997). *What Works for Whom? A Critical Review of Psychotherapy Research.* London: Guildford press.

Royal College of Psychiatrists (1999). *Patient Advocacy: Council Report CR74.* London: RCP.

Royal Society of Great Britain (1997). *From compliance to concordance: achieving shared goals in taking medication.* London: The Society.

Rutter, D., Manley, C., Weaver, T., Crawford, M. and Fulop, N. (2004). Patients or partners?

Case studies of user involvement in the planning and delivery of adult mental health services in London. *Social Science and Medicine,* 58, 1973-1984.

Sainsbury Centre for Mental Health (2002). *Breaking the Circles of Fear: A Review of the Relationship between Mental Health Services and the African and Caribbean Communities.* London: SCMH.

Sainsbury Centre for Mental Health (2003). *On Our Own Terms: Users and Survivors of Mental Health Services Working Together for Support and Change.* London: SCMH.

Scaife, J. (2001) *Supervision in the Mental Health Professions A Practitioner's Guide.* Hove: Bruner-Routledge.

Schön, D. (1987). *Educating the Reflective Practitioner: How Professionals Think In Action.* New York: Basic Books.

Segal, S.P., Silverman, C. and Temkin, T. (1993). Empowerment and self-help agency practice for people with mental disabilities. *Social Work,* 38 (6), 708.

Semple, M. and Cable, S. (2003). The New Code of Professional Conduct. *Nursing Standard,* 17, 23, 40-48.

Silgrove, D. and Manicavasagar, V. (2000). *Overcoming Panic. A self-help guide using Cognitive Behavioural Techniques.* London: Robinson.

Sim, A. (1987). Why the excess mortality from psychiatric illness? *British Medical Journal,* 294, 986-987.

Simnett, I. (1995). *Managing Health Promotion: Developing Healthy Organisations and Communities.* Chichester: Wiley.

Simon, G.E., Ludman, E.J., Tutty, S., Operskalski, B. and Von Korff, M. (2004). Telephone psychotherapy and telephone care management for primary care patients starting antidepressant treatment: A randomised trial. *JAMA,* 292 (8), 935-942.

Simon, G.E. and Von Korff, M. (1995). Recognition and management of depression in primary care. *Archives of Family Medicine,* 4, 99-105.

Simon, G. E., Von Korff, M., Rutter, C. and Wagner, E. (2000). Randomised trial of monitoring, feedback and management of care by telephone to improve treatment of depression in primary care. *British Medical Journal.* 320, 550-554.

Smith, A.P., Brice, C., Collins, A., Matthews, V. and McNamara, R. (2000). *The scale of occupational stress: A further analysis of the impact of demographic factors and type of job.* Caerphilly: Health and Safety Executive.

Smith, A.P., Wadsworth, E., Johal, S.S., Davey Smith, G. and Peters, T. (2000). *The scale of occupational stress: The Bristol Stress and Health at Work Study.* Caerphilly: Health and Safety Executive.

Social Exclusion Unit (2001). *Preventing Social Exclusion: Report by the Social Exclusion Unit.* London: SEU.

Social Exclusion Unit (2003). *Mental Health and Social Exclusion: Consultation Document.* London: SEU.

Social Exclusion Unit (2004). *Action on Mental Health.* London: SEU.

Social Exclusion Unit (2004). *Action on Mental Health: A guide to promoting social inclusion* London: SEU.

Sofarelli, D. and Brown, D. (1998). The need for nursing leadership in uncertain times. *Journal of Nursing Leadership,* 6, 201-207.

Taylor, B. (ed) (1994). *Successful Change Strategies: Chief Executives in Action.* Hemel Hempstead: Fitzwilliam Publishing.

The Long-term Medical Conditions Alliance (2001). *Supporting Expert Patients: how to develop lay led self-management programmes for people with long-term medical conditions.* London: LMCA.

The National Prescribing Centre (2000). The drug treatment of depression in primary care. *MeRec Bulletin.* 11, 9, 33-36.

Tingle, J. (1998). Nurses must improve their record keeping skills. *British Journal of Nursing,* 7, 5, 245.

Tones, K. and Tilford, S. (1995). *Health Education: Effectiveness, Efficiency and Equity* (Second Edition). London: Chapman and Hall.

United Nations (1993). *Earth Summit Agenda 21: the United Nations programme of action from Rio.* New York: The United Nations Department of Public Information.

Untied Kingdom Advocacy Network (UKAN) (1997). *Advocacy – A Code of Practice.* London: NHS Executive Mental Health Task Force User Group.

Walsh, K., Nicholson, J., Keough, C., Pridham, R., Kramer, M. and Jeffrey, J. (2003). Development of a group model of clinical supervision to meet the needs of a community mental health nursing team. *International Journal of Nursing Practice,* 9, 33-39.

Ward, M. (1994). *Why your Corporate Culture Change isn't working and what to do about it.* Aldershot: Gower.

Weingarten, S.R., Henning, J.M., Badamgarav, E., Knight, K., Hasselblad, V., Gano, A. and Ofman, J.J. (2002). Interventions used in disease management programmes for patients with chronic illness – which ones work? Meta-analysis of published reports. *British Medical Journal,* 325, 925-940.

Wells, A. (1997). *Cognitive Therapy of Anxiety Disorders. A Practice Manual and Conceptual Guide.* Chichester: John Wiley and Sons.

Wells, K.B., Schoenbaum, M., Unutzer, J., Lagomasino, I.T. and Rubenstein,L.V. (1999). Quality of care for primary care patients with depression in managed care. *Archives of Family Medicine,* 8, 529-536.

Wilber, K. (2000). *Sex, Ecology and Spirituality: The spirit of evolution.* Boston MA: Shambhala.

Wilbourn, M. and Prosser, S. (2003). The Pathology and pharmacology of mental illness. Cheltenham: Nelson Thornes Ltd.

Wilkinson, R. (1996). *Unhealthy Societies: the Afflictions of Inequality.* London: Routledge.

Williams, C.J. (2001). *Overcoming Depression: A Five Areas Approach.* London: Arnold.

Wilson, J. (1999). Acknowledging the expertise of patients and their organisations. *British Medical Journal,* 319, 18 Sept, 771-774.

Wilson, P.M. (2001). A policy analysis of the Expert Patient in the United Kingdom: self care as an expression of pastoral power? *Health and Social Care in the Community,* 9 (3), May, 134-142.

World Health Organisation (WHO) (1946). *World Health Organisation Constitution.* Geneva: WHO.

World Health Organisation (WHO) (1986). *Ottawa Charter for Health Promotion.* Geneva: WHO.

World Health Organisation (WHO) (1994). *ICD-10 International Statistical Classification of Diseases and Related Health Problems.* Geneva: World Health Organisation. www.who.int.

World Health Organisation (WHO) (1998). *Health Promotion Glossary*, Geneva: WHO.

World Health Organisation (WHO) (2000). *WHO Guide to Mental Health in Primary Care.* London: The Royal Society of Medicine Press Ltd. www.who.int.

World Health Organisation Collaborating Centre for Research and Training for Mental Health (2000) *WHO Guide to Mental Health in Primary Care.* London: Royal Society of Medicine Press.

Wykurz, G. and Kelly, D. (2002). Learning in practice - developing the role of patients as teachers: literature review. *British Medical Journal,* 325 (12 Oct), 818-821.

Young, A. (1995). Law Series 3: Record Keeping. *British Journal of Nursing,* 4, 3, 179.

Index